Diseases of the Brain, Head and Neck, Spine
Diagnostic Imaging and Interventional Techniques

Springer-Verlag Italia Srl.

G.K. von Schulthess • Ch.L. Zollikofer (Eds)

DISEASES OF THE BRAIN, HEAD AND NECK, SPINE

DIAGNOSTIC IMAGING AND INTERVENTIONAL TECHNIQUES

36th International Diagnostic Course in Davos (IDKD)
Davos, March 27-April 2, 2004

presented by the Foundation for the
Advancement of Education in Medical Radiology, Zurich

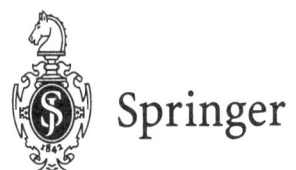

Springer

G. K. von Schulthess
Universitätsspital
Nuklearmedizin
8091 Zürich, Switzerland

Ch. L. Zollikofer
Kantonsspital
Institut für Radiologie
8401 Winterthur, Switzerland

© Springer-Verlag Italia 2004
Originally published by Springer-Verlag Italia, Milano in 2004

springeronline.com

ISBN 978-88-470-0251-7   ISBN 978-88-470-2131-0 (eBoook)
DOI 10.1007/ 978-88-470-2131-0

Typesetting: Color Point Srl, Milan

Cover design: Simona Colombo

Preface

The International Diagnostic Course in Davos (IDKD) offers a unique learning experience for imaging specialists in training as well as for experienced radiologists and clinicians wishing to be updated on the current state of the art and the latest developments in the fields of imaging and image-guided interventions.

This annual course is focused on organ systems and diseases rather than on modalities. This year's program deals with neuroradiology and radiology of the spine. During the course, the topics are discussed in group seminars and in plenary sessions with lectures by world-renowned experts and teachers. While the seminars present state-of-the-art summaries, the lectures are oriented towards future developments.

These proceedings represent a condensed version of the contents presented under the 20 topics dealing with imaging and interventional therapies in the neuroradiology and radiology of the spine. The topics encompass all the relevant imaging modalities including conventional x-rays, computed tomography, nuclear medicine, ultrasound and magnetic resonance angiography, as well as image-guided interventional techniques.

The volume is designed to be an "*aide-mémoire*" for the course participants so that they can fully concentrate on the lectures and participate in the discussions without the need of taking notes. Additional information is found on the web page of the IDKD (http//:www.idkd.ch).

G.K. von Schulthess
Ch.L. Zollikofer

Table of Contents

Brain Tumors
E.A. Knopp, W. Montanera 3

**Neuroimaging of Cerebral Vessel: Evidence-based Medicine
in the Evaluation of Acute Stroke and Aneurysm Detection**
M. E. Jensen 11

Evaluation of the Cerebral Vessels
R. Willinsky 14

Imaging and Management of Acute Stroke
W.T.C. Yuh, T. Taoka, T. Ueda, M. Maeda 20

Brain Ischemia
R. von Kummer 27

Haemorrhagic Cerebral Vascular Disease
J. Byrne 34

Hemorrhagic Vascular Phatology
M. Forsting, I. Wanke 36

Demyelinating Discascs
K.K. Koeller, R.G. Ramsey 44

Brain Degeneration and Aging
M.A. van Buchem 50

Imaging the Effects of Systemic Metabolic Diseases on the Brain
M. Castillo 55

**Neuroradiological Diagnosis of Craniocerebral and Spinal Trauma:
Current Concepts**
P.M. Parizel, C.D. Phillips 60

Nontraumatic Neuroemergencies
J.R. Hesselink, S. Atlas 73

Imaging the Patient with Seizures
P. Ruggieri, A. Nusbaum 77

Infectious Diseases of the Central Nervous System
V. Dousset 85

Cerebral Infections
D. Mikulis 93

Diseases of the Sella
J.F. Bonneville, W. Kucharczyk 100

Neuroimaging Diagnosis of Primary Brain Neoplasms in Childhood
W.S. Ball 107

Central Nervous System Diseases in Children
C. Raybaud 112

Orbit and Visual Pathways
M.F. Mafee, D.M. Yousem 118

Temporal Bone and Auditory Pathways
J.W. Casselman 124

Imaging the Temporal Bone
F. Veillon, S. Riehm 130

Imaging the Pharynx and Oral Cavity
B. Schuknecht, A.N. Hasso 136

Imaging of the Larynx
H.D. Curtin 146

Imaging the Larynx and Hypopharynx
M. Becker 149

Paranasal Sinuses and Nose: Normal Anatomy and Pathologic Processes
L.A. Loevner 158

Nose, Paranasal Sinuses and Adjacent Spaces
R. Maroldi, D. Farina, P. Nicolai 165

Degenerative Diseases of the Spine
B.C. Bowen 174

Degenerative Diseases and Pain Syndromes
J.L. Drapé 181

Neoplastic Spinal Cord Disease
D.L. Balériaux 184

Spinal Trauma and Spinal Cord Injury
A.E. Flanders 189

Spinal Inflammation and Demyelinating Diseases
C. Manelfe 193

Spinal Inflammation and Demyelinating Diseases
M. Leonardi, M. Maffei 197

SEMINARS

Brain Tumors

E.A. Knopp[1], W. Montanera[2]

[1] Section of Neuroradiology, Department of Radiology and Neurosurgery, NYU School of Medicine, New York, NY, USA
[2] Department of Medical Imaging, St. Michael's Hospital, University of Toronto, Toronto, Canada

Introduction

The designation "brain tumor" is commonly applied to a wide variety of intracranial mass lesions, each distinct in location, biology, treatment, and prognosis. Since many of these lesions do not arise from brain parenchyma, the more appropriate term is "intracranial tumor". Since the category encompasses both neoplasms and non-neoplastic mass lesions, the word "tumor" is used in its broadest sense to indicate a space-occupying mass.

Epidemiological data indicate that the annual incidence of intracranial tumors is 11-19 per 100000 persons. Metastases to the brain from a systemic primary cancer outside the central nervous system are even more common. Intracranial tumors can cause focal or generalized neurological symptoms. Headache, nausea, vomiting and occasional cranial nerve palsy (especially involving the sixth cranial nerve) may result from increased intracranial pressure. Focal symptoms and signs (e.g. paresis, visual deficit, aphasia) usually reflect the intracranial location of the tumor and the affected area of the brain. The frequency and duration of symptoms and signs also vary with the type of tumor. Rapidly growing tumors may exhibit symptoms earlier, with less overall tumor bulk than a more slowly growing tumor.

Headache occurs in about half of patients with brain tumors and is typically worse in the morning and improves after erect posture. Seizures are common (in 15%-95% of cases) and may be focal or generalized. Focal symptoms like hemiparesis and dysphasia are usually subacute in onset and progressive.

The only unequivocal risk factor for intracranial tumors, past cranial radiation, has been linked to both glial and meningeal neoplasms. Primary central nervous system lymphoma has tripled in incidence over the past two decades, largely due to the increased incidence in patients with acquired immunodeficiency syndrome. However, the incidence of lymphoma has also risen in the immunocompetent population with no known environmental exposure or behavioral risk factor [1-9].

Imaging Features of Intracranial Tumors

Prognosis and treatment of intracranial tumors are highly dependent on tumor histology. Predicting histology from preoperative imaging procedures depends largely on establishing the correct location of the origin of the mass. Specifically, the radiologist must first establish if the mass arises from within the brain parenchyma (intra-axial) or arises outside the brain parenchyma (extra-axial), whereby symptoms are usually due to brain compression. Radiologically identifiable anatomical clues that a tumor is extra-axial in location include the following:
(a) Widening of the ipsilateral subarachnoid space
(b) Cerebrospinal fluid (CSF) cleft between mass and brain parenchyma
(c) Deviation of pial vessels between mass and brain tissue
(d) Buckling of white matter
(e) Bony changes (e.g. hyperostosis in meningioma)

Once established as intra-axial or extra-axial, the specific location of the mass becomes equally important in imaging analysis since certain histological types of intracranial tumor tend to occur with higher frequency in specific locations. Thus, accurate compartmentalization of the mass limits the differential diagnosis to a relevant few tumors (Table 1) and helps direct further imaging evaluation and treatment [1-5].

Beyond the location of the mass, it is important to note other features in the imaging analysis of intracranial tumors further increase the likelihood of arriving at an accurate diagnosis and evaluating accurately the effect of the mass on adjacent brain tissue. Histologic features such as calcium or fat can be easily seen on cross-sectional imaging. The density of the mass on computed tomography (CT) and the signal intensity on T2-weighted magnetic resonance images can offer clues to cell composition and relative water content (e.g. nucleus-cytoplasm ratio). Compressive effects on adjacent brain tissue, extent of vasogenic edema accompanying the mass, and complicating hydrocephalus are easily and noninvasively assessed. Certain tumors have a higher likelihood

Table 1. Regional classification of common intracranial tumors

Intraventricular	Cavernous sinus
Ependymoma	Meningioma
Subependymoma	Schwannoma
Choroid plexus papilloma	Pituitary adenoma
Central neurocytoma	Metastasis
Colloid cyst	Cerebellopontine angle
Giant cell astrocytoma	Schwannoma
Pineal region	Meningioma
Pineocytoma	Epidermoid
Germ cell tumor	Arachnoid cyst
Primitive neuroectodermal	Paraganglioma
tumor (PNET)	Metastasis
Tectal glioma	Skull base
Meningioma	Chordoma
Dermoid	Chondrosarcoma
Arachnoid cyst	Paraganglioma
Sella and suprasellar region	Metastasis and myeloma
Pituitary adenoma	Sinonasal carcinoma
Craniopharyngioma	Esthesioneuroblasoma
Meningioma	Lymphoma and leukemia
Rathke's cyst	Foramen magnum
Chiasmatic glioma	Meningioma
Dermoid and epidermoid	Schwannoma
Germ cell tumor	Brainstem glioma
	Ependymoma

of presenting with hemorrhage that can be readily diagnosed on CT or magnetic resonance imaging (MRI). Furthermore, these conventional imaging tools can be used to predict vascularity of intracranial tumors that have not presented with hemorrhage. Intravenous contrast agents add further to the conventional imaging analysis of intracranial tumors by increasing conspicuity and demonstrating enhancement characteristics that help increase specificity.

Advanced Imaging Techniques in Intracranial Tumors

With the advent of faster imaging techniques, MRI can now depict various aspects of brain function in addition to brain anatomy.

Brain Diffusion

Diffusion imaging uses echo planar sequences. What is being imaged is the macromolecular motion of water within the extracellular space. In the normal brain this space is defined by the boundaries of axonal pathways. The axon bundles restrict the patterns of motion of water. This restriction occurs in a variety of directions in normal brain. In abnormal brain, these patterns are perturbed. Diffusion imaging relies on these perturbations. The most significant limitation is due to motion. Since what is being imaged in the first place is motion, the sequences

have to be inherently motion sensitive. The echo planar methods do limit the amount of extrinsic motion but they do not completely eliminate it.

The principle application for diffusion imaging is in the identification of hyperacute infarct. This determination can be made well in advance of T2 changes (minutes rather than hours). We use infarct as an example to explain the principles involved. With the onset of ischemia, there is breakdown of cell membrane Na-K ATPase pumps. This results in an influx of sodium ions into the cell. Water then follows, resulting in cell swelling. All this occurs within minutes of cessation of blood flow. At this time, the cells are still viable, however the extracellular space is compressed secondary to the swollen cells. The water in this compressed extracellular space is restricted in its ability to move. It is this restriction that the diffusion sequence detects. One can therefore see how diffusion imaging can detect hyperacute infarct.

The major problem with the interpretation of these images lies in the anisotropic patterns of motion; one therefore has to image in 3 orthogonal planes in order to achieve anisotropy. Once this is achieved, the method is inherently reproducible and easy to interpret.

A second application of diffusion techniques is in the differentiation of edema (vasogenic) from gliotic change. This has implication in tumor imaging and subsequent follow-up. Although infiltrative brain parenchyma has a diffusion abnormality, it does not give as significant a signal change on a diffusion-weighted image as does vasogenic edema. By using more advanced diffusion techniques, diffusion-tensor imaging and tractography, one can see more subtle infiltrative changes based upon the distortions in normal brain anisotropy. As glial neoplasms infiltrate along axonal pathways, they cause an inherent change in the fractional anisotropy along with visible changes seen on tractography.

Diffusion techniques readily enable one to differentiate solid from true cystic lesions. This in certain instances can aid in preoperative surgical planning [10-13].

Brain Perfusion

Perfusion imaging of the brain is a means to define the cerebral (capillary) blood volume by imaging during a bolus of contrast medium. This is different from conventional spin echo (SE) post-contrast imaging. In SE imaging, one is looking at the breakdown of the blood-brain barrier (in a similar fashion to CT). With perfusion imaging, the imaging is carried out during the first pass of contrast medium through the capillary bed. The imaging is finished before a significant amount of contrast medium crosses a disturbed blood-brain barrier.

The echo planar sequences routinely employed rely on the susceptibility changes in the image due to the presence of gadolinium. These changes manifest as a signal intensity drop. The drop is proportional to the "volume" of capillaries present. This method can be used in two major areas of imaging.

The first one we discuss is in tumor imaging. In this instance, perfusion "maps" enable one to determine the volume of the capillaries in the lesion in question as well as in normal brain. This is useful in the differentiation of areas of higher-grade disease within neoplasms. This has implications in choosing biopsy sites. Tumor boundaries may also be better characterized. Perfusion methods also allow one to differentiate therapeutic necrosis (secondary to radiation as well as high-dose chemotherapy). In these instances, the contrast-enhancing mass, while not having an intact blood-brain barrier, does not have any increase in capillary volume: in fact this is significantly reduced (if not absent). This fact manifests as a "cold" region with perfusion techniques.

The second (and more widely used) application is in the determination of hyperacute infarct. This is mentioned here only for the sake of completeness. With infarct, there is diminution of blood flow and an overall decrease in the affected capillary blood volume. These changes occur prior to any significant T2 abnormality. In this regard, the perfusion map shows the infarct as a "cold spot".

There are, however, limitations in perfusion scanning. The primary limitation reflects the need to administer gadolinium. In order to achieve a high intravascular level of gadolinium in a short, finite period of time, the contrast medium must be administered in a rapid bolus and flush fashion. Standard rates of administration are on the order of 5 ml/s. This rate is difficult to standardize with a hand injection. The use of a power injector does simplify this, but instead adds significantly to the cost. A large-bore intravenous needle (20 gauge) is needed. The second major limitation has to due with the necessity to post-process the data. Perfusion maps based upon statistical significance need to be calculated.

Previous work suggests that within a given tumor various grades of malignancy can co-exist. It has also been shown that tumor grade is related to the integrity of the blood-brain barrier and to the density and character of the tumor neovascularity. Although the integrity of the blood-brain barrier has been studied with both CT and MRI, this characteristic alone has not been sufficient to predict tumor grade. With the advent of MRI methods that measure relative cerebral blood flow (perfusion), it should be possible to explore the degree of neovascularity. Aronen et al. [14] used MRI perfusion techniques to obtain a cerebral blood volume map of gliomas and demonstrated that there is a correlation between the degree of perfusion (maximal cerebral blood volume) and the tumor mitotic activity and vascularity. In their study, however, one sample was randomly obtained from each tumor via either biopsy or resection, and they were unable to directly correlate tumor pathology with the radiographic features. In contrast, our methodology of stereotactic serial biopsy assures precise sampling of the lesion and allows for targeting based upon imaging features [12, 14-18].

Clinical MR Spectroscopy

Proton spectroscopy extends the diagnostic utility of the MRI brain examination beyond the typical structural images of anatomy and provides another functional dimension based on biochemical information. In a noninvasive manner, MRS provides valuable functional information that adds diagnostic value to the traditional MRI exam. The functional nature of the spectroscopy examination augments other functional MRI techniques such as diffusion, perfusion and blood oxygen level-dependent (BOLD) MRI studies. Together, these new diagnostic techniques are expanding the role of diagnostic MRI in the brain.

The major biochemical compounds detected using proton MRS in normal and pathological brain as summarized in Table 2 and as follows:
- N-Acetylaspartate (NAA) is a marker of neuronal viability and density. It is synthesized in neurons and transported along axons. NAA gives the highest metabolic peak on proton MRS with a frequency shift of 2.0 ppm. NAA concentration increases in Canavan's disease and decreases in physiologic conditions of birth (low concentration) and aging, neoplasia, hypoxia, ischemia, infarct, epilepsy, infection, inflammation and neurodegenerative states.
- Creatine (Cr) is generally used as an internal standard (reference) because its signal amplitude remains constant in most situations. Creatine, creatine kinase and phosphocreatine are central to the ADP/ATP energy pathway. The Cr peak, assigned at 3.03 ppm, is the second highest in proton MRS. Creatine concentration increases in trauma and aging, while it decreases with metastases.
- Choline (Cho) is involved in synthesis of phospholipids and thus it is a membrane compound and indicator of cellular turnover. Cho gives the third highest peak on proton MRS, assigned at 3.2 ppm. Choline concentration increases in a wide variety of conditions: physiologic, recovery from insult, gliosis, neoplasia, demyelination, inflammation and infection. It decreases in dementia, stroke and asymptomatic liver disease.
- Glutamine (Gln) and glutamate (Glu) are astrocyte markers. Glutamate is an excitatory neurotransmitter, which in excess concentration is a neurotoxin. Disruption of Gln/Glu regulatory mechanisms has been implicated in the initiation of a cascade leading to neuronal damage and death. These amino acids are increased in ischemia, recovery from ischemia, and liver disease. They are decreased primarily in Alzheimer's disease.
- Lactate (Lac) is seen in processes with cellular necrosis; normally it is not found in brain. Lactate is observed in pathologic processes with increased anaerobic metabolism. In proton MRS, lactate appears as a doublet configuration, with a peak assigned at 1.32 ppm.

Table 2. Common biochemical compounds in brain detected by proton magnetic resonance spectroscopy (MRS) and their significance to brain imaging

Compound	Resonating structure	Clinical significance
N-Acetylaspartate (NAA)	-CH$_3$ moiety of NAA	Marker for active neuronal tissue
Lactate (Lac)	-CH$_3$ moiety of lactate	Marker for low tissue oxygen and anaerobic glycolysis
Creatine (Cr)	-CH$_2$ and -CH$_3$ moieties of creatine and creatine phosphate	Important bioenergetic compounds in all living cells
Choline (Cho)	-N$^+$(CH$_3$)$_3$ moiety of all choline compounds, including choline, acetylcholine, phosphatidyl choline and others	Important cell membrane components
Lipid	-CH$_2$ and -CH$_3$ moieties of adipose tissue storage fats (triglycerides)	The fatty acyl groups in phospholipid membrane bilayer appear as broad components in the baseline
Myoinositol (MI)	-CH moieties of inositol isomers	
Glutamine (Glu), glutamate (Gln)	-CH$_2$ moieties of glutamate and glutamine	
Glucose (Glc)	-CH moieties of glucose	

- Lipids are elevated in brain in pathologic processes such as infection, inflammation, tumor necrosis and stroke. Lipids within brain are associated with myelin, sphingomyelins, phospholipids, and lecithins. Be aware that extracerebral lipids can contaminate volumes of interest (VOI).
- Myoinositol is almost exclusively found in astrocytes. Its major role is as an osmolyte. Chemically it looks like glucose, having a variable amplitude, assigned to 3.56 ppm. Its concentration is increased in patients with Alzheimer's disease, in neonates (compared to adults), and in hyperosmolar states. It is decreased in hepatic encephalopathy and hyponatremia.

The basic patterns observed in MRS are as follows:
- *CSF*. Cerebral metabolites are virtually absent from CSF. Lactate and glucose are present in normal CSF; if included in VOI, they reduce the signal to noise ratio (SNR) of cerebral metabolites.
- *Hypoxic-ischemic cascade*: loss of NAA; appearance of lactate; increased glutamine and glutamate; excess lipid is frequently found; and ultimately loss of creatine.
- *Abscess*: metabolites not usually detected but acetate peak is at 1.92 ppm; leucine, isoleucine, valine, succinate, pyruvate and lactate and lipids can be found.
- *HIV toxoplasmosis*: increased lactate and lipids at 1.3 and 0.9 ppm, respectively; decreased myoinositol, NAA, Cr, Cho. The diagnostic accuracy is approximately 100%.
- *HIV CNS lymphoma*: increased choline, lactate and lipids; decreased myoinositol, NAA and Cr. The diagnostic accuracy is 75%.
- *PML*: increased myoinositol and Cho; decreased Cr and NAA; lower levels of lactate and lipids. The diagnostic accuracy is 83%.
- *Cerebral neoplasms*, generally: low or absent NAA; low Cr; elevated Cho and lipid; lactate levels are variable.

Neuropathological applications of proton MRS include histological grading of tumors based on the Cho/Cr ratio [19]:
- Low grade hamartomas, <1.5
- Intermediate gliomas, 1.5-2.0
- High-grade gliomas, >2.0

The Cho/NAA ratio can be used in the differential diagnosis of intracranial tumors [20]:
- Normal, 0.75
- Low-grade glioma, 1.86
- Ependymoma, 1.8
- PNET, 7.5
- Choroid plexus carcinoma, 8.4
- High-grade glioma, 16.6

In radiation necrosis, the proton MRS profile is low in all metabolites, especially lactate and lipids (in contrast to recurrent tumor); however choline is increased. These observations correlate with those on positron emission tomography (PET).

Finally, proton MRS can be used to distinguish primary and secondary neoplasms. In primary glial tumors, the peritumoral MRS spectra demonstrate elevated choline. In secondary tumors or metastases, choline is not elevated in peritumoral tissue. This correlates with MR perfusion findings in which there is increased relative cerebral blood volume (rCBV) in the peritumoral region of primary neoplasms but not of secondary tumors. The basis for this difference is the presence of infiltrative tumor cells in the first instance and the presence of edema in the second case [10, 18, 21].

Technical Aspects of Proton MRS

The *single voxel technique* (one-dimensional single voxel spectroscopy, SVS) permits interrogation of brain metabolites in a single location selected by the operator. Typical imaging time is 2-8 min, depending on voxel dimensions. SVS pulse sequences include stimulated echo acquisition mode (STEAM) and point-resolved spectroscopy (PRESS).

- STEAM can be performed as 90°-90°-90°-echo, as well as gradient echo with low signal-to-noise ratio (SNR). Advantages are the short echo time (TE) that allows detection of metabolites with short T2 relaxation times (e.g. glutamine, glutamate, myoinositol, lipids), and more effective water suppression. Disadvantages are lower SNR and extreme sensitive to motion.
- PRESS is performed as 90°-180°-180°-echo, as well as spin echo with high SNR. Advantages are higher SNR. Disadvantages are long TE (135 ms), longer acquisition times and the possibility to "miss" metabolites with short TE.

Chemical shift imaging (CSI) extends the spectroscopic technique to multivoxel arrays covering a large volumes of interest in a single measurement. This two-dimensional technique permits the localization of chemical changes relating to various disease states. An important note is that the spectral data can be examined as single spectra, spectral maps or metabolite images. Typical imaging time is 6-12 min.

Three-dimensional (3D) CSI is similar to CSI but offers volumetric coverage; this technique can be done in true 3D fashion or with multislice 2D approaches.

Intracranial Tumors and Age of Presentation

Central nervous system tumors rank second in incidence only to lymphoreticular neoplasms during childhood. Approximately 15%-20% of all intracranial tumors occurs in children below 15 years. Most intracranial tumors in children represent primary lesions, while cerebral metastases are rare. The histologic spectrum of intracranial tumors and their location in children vary considerably from those of adults (Table 3). A higher proportion of childhood intracranial tumors occurs in the posterior fossa where they form the majority of intracranial tumors in the 2-10 year age group. Any analysis of intracranial

tumors must include a consideration of patient age in recognition of the most frequent histologies that occur in various age groups [1-4, 7, 22].

Common Intra-Axial Tumors

Astrocytoma is the most common primary intra-axial mass in the adult population. While there are various grading schemes in use throughout the world, the basic premise is the same. These tumors range from low-grade lesions to highly aggressive malignant neoplasms. The differences reflect the degree of cellularity along with the presence of mitotic activity, vascular hyperplasia and necrosis. These lesions grow by a pattern of infiltration: as they infiltrate, they secrete a wide variety of substances whose purpose is to promote the survival of the tumor cells. Hence they are capable of recruiting their own blood supply. As they dedifferentiate, they are seen to enhance. If we use the World Health Organization's 3-tier classification scheme, grade I tumors are termed either pilocytic or fibrillary. Grade II tumors are anaplastic; these have vascular hyperplasia and mitosis. Grade III tumors are glioblastoma multiforme; in addition to meeting the criteria for grade II tumors, they also exhibit necrosis. They are so aggressive as to "out-grow" their own blood supply [1, 3-5, 9, 23-26].

Oligodendrogliomas, as the name implies, take origin from oligodendroglia. They are significantly less common than astrocytomas, and comprise under 10% of primary intra-axial tumors. Typically they are seen to contain CT-visible calcification in upwards of 80% of cases. They tend to be located subcortically. As is the case with astrocytomas, they also vary from low grade to high grade. These tumors, though, tend to have a better prognosis as they are somewhat more chemosensitive than their pure astrocytic counterparts. They also exist in a mixed form, where there are varied proportions of oligodendroglial cells and astrocytes. As the degree of the oligocomponent increases, so does the prognosis [1, 3-5, 24-28].

Table 3. Common primary intra-axial brain tumors

Pediatric	Supratentorial	Pleomorphic xanthoastrocytoma (PXA) Primitive neuroectodermal tumor (PNET) Dysembryoplastic neuroectodermal tumor (DNET) Ganglioglioma
	Infratentorial	Juvenile pilocytic astrocytoma Primitive neuroectodermal tumor (PNET) Brainstem astrocytoma
Adult	Supratentorial	Fibrillary astrocytoma Anaplastic astrocytoma Glioblastoma multiforme Oligodendroglioma
	Infratentorial	Hemangioblastoma

Gangliogliomas are tumors of a mixed cell population taking origin from both glial and neuronal cell lines. These are the most common of the so-called mixed tumors. They tend to be low grade with a good prognosis. However, they can be somewhat more aggressive and dedifferentiate into higher grade lesions. Typically the patient presents with a seizure and is found to have a lesion in a cortical location. Most commonly, they are found in the temporal lobes. In addition, you can see thinning of the overlying bony calvarium, an indicator of the long-standing nature of these lesions [1, 3-5, 27].

In adults, *hemangioblastomas* are the most common primary infratentorial tumors. They are low grade, essentially benign neoplasms. Incomplete resection, however, can lead to recurrence. Typically they form a cystic mass with a solid mural nodule which is highly vascular. The cyst wall is not seen to enhance. Their appearance is similar to that of juvenile pilocytic astrocytoma. The principal differentiating feature is age. Hemangioblastomas tend to present in young, middle-age males (30-40 years). They can be multiple, in which case they are typically associated with von Hippel-Lindau syndrome [1, 3-5].

PNET has been previously referred to as medulloblastoma. However given its primitive nature along with the neuroectodermal cell origin, this tumor has been renamed. PNET is the most common posterior fossa neoplasm in children. It does, however, have a second peak of incidence in adults. While classically occurring in relation to the cerebellum, PNET does occur in the supratentorial brain as well. It represents a spectrum of diseases with a varied degree of aggressiveness, the most aggressive being the atypical teratoid rhabdoid tumor [1, 3-5, 7].

Juvenile pilocytic astrocytomas or, more commonly, pilocytic astrocytomas, classically have been separated out from the more infiltrative low-grade astrocytomas. In fact, they are histopathologically distinct. They are nonaggressive tumors in which gross surgical resection should be curative. Their imaging features are a combination of low- and high-grade lesions. They are well circumscribed yet enhance. Advanced imaging characteristics (perfusion and spectroscopy) tend to mimic higher grade lesions. Thus it is paramount that in this instance (and in fact in all instances) the advanced MRI data be interpreted along with the conventional images. Obviously, the patient's history helps as well [1, 3-5, 7].

By far and away, *metastases* are the most common supratentorial (infratentorial as well) neoplasms in the adult. They comprise upwards of 40% of all tumors. About half of these lesions are reported to be solitary, however, with the use of higher doses of gadolinium (as well as higher field strength) this number is decreasing. In decreasing order in numbers, they tend to arise from lung, breast (in women), melanoma, kidney and gastrointestinal primary tumors. They tend to be located at the gray-white junction with a fair amount of vasogenic edema (recognized by the sparing of the arcuate fibers along with its frond-like appearance). Increased T1 signal can mean either melanin or blood products. Mucinous primary tumors tend to have low signal on both T2-weighted and FLAIR images. Calcification is observed typically with lung or breast primary tumor [1, 3-5, 9, 18].

Common Extra-Axial Tumors

Meningioma is the most common extra-axial neoplasm of adults. Its incidence is highest in middle-aged women. Meningiomas are thought to originate from arachnoid cap cells and their distribution parallels that of the cap cells that are most abundant in arachnoid granulations. The parasagittal and convexity dura, sphenoid ridge, parasellar and cerebellopontine (CP) angle are common locations. Varying histologic types and varying compositions lead to some variability of imaging features. Meningiomas are usually hyperdense relative to brain on CT. Calcification can be detected in roughly 20% of cases and a bony reaction in the adjacent skull is relatively common. If present, this bony reaction usually consists of hyperostosis (due to stimulation of a bony reaction with or without tumor invasion) and less frequently consists of bone destruction. Enhancement on CT or MRI is usually relatively homogeneous with occasional cystic components, areas of necrosis, or calcium. Meningiomas have a propensity for invasion of dural venous sinuses and encasement of carotid arteries when originating in the cavernous sinus. When located in the cavernous sinus, meningioma can also cause caliber narrowing of the vessel as well as encasement. Edema in the brain adjacent to meningioma is variable and more frequent in larger lesions [2-4, 29, 30].

The tem "neurogenic tumor" refers primarily to *schwannoma* and much less commonly to neurofibroma. Schwannomas originate from Schwann cells, whose myelin processes surround axons of cranial nerves. They are most frequently found at the transition zone between oligodendroglial and Schwann cell coverings of the axons. They originate much more frequently from sensory than from motor nerves. Schwannomas represent 6%-8% of primary intracranial neoplasms, are more frequent in adulthood (peaking in the fifth and sixth decades), and are slightly more common in women. Presenting symptoms depend upon the nerve affected. As these tumors are well delineated and encapsulated, they affect the cranial nerve of origin and adjacent brain by compression rather than invasion. The vestibular division of the eighth cranial nerve is the most frequent origin (internal auditory canal and cerebellopontine angle), followed by the fifth and seventh cranial nerves. On CT, schwannomas are iso-dense or slightly hypodense relative to brain. Calcification and hemorrhage are rare. MRI usually demonstrates an iso- to hypointense extra-axial mass on T1-weighted sequences, becoming hyperintense on T2-weighted sequences. Schwannomas usually enhance intensely on both CT and MRI. Smaller tumors usually enhance homogeneously, whereas heterogeneity is more common in larger tumors due to intralesional necrosis or cyst formation. Arachnoid cysts can also be seen in association with the surface of these lesions. In most cases, cerebellopontine angle tumors form acute angles with the porus acusticus and the tumor extends into the internal auditory canal, often with canal expansion, allowing distinction from meningiomas which are also common in this location. Schwannomas may affect bony foramina by slowly expanding and remodeling them [2-4, 6].

Several intracranial mass lesions are not true neoplasms, but are traditionally included among brain tumors because they represent space-occupying intracranial lesions. Dermoids and epidermoids are included in this group. Each represents a non-neoplastic "inclusion cyst" presumably arising from ectodermal cell rests during embryogenesis.

- *Epidermoids* consist of an ectoderm-derived epithelial lining (without ectodermal appendages). As the cyst wall desquamates, this material collects within the cyst. The cyst slowly expands and insinuates within cisternal spaces and fissures. Epidermoids are most frequently found off midline and most often in the cerebellopontine angle, less frequently around the sella. Epidermoids may show CT and MRI characteristics similar to CSF, and they typically do not enhance following contrast medium administration. Use of diffusion-weighted imaging can reliably distinguish these lesions from arachnoid cysts.
- *Dermoids* are similar inclusion cysts, but their lining may also contain ectodermal derived appendages (hair, teeth, sweat glands, etc). They are more typically found near the midline and may be associated with a dermal sinus. Secretions and their breakdown products often result in contents that are oily and contain lipid metabolites, giving rise to imaging features similar to fat. CT usually shows a low density extra-axial mass, often with peripheral calcification. Ectodermal appendages (hair, teeth, etc.) can contribute to heterogeneity. Although the cyst wall may show some enhancement, the center of the mass should not enhance with contrast medium. Dermoids may occasionally rupture intracranially and release their oily contents into the subarachnoid space. The clinical presentation may simulate acute subarachnoid hemorrhage and imaging demonstrates dispersal of the oily contents into the subarachnoid space.
- Other non-neoplastic extra-axial lesions include: arachnoid cyst (CSF-filled cavity within arachnoid membrane); colloid cyst (anterior third ventricle at foramen of Monro); neuroepithelial cyst (most likely intraventricular of choroidal origin); and neurenteric cyst (cyst wall composed of gut or respiratory epithelium, remnant of neurenteric canal during embryogenesis) [2-4, 6, 31].

Cranial *paragangliomas* may arise at the jugular foramen (glomus jugulare) or in the middle ear cavity (glomus tympanicum). These tumors arise from glomus bodies (neural crest derivatives) and often present with pulsatile tinnitus. Glomus jugulare tumors originate in the adventitia of the jugular foramen and occlude the jugular vein with growth. At the time of diagnosis, there is usually infiltration of tumor into the bony margins of the jugular foramen with a pattern of permeative bone destruction. CT and MRI show an enhancing soft-tissue mass centered on the jugular foramen (jugulare) or inferior portion of the middle ear cavity (tympanicum). A soft tissue component may grow intracranially toward the cerebellopontine angle. Highly vascular tumors, these are characterized by direct visualization of prominent vessels within mass evidenced by MRI flow voids or a "salt and pepper" appearance [2-4, 6].

Craniopharyngiomas, thought to arise from metaplasia of squamous epithelial remnants of Rathke's pouch, are usually centered in the suprasellar cistern. They may extend into the sella and retroclival region, or up into the third ventricle. Although most common in children, these tumors occur scattered throughout the age spectrum. As well as their characteristic location, these tumors often exhibit cyst formation, calcification, and solid enhancing components [2-4, 7, 22, 31].

Chordomas arise from remnants of the notochord. They are most common in the sacrum. Cranial chordomas occur almost exclusively in the clivus. They are locally aggressive tumors that destroy bone and may grow into nasopharynx, parasellar region or prepontine cistern. MRI and CT demonstrate an enhancing soft-tissue mass centered on the clivus, exhibiting bone destruction and areas of calcification. They are almost always hyperintense on T2-weighted MR sequences and may exhibit internal "septations" [2-4, 29].

Tumor Follow-up

Follow-up of patients with intracranial neoplasms tends to be dictated by the clinical situation and to fall into two general groups: medical and surgical.

In patients undergoing surgical resection, we perform imaging within 24 hours of surgery using routine protocols. In this timeframe, the postoperative changes affecting the blood-brain barrier are not manifest and any enhancement is thought to represent residual enhancing tumor. It is imperative that a noncontrast T1-weighted image is obtained, as there can be a fair amount of hyperintense blood products present. After this, our first conventional follow-up is 6 weeks later. Scanning between these intervals can be fraught with difficulty due to the exuberant contrast enhancement present. Remember, though, if the lesion was nonenhancing preoperatively it will not enhance in the month following surgery. Further follow-up is dictated by the therapeutic protocol the patient is receiving. Pure surgical lesions (with gross total resection) tend to be followed at 6 weeks, 3 , 6 , 12 and 18 months, and then yearly.

In patients undergoing further medical therapy, precise follow-up timing depends upon treatment. Typically in patients actively receiving chemotherapy, follow-up is between 4 and 6 weeks, with courses of chemotherapy in between. In this instance, follow-up should include at least 1 advanced method (perfusion or spectroscopy) in case the therapeutic effect mimics disease progression and needs to be differentiated. The same holds true for radiation therapy. When patients are no longer actively receiving aggressive treatment, follow-up occurs in 3-month intervals.

In all instances, the presence of any imaging changes with mass effect should prompt further investigation with advanced methods. It is also important to realize the patterns of tumor spread when looking at follow-up images. Primary lesions, being so highly infiltrative, spread along paths of less resistance, e.g. along axonal bundles and more importantly in a subependymal fashion. If we have a lesion which is adjacent to the ventricular system, we must take care to assess the subependymal surfaces for subtle linear FLAIR abnormalities tracking around the ventricular system, which may eventually enhance as well. Do not assume it's just "white matter disease".

When a suspicious finding is made, there are two roads to follow: if it is obvious, then it is a tumor recurrence that must be acted upon. If however, you are not 100% convinced, then closer follow-up in 4-6 weeks is warranted [17, 23, 25-28].

References

1. Atlas SW, Lavi E, Fisher PG (2002) Intraaxial brain tumors. In: Atlas SW (ed) Magnetic resonance imaging of the brain and spine. Lippincott Williams Wilkins, Philadelphia, pp 565-693
2. Altas SW, Lavi E, Golberg HI (2002) Extraaxial brain rumors. In: Atlas SW (ed) Magnetic resonance imaging of the brain and spine. Lippincott Williams Wilkins, Philadelphia, pp 695-772
3. Grossman RI, Yousem DM (2003) Neoplasms of the brain. In: Thrall JH (ed) Neuroradiology: the requisites. Mosby Elsevier, Philadelphia, pp 97-172
4. Osborn AG, Rauschning W (1994) Brain tumors and tumorlike masses: classification and differential diagnosis. In: Patterson AS (ed) Diagnostic neuroradiology. Mosby Year Book, St. Louis, pp 401-528
5. DeAngelis LM (2001) Brain tumors. N Engl J Med 344:114-123
6. Zamani AA (2000) Cerebellopontine angle tumors: role of magnetic resonance imaging. Top Magn Reson Imaging 11:98-107
7. Luh GY, Bird CR (1999) Imaging of brain tumors in the pediatric population. Neuroimaging Clin N Am 9:691-716
8. Koeller KK, Smirniotopoulos JG, Jones RV (1997) Primary central nervous system lymphoma: radiologic-pathologic correlation. Radiographics 17:1497-526
9. Lassman AB, DeAngelis LM (2003) Brain metastases. Neurol Clin 21:1-23
10. Kauppinen RA (2002) Monitoring cytotoxic tumour treatment response by diffusion magnetic resonance imaging and proton spectroscopy. NMR Biomed 15:6-17
11. Castillo M, Mukherji SK (2000) Diffusion-weighted imaging in the evaluation of intracranial lesions. Semin Ultrasound CT MR 21:405-416
12. Le Bihan D, Douek P, Argyropoulou M, Turner R, Patronas N, Fulham M (1993) Diffusion and perfusion magnetic resonance imaging in brain tumors. Top Magn Reson Imaging 5:25-31
13. Chenevert TL, Meyer CR, Moffat BA, Rehemtulla A, Mukherji SK, Gebarski SS, Quint DJ, Robertson PL, Lawrence TS, Junck L, Taylor JM, Johnson TD, Dong Q, Muraszko KM, Brunberg JA, Ross BD (2002) Diffusion MRI: a new strategy for assessment of cancer therapeutic efficacy. Mol Imaging 1:336-343
14. Aronen H, Glass J, Pardo F, Belliveau J, Gruber M (1995) Echo-planar MR cerebral blood volume mapping of gliomas. Clinical utility. Acta Radiologica 86:520-528
15. Knopp EA, Cha S, Johnson G, Mazumdar A, Golfinos JG, Zagzag D, Miller DC, Kelly PJ, Kricheff II (1999) Dynamic contrast-enhanced T2*-weighted MR imaging of glial neoplasms. Radiology 211:791-798
16. Cha S, Knopp EA, Johnson G et al (2002) Intracranial mass lesions: dynamic contrast-enhanced susceptibility-weighted echo-planar perfusion MR imaging. Radiology 223:11-29
17. Cha S, Knopp EA, Johnson G et al (2000) Dynamic, contrast-enhanced T2*-weighted MR imaging of recurrent malignant gliomas treated with thalidomide and carboplatin. AJNR Am J Neuroradiol 21:881-890
18. Law M, Cha S, Knopp EA, Johnson G, Arnett J, Litt AW (2002) High-grade gliomas and solitary metastases: differentiation using perfusion MR imaging and proton spectroscopic MR imaging. Radiology 222:715-721
19. Norfray JF, Darling C, Byrd S, Ross B et al (1999) Short TE proton MRS and neurofibromatosis type 1 intracranial tumors. J Comp Assist Tomogr 23(6):994-1003
20. Zimmerman R et al (1994) CHOP, Philadelphia3
21. Nelson SJ, McKnight TR, Henry RG (2002) Characterization of untreated gliomas by magnetic resonance spectroscopic imaging. Neuroimaging Clin N Am 12:599-613
22. Poussaint TY (2001) Magnetic resonance imaging of pediatric brain tumors: state of the art. Top Magn Reson Imaging 12:411-433
23. Earnest F 4th, Kelly PJ, Scheithauer BW, Kall BA, Cascino TL, Ehman RL, Forbes GS, Axley PL, Earnest F (1988) Cerebral astrocytomas: histopathologic correlation of MR and CT contrast enhancement with stereotactic biopsy. Radiology 166:823-827
24. Kelly PJ, Daumas-Duport C, Scheithauer BW, Kall BA, Kispert DB (1987) Stereotactic histologic correlations of computed tomography- and magnetic resonance imaging-defined abnormalities in patients with glial neoplasms. Mayo Clin Proc 62:450-459
25. Schiffer D (2000) Glioma malignancy and its biological and histological correlates. J Neurosurg Sci 34:163-165
26. Schiffer D (1991) Pathology of brain tumors and its clinicobiological correlates. Dev Oncol 66:3-9
27. Kleinman G, Zagzag D, Miller D (1994) Diagnostic use of immunohistochemistry in neuropathology. Neurosurg Clin N Am 5:97-126
28. Fine HA (1995) Novel biologic therapies for malignant gliomas. Antiangiogenesis, immunotherapy, and gene therapy. Neurol Clin 13:827-846
29. Sheporaitis LA, Osborn AG, Smirniotopoulos JG et al (1992) Intracranial meningioma. AJNR Am J Neuroradiol 13:29-37
30. Maiuri F, Iaconetta G, de Divitiis O et al (1999) Intracranial meningiomas: correlations between MR imaging and histology. Eur J Radiol 31:69-75
31. Fitzpatrick M, Tartaglino LM, Hollander MD et al (1999) Imaging of sellar and parasellar pathology. Radiol Clin North Am 37:101-21

Neuroimaging of Cerebral Vessels: Evidence-based Medicine in the Evaluation of Acute Stroke and Aneurysm Detection

M.E. Jensen

Interventional Neuroradiology Unit, Department of Radiology, University of Virginia Health Sciences Center, Charlottesville, VA, USA

Introduction

As neuroimaging becomes more complex and widely available, the cost of health care is rising rapidly for both the individual and society as a whole. A continuous flow of medical literature makes it difficult to elucidate the true science from the merely descriptive. The current trend towards evidence-based medicine is an attempt to find those diagnostic and therapeutic imaging studies that provide the best information at the most reasonable cost. The best information comes from randomized controlled trials that are prospectively designed to determine performance and efficacy (Level 1 evidence) [1]. It is more likely, however, that Level 2 (clinical non-randomized studies, cohort and case-controlled studies, uncontrolled prospective studies) or Level 3 (descriptive studies, case series, expert committee reports) evidence will be more readily available. Readers are referred to the recent Neuroimaging Clinics of North America monograph [2] for more in-depth information. A synopsis of the evidence-based medicine as it pertains to the neuroimaging of common clinical conditions follows here.

Intracranial Vascular Assessment in the Treatment of Acute Stroke

One of the pitfalls of the NINDS intravenous thrombolysis trial was the lack of information regarding the degree and location of vascular occlusion. In a large, randomized controlled trial of intra-arterial thrombolysis (PROACT), arterial occlusions were demonstrated by digital subtraction angiography (DSA) in only 38% of patients with major neurological deficits [3]. Del Zoppo and colleagues performed angiography before and after the intravenous administration of recombinant tissue plasminogen activator (rtPA), and found improved recanalization rates in the more distal middle cerebral artery (MCA) branches compared the internal carotid artery (ICA) [4]. These two studies suggested that an intra-arterial approach to large proximal thrombi and an intravenous approach to distal emboli may be the best therapeutic strategies in acute stroke [5]. Reliable imaging information regarding clot burden and location must be obtained prior to therapeutic selection.

Angiography remains the gold standard in evaluation of the arterial tree although it does not define the status of the brain parenchyma. It allows evaluation in multiple projections, depicts the morphology of the vessel lumen, assesses the collateral circulation and visualizes the most distal vasculature. The disadvantages include risks of stroke and nephrotoxicity, expense, invasiveness, and procedural time.

An advantage of computed tomographic angiography (CTA) is that it can be performed immediately after routine non-contrast CT, shortening the time to diagnosis by eliminating the need to move the patient. Perfusion data can be collected at the same time, which may influence therapeutic options. CTA images are easy to interpret and, in my experience, clinician acceptance is high. The images are acquired rapidly, so even uncooperative patients can be scanned. There are disadvantages, including rapid injection of a large bolus of contrast medium that requires a large-bore intravenous line and good renal function. Evaluation of the extracranial vessels may also yield important diagnostic and therapeutic information; however imaging the cervical vessels results in significant intracranial venous opacification that can interfere with interpretation and image reconstruction [6].

Several studies have reported the sensitivity and specificity of CTA for detecting occlusions in the circle of Willis. Lev et al. [7] recently evaluated the accuracy of CTA for the detection of large vessel intracranial thrombus in clinically suspected hyperacute stroke patients. In this study, 44 consecutive intra-arterial thrombolysis candidates underwent CTA as part of the imaging protocol. Acquisition, reconstruction, and analysis of CTA images took approximately 15 minutes. Using axial source and maximum intensity projection (MIP)-reformatted images, the studies were evaluated for the presence or absence of large vessel occlusion. A total of 572 circle of Willis vessels were examined; arteriographic correlation was available for 224 vessels. Sensitivity and specificity for the detection of large vessel occlusion were 98.4% and 98.1%, respectively. Accuracy, calculated using receiver operating characteristics analysis, was 99%. Other older series have also shown sensitivities and specificities of 83%-100% and 99%-100%, respectively, compared to DSA [5].

The sensitivity and specificity of magnetic resonance angiography (MRA) is limited compared to that of DSA. One study evaluated the reliability of MRA source images and MIP images in showing the arterial segments of the circle of Willis [8]. MRA source images and MIP images were evaluated in 526 arterial segments and compared to DSA. MRA MIP images had a sensitivity of 87% and a specificity of 88%. MRA source images had a sensitivity of 89% and a specificity of 63% in depicting the presence of a vessel segment. In an earlier study of 50 patients [9], the same authors found that MRA had a sensitivity of 100% and specificity of 95% for vascular occlusion, and a sensitivity of 89% and a specificity of 89% for stenosis of the intracranial vessels, when compared to DSA. A more recent study compared the value of three-dimensional (3D) time-of-flight (TOF) and phase-contrast (PC) MRA for the detection and grading of intracranial vascular steno-occlusive disease [10]. Eighteen patients were studied with both techniques, and the results were compared to those of DSA (performed in 15 patients) and transcranial Doppler sonography (TCD). 3D-TOF MRA was more specific than 3D-PC MRA (for two observers, 87% and 86% vs. 65% and 60%) and had a higher negative predictive value (96% vs. 89%). Correct grading of stenosis was achieved by 3D-TOF in 78% of patients and by 3D-PC MRA in 65%.

Although technical advances in MRA have improved the sensitivity and accuracy of this technique in the evaluation of vascular steno-occlusive disease of the brain, technical limitations still exist. Relative disadvantages include study time when the patient is required to remain motionless. Movement may result in slice misrepresentation on 2D TOF images and can blur images in all studies [6]. In addition, turbulent flow in highly stenosed lesions leads to overestimation of the true lumen size. This problem is particularly crucial when surgical decisions are to be made using specific operative criteria involving the exact measurement of the stenosis.

In summary, CTA and MRA are currently used to assess the intracranial vasculature in patients suffering from acute stroke. There is some Level 2 and Level 3 evidence that shows favorable comparison with DSA in the detection of circle of Willis occlusions, particularly for CTA. The literature is lacking in the evaluation of smaller branches. In addition to providing information about the vasculature, these modalities also evaluate the status of the brain parenchyma and play a definitive role in the evaluation of stroke patients. However, strong evidence to support its use as a screening tool for the determination of use and delivery method of thrombolytic therapy is currently lacking [5].

Evaluation of Cerebral Aneurysms

DSA remains the gold standard in the evaluation of intracranial aneurysms. As noted before, small but real risks are associated with angiography, and a noninvasive diagnostic examination would be preferred, if it were sufficiently accurate. A meta-analysis of noninvasive imaging used to detect intracranial aneurysms was performed by White and colleagues in 2000 [11]. These authors analyzed all reports from 1988 to 1998 in which 10 or more patients were studied and the results were compared to DSA. Thirty-eight studies meeting initial criteria and scoring greater than 50% on an intrinsically weighted standardized assessment were included. The rates of aneurysm accuracy for CTA and MRA were 89% and 90%, respectively. The study showed greater sensitivity for aneurysms larger than 3 mm using both modalities: for CTA, sensitivity was 96% for aneurysms >3 mm and 61% for those <3 mm; for MRA, these values were 94% and 38%, respectively. The same authors also performed a prospective blinded study comparing CTA and MRA to DSA for the detection of aneurysms [12]. DSA was performed in 142 patients along with CTA and 3D-TOF MRA and all studies were read by two observers. The accuracy rates per patient for the best observer were 87% for CTA and 85% for MRA. The accuracy rates per aneurysm for the best observer were 73% for CTA and 67% for MRA. The sensitivity of aneurysm detection improved with aneurysms 5 mm or larger, to 94% for CTA and 86% for MRA. Sensitivities were dramatically diminished with aneurysms smaller than 5 mm (57% for CTA and only 35% for MRA).

Overall, CTA and MRA show good sensitivity in cases where aneurysms are 5 mm or larger. Sensitivity drops dramatically with smaller aneurysms. Should either modality be considered a screening tool for the evaluation of ruptured and unruptured aneurysms? Using complex statistical methodology and computer modeling, Van Gelder [13] concluded that clinicians can trust a CTA finding of a large aneurysm (>6 mm) when subarachnoid hemorrhage is present, but the specificity decreases for smaller aneurysms (<2 mm). When hemorrhage is present, the likelihood of an aneurysm increases and clinicians can trust CTA findings of both large and small aneurysms; however, angiography is warranted in patients with hemorrhage and a negative CTA examination. When no hemorrhage is present and no aneurysm is found at CTA, further evaluation by angiography is less warranted than it is in the setting of subarachnoid hemorrhage.

Technical advances have not been limited to noninvasive imaging alone. In the interpretation and treatment of aneurysms, 3D rotational angiography is playing a prominent role. Three-dimensional images are acquired through the use of specialized angiography equipment and special reconstructive computer software. With the patient isocentered in the C-arm, the C-arm rapidly rotates in a 200-degree arc around the patient's head. Acquisition time is approximately 5 s. The first sweep provides the data necessary for acquiring the mask images. The second sweep is done during the injection of contrast medium at a rate of 2.5-3.0 ml/s for a total of 30-35 s. Distortion is automatically corrected. The images are sent to a workstation for reconstruction in volume-rendered technique; however, source images, maximum intensity projection, multiplanar reformatting and surface-shaded display can also be chosen.

The information acquired from 3D angiography has dramatically improved aneurysm evaluation and treatment planning. Important information for both endovascular treatment and surgical clipping is acquired, including the true neck size, morphology of the neck, relationship of the neck to the surrounding vessels, and visualization of vessels arising from the neck [14]. This technique is not without its disadvantages. Patient movement can result in poor image acquisition, and the best images are obtained when general anesthesia is used. Low cardiac output and poor C-arm reproducibility may also affect image quality. In addition, the radiation dose to the patient's skin is significant a routine 14-s acquisition delivers a similar dose as an entire biplane cerebral angiogram. Radiation dose is minimized by diminishing the acquisition time to 5-8 s.

Conclusions

The current movement is towards evaluation of the intracranial circulation using less invasive therapy. Before a technique can replace existing "gold standards," a body of solid evidence-based medicine must exist. To date, some data are available to make confident decisions, but prospective randomized trials are lacking in many areas. To ensure the acceptance of such modalities in the future, we are responsible to our patients and to society for providing the best possible data from which clinical and financial decisions will be made.

References

1. Mendina LS, Aguirre E, Zurakowski D (2003) Introduction to evidence-based medicine. Neuroimaging Clin N Am 13(2):157-165
2. Medina LS (ed) (2003) Evidence-based neuroimaging. Neuroimaging Clin N Am 13(2)
3. Furlan A, Higashida R, Wechsler L et al (1999) Intra-arterial prourokinase for acute ischemic stroke. The PROACT II study: a randomized controlled trial. Prolyse in Acute Cerebral Thromboembolism. JAMA 282:2003-2011
4. del Zoppo G, Poeck K, Pessin MS et al (1992) Recombinant tissue plasminogen activator in acute thrombotic and embolic stroke. Ann Neurol 32:78-86
5. Vo KD, Lin W, Lee JM (2003) Evidence-based neuroimaging in acute ischemic stroke. Neuroimag Clin N Am 13(2):167-183
6. Phillips CD, Bubash LA (2002) CT angiography and MR angiography in the evaluation of extracranial carotid vascular disease. Radiol Clin N Am 40(4):783-798
7. Lev MH, Farkas J, Rodriguez VR et al (2001) CT angiography in the rapid triage of patients with hyperacute stroke to intraarterial thrombolysis: accuracy in the detection of large vessel thrombus. J Comput Assist Tomogr 25(4):520-528
8. Stock KW, Wetzel S, Kirsch E, Bongartz G, Steinbrich W, Radue EW (1996) Anatomic evaluation of the circle of Willis: MR angiography versus intraarterial digital subtraction angiography. AJNR Am J Neuroradiol 17(8):1495-1499
9. Stock KW, Radue EW, Jacob AL et al (1995) Intracranial arteries: prospective blinded comparative study of MR angiography and DSA in 50 patients. Radiology 195:451-456
10. Oelerich M, Lentschig MG, Zunker P et al (1998) Intracranial vascular stenosis and occlusion: comparison of 3D time-of-flight and 3D phase-contrast MR angiography. Neuroradiology 40(9):567-573
11. White PM, Wardlaw JM, Easton V (2000) Can noninvasive imaging accurately depict intracranial aneurysms? A systematic review. Radiology 217:361-370
12. White PM, Teasdale EM, Wardlaw JM, Easton V (2001) Intracranial aneurysms: CT angiography and MR angiography for detection prospective blinded comparison in a large patient cohort. Radiology 219:739-749
13. van Gelder JM (2003) Computed tomographic angiography for detecting cerebral aneurysms: implications of aneurysm size distribution for the sensitivity, specificity and likelihood ratios. Neurosurgery 53(3):597-606
14. Klucznik RP (2002) Current technology and clinical applications of three-dimensional angiography. Radiol Clin N Am 40:711-728

Evaluation of the Cerebral Vessels

R. Willinsky

Toronto Western Research Institute, Clinical Studies Resourse Centre, Toronto, Canada

Introduction

In the last decade there has been a dramatic shift to non-invasive imaging of the cerebral vessels. This is justified since cerebral digital subtraction angiography (DSA) still has a risk of neurological complications despite advances in techniques and safer contrast agents. Carotid Doppler ultrasonography (US) is an excellent screening tool to study the carotid bifurcation in patients with transient ischemic attacks and stroke. Transcranial Doppler US is useful to detect early vasospasm in patients with subarachnoid hemorrhage. Multislice computed tomography (CT) and magnetic resonance imaging (MRI) have become effective methods to image the cerebral arteries and veins. DSA is now used selectively in treatment planning after noninvasive imaging has been used for diagnosis.

CT Angiography

With the advent of multislice CT and improved post-processing, CT angiography (CTA) and venography (CTV) play important roles in the evaluation of the cerebral vessels. CTA can be used to evaluate patients with carotid stenosis. CTA can detect a hairline residual lumen ("string sign") in patients with near occlusion. Typically, the string sign, which was described on DSA, has been difficult to show by MRA.

CTA is a fast and reliable method to evaluate patients with subarachnoid hemorrhage. CTA shows most cerebral aneurysms that are detected using DSA. CTA may also show thrombosis or calcification in the wall of a large or giant aneurysm. Post-processing allows assessment of the aneurysm with maximum intensity projections (MIP) and surface rendered three-dimensional (3D) projections in multiple planes (Fig. 1). In many cases, CTA is sufficient to allow treatment planning. If the aneurysm is unsuitable for endovascular treatment, the patient can be treated surgically without the need for DSA. In patients with subarachnoid hemorrhage, CTA is often more suitable than MRA since patients may be uncooperative. CTA can also be used for aneurysm screening in high-risk groups such as those with familial aneurysms and polycystic kidney disease. CTV can be used to evaluate patients with suspected sinovenous thrombosis.

MR Angiography

MRA plays a major role in cerebrovascular imaging. Gadolinium-enhanced auto-triggered elliptic centric-ordered MRA (ATECO) has superior resolution compared to time-of-flight (TOF) MRA. This has been shown in the evaluation of the carotid bifurcation and the intracranial arteries and veins. MRA to evaluate carotid stenosis has eliminated the need for DSA in the majority of patients. MRA of the extracranial and intracranial arteries is a standard part of the MR evaluation of patients with stroke (Fig. 2). Since ATECO is not dependent on the direction of flow, this technique gives excellent visualization of tortuous vessels and vessels with slow or turbulent flow. ATECO can determine if there is an intracranial arterial occlusion in patients being evaluated for possible intra-arterial thrombolysis.

MRA is a good technique to screen high-risk individuals for aneurysms. The ATECO technique is far superior to TOF MRA since the turbulent flow in an aneurysm may not be detected using the TOF method. ATECO is useful in detecting neck remnants in patients previously treated by coiling.

ATECO MRV is the imaging modality of choice to evaluate the cerebral veins and venous sinuses in patients with sinovenous thrombosis. It is far superior to TOF and phase contrast methods. In addition, the brain parenchyma can be assessed at the same time.

Digital Subtraction Angiography

Traditionally DSA has been the gold standard to evaluate the cerebral vessels. This remains true for the evaluation of the cerebral arteries, circulation time and collateral flow. This is no longer true for the evaluation of the venous sys-

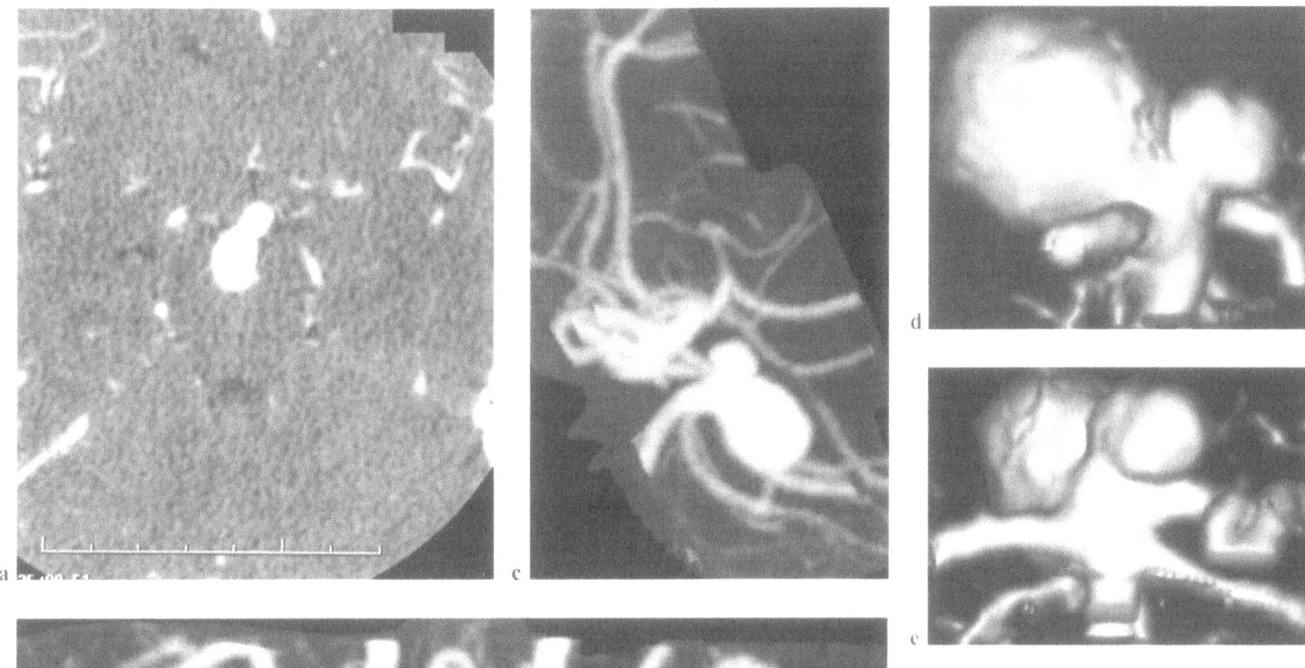

Fig. 1a-e. *Incidental aneurysm in a 44-year-old woman.* **a** Source image from CTA shows a basilar tip aneurysm projecting posteriorly. **b, c** Sagittal and axial collapsed MIP images show two lobules and the neck of the aneurysm. **d, e** Surface-rendered 3D images (posterior and anterior views) from CTA better define the relationship of the neck of the aneurysm to the parent vessel

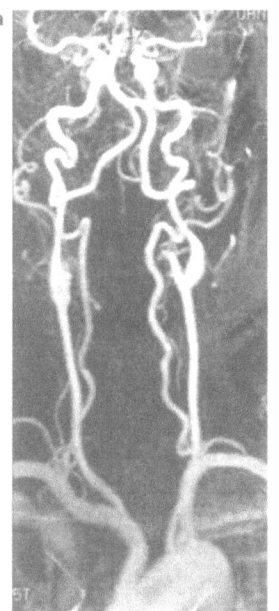

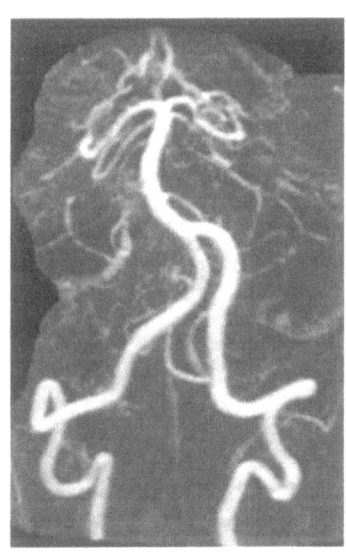

tem. ATECO MRV is superior to DSA. Since DSA uses selective arteriograms, there is washout of the cerebral veins and venous sinuses from unopacified blood. In ATECO MRV all the veins are opacified equally (Fig. 3).

DSA allows assessment of the circulation time. This is helpful in arterial occlusive disease, arteriovenous shunts,

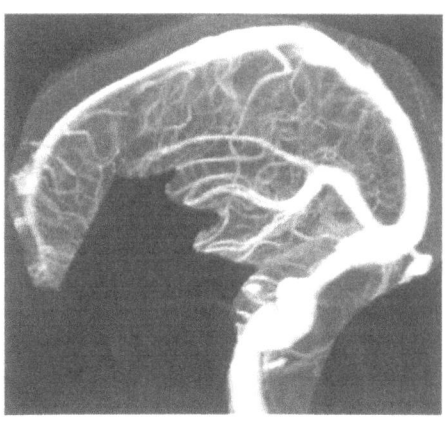

Fig. 2a, b. *Normal craniocervical ATECO MRA.* **a** Frontal view from the aortic arch to the circle of Willis. **b** Post-processing allows better visualization of the posterior fossa arteries

Fig. 3. Normal ATECO MRV gives a robust signal from the deep and superficial veins

venous occlusive disease and the venous congestion related to dural arteriovenous fistula with cortical venous reflux. In the case of brain micro-arteriovenous malformations, the only clue to detect the shunt is the presence of an early draining vein. This would be difficult to detect using CTA or ATECO MRA.

Collateral flow develops in response to occlusive disease in the arteries and veins. Collateral flow and the direction of flow are best assessed using DSA. Noninvasive imaging with CTA or MRA may detect the presence of a vessel but not the direction of flow. Assessment of collateral flow and circulation time is important in arterial stenosis and chronic venous occlusive disease. When venous collaterals enlarge and become tortuous, they may be evident on noninvasive imaging. These venous collaterals have been referred to as the pseudophlebitic pattern on DSA.

CTA and MRA are now used extensively to diagnosis cerebral aneurysms. Rotational DSA with 3D reconstruction gives the best details of the morphology of the aneurysm and the adjacent vessels (Figs. 4, 5). Rotational

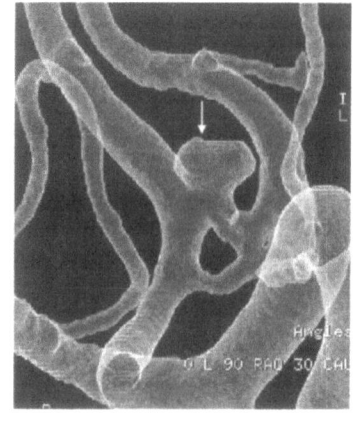

Fig. 5. Transparent shading of a 3D image from right internal carotid rotational DSA. Note the anterior communicating aneurysm (*arrow*) and duplication of the anterior communicating artery

DSA may reveal an aneurysm not evident on standard DSA projections. Treatment planning of complex and wide neck aneurysms is best determined after analysis of the rotational DSA and 3D reconstruction.

Cavernous Malformations

Cavernous malformations (CMs), or cavernomas, are vascular malformations of the central nervous system composed of well-circumscribed sinusoidal vascular channels containing blood in various stages of thrombosis. They affect 0.4%-0.9% of the general population according to large autopsy studies. They constitute 5%-16% of all vascular malformations. Multiple lesions are found in 17%-54% of patients, and in 50%-85% of these cases the multiple CMs are familial (autosomal dominant). Cavernous malformations often present in the second to fifth decades. Presentation includes seizures (31% of cases), hemorrhage (18.4%) and focal neurologic deficits (15%); the rest are incidental.

Developmental venous anomalies (DVAs) are associated with CMs. DVAs represent an extreme variant of the normal venous drainage. DVAs drain normal brain and must be preserved when CMs are excised. On MRI, CMs appear as radiating, linear flow voids (a "caput medusa" pattern) centered on a large collecting vein.

MRI is the diagnostic tool of choice for detecting and identifying cavernous malformations. On noncontrast CT, CMs frequently appear as focal areas of increased density within the brain often without mass effect. The differential diagnosis on CT includes low grade calcified neoplasms, hemorrhage and vascular malformations. The characteristic MRI appearance is a well-defined, lobulated lesion with a reticulated core of heterogeneous signal intensity on both T1- and T2-weighted sequences resulting from thrombosis, fibrosis, calcification and hemorrhage. On T2-weighted or gradient echo images, there is a peripheral ring of hypointensity that corresponds to the deposition of hemosiderin in the surrounding brain parenchyma. Cavernous malformations are angiographically occult.

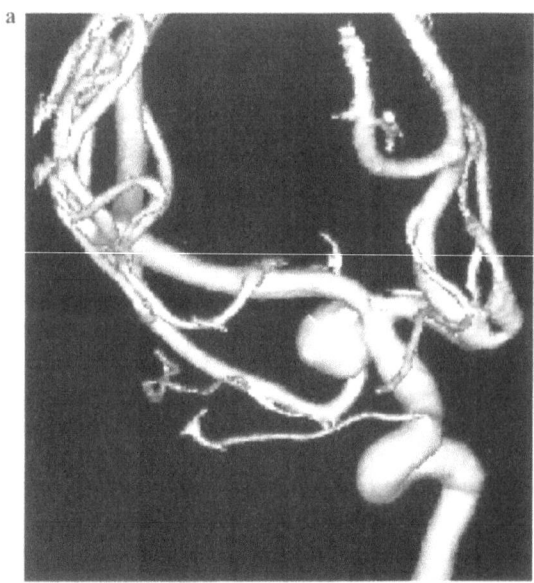

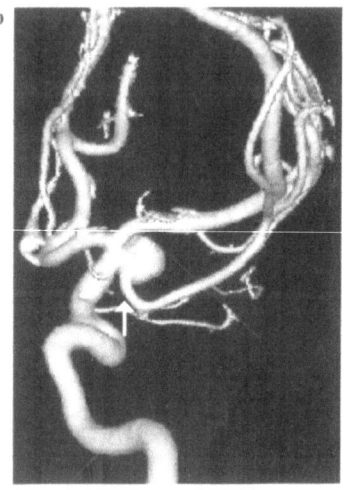

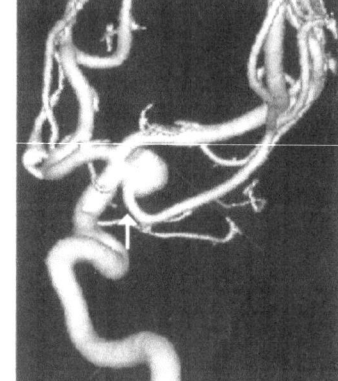

Fig. 4a, b. *Surface-rendered 3D images from right internal carotid rotational DSA.* **a** Frontal view shows an aneurysm at the accessory middle cerebral artery bifurcation. **b** Posterior view shows that the branch arises from the aneurysm

In cases where a CM is suspected but the radiologic image is not pathognomonic, serial imaging is of value if immediate surgical intervention is not warranted. Differential diagnoses include neoplasms and hematomas. If there is a recent bleed or thrombosis in a CM, the typical features of a CM may not be evident. Perilesional and extralesional hemorrhage may be evident outside the hemosiderin ring.

Dissection of the Extracranial Cervical Arteries

Dissection of the carotid or vertebral artery can be spontaneous or traumatic. Spontaneous dissections of the carotid or vertebral artery account for 2% of all ischemic strokes but in young and middle-aged patients they account for 10%-25% of cases. Spontaneous dissections occur in all ages but there is a peak incidence in the fifth decade.

Dissections are more common in patients with heritable connective tissue disorders including Ehlers-Danlos syndrome type IV, Marfan's syndrome, polycystic kidney disease and osteogenesis imperfecta. Angiographic changes of fibromuscular dysplasia are found in 15% of patients with spontaneous dissections of the carotid or vertebral artery. Bilateral dissections, either carotid or vertebral, are not rare (Fig. 6).

Dissections of the carotid or vertebral artery arise from a tear of the intima. The intramural hematoma may be subintimal or subadventitial. The typical patient with carotid dissection presents with pain on one side of the face or neck, a partial Horner's syndrome (miosis, ptosis) and the delayed onset of stroke. Patients with vertebral dissection often have pain in the back of the neck, an occipital headache and the delayed onset of posterior fossa ischemic symptoms. A lateral medullary syndrome (Wallenberg's syndrome) is a commonly found.

DSA has been the traditional diagnostic test to detect a dissection. Definitive signs of dissection are the presence of two lumens or demonstration of an intimal flap. Indirect signs are more commonly seen and include a long, irregular tapered stenosis, long tapered occlusion, or a dilatation (pseudoaneurysm) with a proximal stenosis. Carotid dissections tend to start beyond the bulb and often stop at the skull base. Vertebral dissections often occur at the C1-C2 vertebral levels and may be extend into the intradural segment.

MRI is replacing DSA as the primary investigation of carotid or vertebral artery dissections. MRI can show the

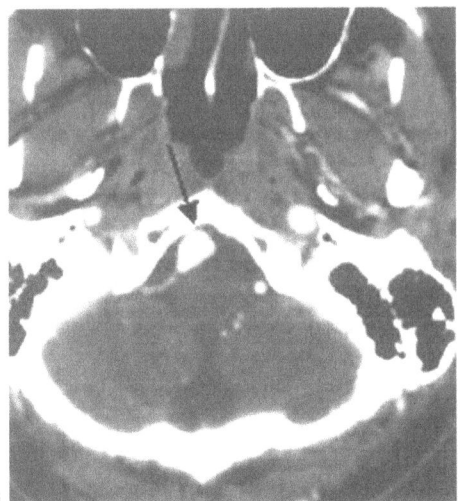
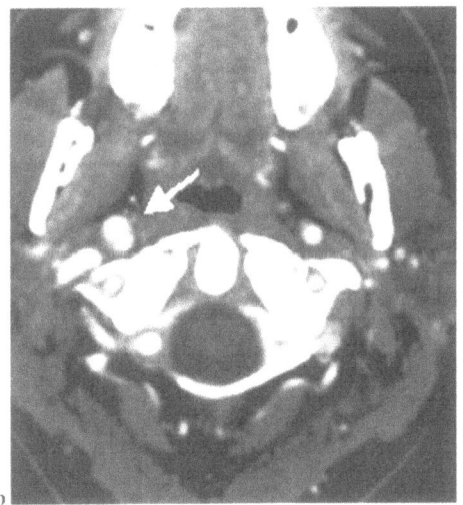
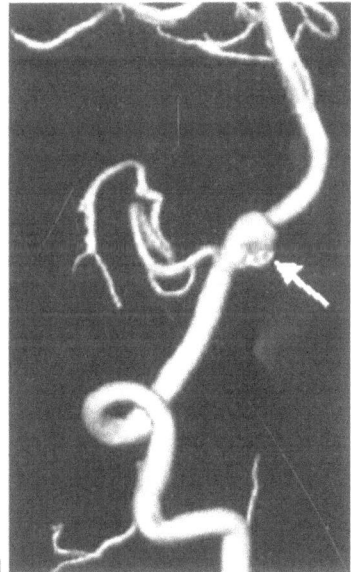
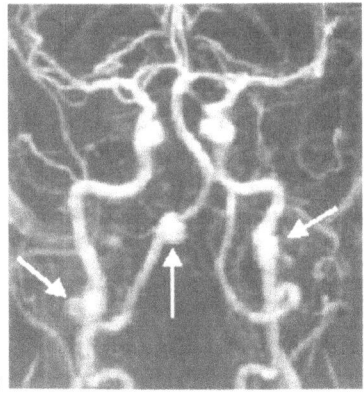

Fig. 6a-d. *Bilateral internal carotid and right vertebral artery dissections in a 44-year-old woman who presented with a posterior fossa stroke.* **a, b** Axial source images from CTA show an aneurysm of the right vertebral artery (*arrow* in **a**) and an intimal flap in the right internal carotid artery (*arrow* in **b**). **c** ATECO MRA shows bilateral internal carotid aneurysms and the right vertebral artery aneurysm (*arrows*). **d** 3D image from right vertebral rotational DSA shows an irregular, fusiform aneurysm just beyond the right posterior inferior cerebellar artery

intramural hematoma especially if fat saturation techniques are used. ATECO MRA can be used to clarify the extent of the abnormality and to detect pseudoaneurysms.

Dissection of the Intracranial Arteries

Intracranial dissections are often spontaneous and may present with subarachnoid hemorrhage or stroke. The commonest location is the intradural vertebral artery. Other common sites include the proximal posterior cerebral artery and the proximal posterior inferior cerebellar artery. Patients who present with hemorrhage have high risk for re-bleeding. Noninvasive imaging may reveal an aneurysm or a long irregular stenosis. DSA is critical for diagnosis and treatment planning. DSA often shows an irregular fusiform dilatation with a stenosis proximal to the dilatation. Assessment of collateral flow is critical since treatment often involves sacrifice of the diseased segment.

Cerebral Sinovenous Thrombosis

The clinical presentation of cerebral sinovenous thrombosis (CVT) is closely related to the location and the extent of the thrombosis (cortical vs. dural sinus, superficial vs. deep). The clinical sequelae of CVT are related to the temporal evolution of the disease, the patient's venous anatomy and the effectiveness of collateral venous pathways. The most frequent symptoms and signs of CVT are headaches, vomiting, and papilledema reflecting increased cerebral venous pressure. Patients may go on to develop seizures, decreased level of consciousness or focal neurologic deficit. Tissue damage and stasis (trauma, surgery and immobilization), hematologic disorders (proteins C and S deficiencies; increased resistance to activated protein C), malignancies, collagen vascular disease (systemic lupus erythematosus, Behçet's syndrome), pregnancy and some medications (oral contraceptives, hormone replacement therapy, corticosteroids) are predisposing factors for CVT.

Imaging findings of CVT can be categorized as direct, when there is visualization of cortical or dural sinus thrombus, or indirect when there are ischemic changes related to the venous outflow disturbance. Thrombus within the dural sinus or cortical vein can be identified as an elongated high-attenuation lesion on nonenhanced CT (*cord sign*). If the thrombus is located in the superior sagittal sinus, then a triangular filling defect (*empty delta sign*) can be demonstrated on post-contrast images. MRI is the modality of choice in dural sinus thrombosis. Acute thrombus is isointense to brain on T1-weighted images and hypointense on T2-weighted images. From 3-7 days after thrombus formation, the clot on MRI becomes hyperintense on T1-weighted images. The combination of MRI and ATECO MRV allows for an accurate diagnosis of CVT.

Venous infarction may be evident on CT as a diffuse, low-attenuating lesion. Mass effect is common and 40% of symptomatic patients show CT evidence of hemorrhage. Bilateral, parasagittal, hypoattenuating lesions on CT is a common feature of venous thrombosis in the superior sagittal sinus. These lesions do not conform to an arterial distribution but do involve the cortex. Isolated involvement of the temporal lobe is common and found in CVT of the transverse sinus. Bilateral thalamic hypoattenuating lesions on CT may be evident in deep venous thrombosis and, on noncontrast CT, thrombus may be seen in the straight sinus.

MRI is sensitive to the parenchymal changes in CVT. Cortical and subcortical high signal intensity lesions on FLAIR and T2-weighted images are highly suggestive of CVT when the lesions do not correspond to an arterial territory. Restricted diffusion in CVT may not have the same prognostic value as it does in arterial stroke and there may be reversibility of venous ischemia in CVT. This correlates with the important clinical improvement that may occur after an initial major neurological deficit related to CVT.

Intracranial Dural Arteriovenous Fistulas

Dural arteriovenous fistulas (DAVFs) represent 10%-15% of all intracranial arteriovenous lesions. They consist of one or more true fistulas, direct arteriovenous connections without an intervening capillary bed, localized within the dura mater. DAVFs have been categorized as either benign or aggressive based on their venous drainage and clinical symptoms. Benign DAVFs drain into the dural sinuses only, whereas aggressive DAVFs have reflux into the cortical veins. Non-hemorrhagic neurological deficits, hemorrhage and death are considered aggressive, while chronic headache, pulsatile bruit and orbital symptoms including cranial nerve deficit due to cavernous sinus lesions (ophthalmoplegia) are considered benign. Aggressive DAVFs have an annual risk of intracranial hemorrhage or non-hemorrhagic neurological deficits of 8.1% and 6.9% respectively, adding up to a 15.0% annual event rate. Aggressive DAVFs must be treated whereas the benign DAVFs may not require treatment if the symptoms are stable and well tolerated.

The term venous congestive encephalopathy describes a condition of cranial neurological deficits caused by venous hypertension secondary to cortical venous reflux from a DAVF. This entity is analogous to the venous congestive myelopathy of the spinal cord in the presence of a spinal DAVF. On MRI, T2 hyperintensity in the parenchyma can be seen as a result of the venous hypertension and passive congestion of the brain. In the cerebral and cerebellar hemispheres, the deep white matter seems to be the most vulnerable to this phenomenon; after treatment these findings may be partially reversible. The differential diagnosis of the T2 hyperintensity includes a superior sagittal sinus thrombosis with a venous infarction or venous congestion, demyelination or dysmyelination. In the cerebellum, a peripheral diffuse enhancement pattern surrounding the central T2 hyperintensity is characteristic of DAVFs with cortical venous reflux. The combination of central T2 hyperintensity with a surplus of pial vessels is highly suggestive of a vascular malformation and mandates prompt DSA.

Moyamoya Disease

Moyamoya disease is a primary vascular disease characterized by progressive stenosis and eventual occlusion of the supraclinoid portion of the internal carotid artery and the adjacent segments of the middle and anterior cerebral arteries. In response, an abnormal vascular network of small collateral vessels develops to bypass the area of occlusion. This disease affects children as well as adults. Adults tend to present with hemorrhage. The most frequent symptoms in children are multiple transient ischemic attacks and some episodes result in a fixed deficit. Seizures are a common presentation of patients under the age of six years. The disorder is often progressive resulting in a severe motor impairment and intellectual deterioration. The small collateral vessels at the base of the brain are enlarged lenticulostriate vessels. These collaterals may be evident on MRI and on DSA represent the "puff of smoke" appearance characteristic of this disease. DSA may reveal transdural anastomoses and collateral pial vessels crossing the watershed territories.

Central Nervous System Vasculitis

Central nervous system (CNS) vasculitis is inflammation of blood vessel walls that results in symptoms by causing ischemia. Vasculitis affecting the CNS alone is referred to as primary angiitis of the CNS. Secondary vasculitis occurs in association with a variety of conditions, including infections, drug abuse, lymphoproliferative disease and connective tissue diseases. The pathogenesis of vasculitis includes different immunological mechanisms. A wide spectrum of clinical features may occur. The typical clinical presentations of CNS vasculitis are stroke, encephalopathy and seizures.

MRI findings suggestive of vasculitis are multiple, bilateral lesions in the cortex and white matter. The presence of gray matter involvement should help differentiate the white matter lesions from demyelination. In approximately 20% of proven cases, DSA shows abnormalities in the cerebral arteries including segmental narrowing, microaneurysms and vascular beading. The findings may be similar to atherosclerosis, vasospasm and infection. DSA results must be interpreted in conjunction with the clinical and laboratory results.

Suggested Reading

Alvarez-Linera J, Benito-Leon J, Escribano J et al (2003) Prospective evaluation of carotid artery stenosis: elliptic centric contrast-enhanced MR angiography and spiral CT angiography compared with digital subtraction angiography. AJNR Am J Neuroradiol 24:1012-1019

Anderson GB, Findlay JM, Steinke DE, Ashforth R (1997) Experience with computed tomographic angiography for the detection of intracranial aneurysms in the setting of acute subarachnoid hemorrhage: clinical study. Neurosurgery 41:522-528

Farb R, Scott JN, Willinsky R, Montanera W, Wright G, terBrugge K (2003) Intracranial venous system: gadolinium-enhanced three-dimensional MR venography with auto-triggered elliptic centric-ordered sequence – initial experience. Radiology 226:203-209

Fieschi C, Rasura M, Anzini A, Beccia M (1998) Central nervous system vasculitis. J Neurol Sci 153:159-171

Gladstone D, Silver F, Willinsky RA, Tyndel F, Wennberg R (2001) Deep cerebral venous thrombosis: an illustrative case with reversible diencephalic dysfunction. Can J Neurol Sci 28:159-162

Hirai T, Korogi Y, Suginohara K et al (2003) Clinical usefulness of unsubtracted 3D digital angiography compared with rotational digital angiography in the pretreatment evaluation of intracranial aneurysms. AJNR Am J Neuroradiol 24:1067-1074

Lazinski D, Willinsky RA, terBrugge K, Montanera W (2000) Dissecting aneurysms of the posterior cerebral artery: angioarchitecture and review of the literature. Neuroradiology 42:128-133

Lee SK, terBrugge K, Willinsky R, Montanera W (2003) MR imaging of dural arteriovenous fistula draining into cerebellar cortical veins. AJNR Am J Neuroradiol 24:1602-1606

Lev MH, Romero JM, Goodman DNF et al (2003) Total occlusion versus hairline residual lumen of the internal carotid arteries: accuracy of single section helical CT angiography. AJNR Am J Neuroradiol 24:1123-1129

Rivera P, Willinsky R, Porter P (2003) Intracranial cavernous malformations. Neuroimaging Clin N Am 13:27-40

Schievink WI (2001) Spontaneous dissection of the carotid and vertebral arteries. N Engl J Med 344:898-906

Van Dijk M, terBrugge K, Willinsky RA, Wallace C (2002) The clinical course of cranial rural AV fistulas with long-term persistent cortical venous reflux. Stroke 33(5):1233-1236

Van Dijk JMC, Willinsky R (2003) Venous congestive encephalopathy related to cranial dural arteriovenous fistulas. Neuroimaging Clin N Am 13:55-72

Wetzel SG, Kirsch E, Stock KW et al (1999) Cerebral veins: comparative study of CT venography with intrarterial digital subtraction angiography. AJNR Am J Neuroradiol 20:249-255

Willinsky RA, Taylor SM, ter Brugge K, Montanera W, Farb R (2003) Neurologic complications of cerebral angiography: a prospective analysis of 2899 procedures. Radiology 227(2):522-528

Willinsky RA, Harper W, Wallace MC, Kucharczyk W, Montanera W, Mikulis D, terBrugge K (1996) Follow-up MR of intracranial cavernomas, the relationship between hemorrhage events and morphology. Interv Neuroradiol 2:127-135

Willinsky RA, terBrugge K, Montanera W, Mikulis D, Wallace MC (1994) Venous congestion: an MR finding in dural arteriovenous malformations with cortical venous drainage. AJNR Am J Neuroradiol 15:1501-1507

Willinsky RA, Goyal M, terBrugge K, Montanera W (1999) Tortuous, engorged pial veins in intracranial dural arteriovenous fistulas: correlation with presentation, location, and MR findings in 122 patients. AJNR Am J Neuroradiol 20:1031-1036

Imaging and Management of Acute Stroke

W.T.C. Yuh[1], T. Taoka[2], T. Ueda[3], M. Maeda[4]

[1] University of Oklahoma Health Sciences Center, Oklahoma City, OK, USA; [2] Department of Radiology, Nara Medical University, Kashihara, Japan; [3] Department of Neurosurgery, Yokohama Stroke and Brain Center, Isogo-ku, Yokohama, Japan; [4] Department of Radiology, Mie University School of Medicine, Tsu, Mie, Japan

Introduction

With recent advances in both imaging techniques and reperfusion therapies, patients with acute stroke now have a realistic window of opportunity for effective intervention and treatment outcome. It is generally believed that "time is brain," i.e. the maximum benefit can only be achieved when intervention is initiated within the first 3-6 hours after the onset of symptoms, depending upon the treatment (e.g. intravenous administration of tissue plasminogen activator or endovascular recanalization).

Since the US Food and Drug Administration (FDA) approved the intravenous administration of tissue plasminogen activator (tPA) for stroke therapy in 1996, there has been only a limited overall impact (estimated ≤1%) to stroke victims [1]. This limited impact of tPA has been mostly attributed to two major factors. First, there is a relatively low rate of recruitment of eligible patients, likely due to the relatively short therapeutic windows for both intravenous (3 hours) and endovascular (6 hours) recanalization. Second, there is a relatively low rate of therapeutic efficacy (12%-30%) as reported by the recent intravenous thrombolysis trial, likely due to the lack of an effective and validated strategy for patient selection [1-3]. Despite the potential benefits of both intravenous (tPA) and endovascular recanalization procedures, to date only about 1% and 16% of patients are eligible for treatment based upon the conventional 3- and 6-hour therapeutic windows, respectively.

Currently, stroke patients seek medical attention an average of 13 hours after the onset of symptoms. This means that the vast majority do not have an opportunity to benefit from thrombolytic therapy as currently prescribed. The Stroke Council of the American Heart Association (AHA) is increasing its efforts to educate the general public in both the recognition of early signs and symptoms of acute stroke, as well as the need to seek immediate medical attention. The expectation is to significantly increase the number of potentially eligible patients up to 20% [4]. Although the AHA expects that the average time at which patients seek medical attention will shorten, realistically most patients still will not be eligible for intravenous or in-tra-arterial revascularization interventions unless there are ways to identify a subgroup of patients with a therapeutic window longer than the presumed 3 or 6 hours. Therefore, there is a need to apply these useful imaging parameters in triaging patients who may be at risk for reperfusion hemorrhage or who are likely to benefit from arterial reperfusion within or beyond the traditional therapeutic window.

Therapeutic Window after Ischemic Stroke

The true therapeutic window for effective outcome after revascularization in ischemic stroke in humans remains to be defined. Based on both experimental and clinical studies, some have suggested that the maximal time for achieving best treatment outcome after revascularization in the setting of acute stroke is within the first 6 hours after onset of symptoms [5]. This was first confirmed clinically by Zeumer et al. [6] who observed that intra-arterial thrombolytic therapy used in the treatment of acute internal carotid artery or middle cerebral artery occlusion was best performed within 5 hours of symptoms onset. Recently, our group retrospectively evaluated 42 lesions in 30 patients and underwent successful recanalization within the first 12 hours of symptoms [7]. Similar to Zeumer et al.'s work, our study suggested that a 5-hour therapeutic window may be preferable. These studies are consistent with animal experiments that measured the relationship between the severity and duration of ischemia (Fig. 1a). Interestingly, our study also suggested that within the first 5 hours of onset of symptoms, the therapeutic outcome was dependent upon the severity and duration of ischemia (Fig. 1b). However, our findings also pointed out that, after the 5-hour period of ischemia, residual cerebral blood flow appeared to be the most important factor that influenced therapeutic outcome.

Despite conventional wisdom, several studies have provided evidence for an extended therapeutic window up to 36 hours from onset of symptoms [7-11]. In particular, it is well known that the effective therapeutic window for revascularization of posterior circulation of ischemia is

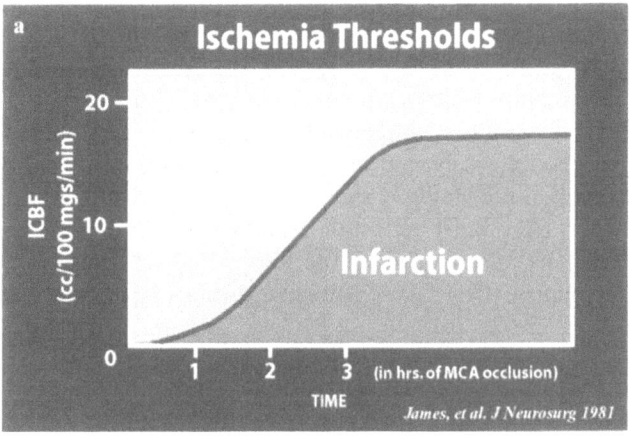
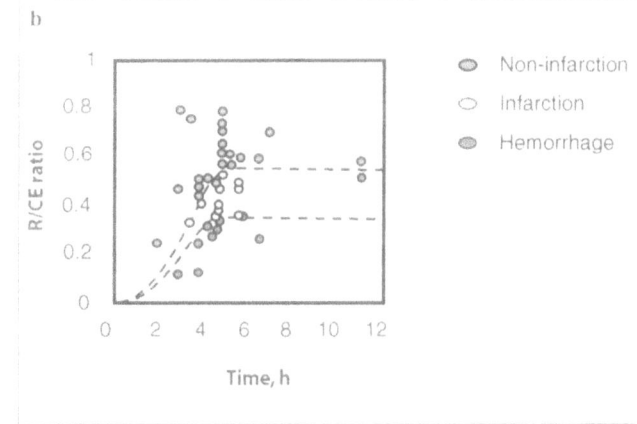

Fig. 1a, b. The relationship between ischemia severity (as determined by the ratio of ischemic regional activity to cerebellar activity, R/CE) and duration **a** Animal study (reproduced from [15] with permission) **b** Our preliminary data from perfusion imaging in human s (reproduced from [7] with permission)

often relatively longer compared to that of the anterior circulation [12, 13]. Conversely, both intravenous and intra-arterial thrombolytic therapies may not always be associated with satisfactory outcomes despite achieving successful recanalization within the conventional 3- or 6-hour therapeutic window. This is often attributed to hemorrhagic complications by reperfusing the ischemic core or a probable lack of reversibility of the ischemic tissue that is located in an eloquent area of the brain.

Cerebral Blood Flow and Assessment of Tissue Viability and Ischemic Reversibility

Cerebral blood flow (CBF) of the normal brain ranges from 45 to 110 ml per minute 100 grams tissue, varying both in time and location within the same individual (Fig. 2a) [14-17]. Below-normal CBF may be broadly

defined as hypoperfusion that includes a range of values arbitrarily defined as oligemic and ischemic. Cerebral oligemia is associated with underperfused brain parenchyma that will spontaneously recover, and is more likely to not be associated with overt neurological symptoms. In contrast, ischemic range reduction of CBF is typically symptomatic and at risk for irreversible infarction if revascularization does not occur. This includes both the core region of CBF reduction as well as the larger surrounding area of so-called penumbra. Animal studies have shown that an ischemic threshold, defined as cessation of normal action potential generation, occurs at approximately $20 \ ml \times min^{-1} \ 100 \ g^{-1}$. For infarction threshold, i.e. the point of irreversible ischemic injury to neurons, the reduction of CBF has been estimated at approximately $10 \ ml \times min^{-1} \ 100 \ g^{-1}$.

It is believed that the ischemic penumbra constitutes a potentially reversible volume of cerebral tissue that has

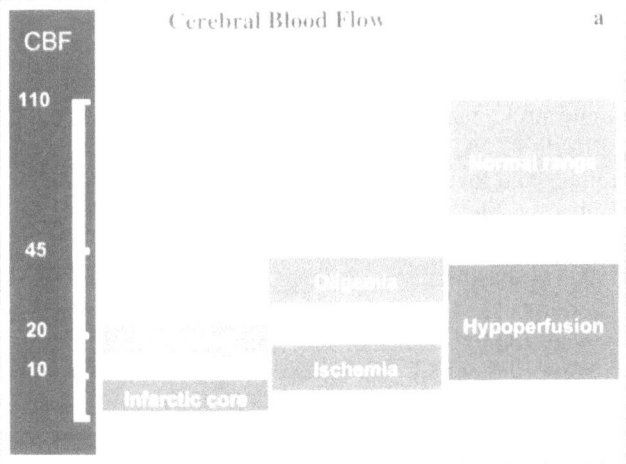
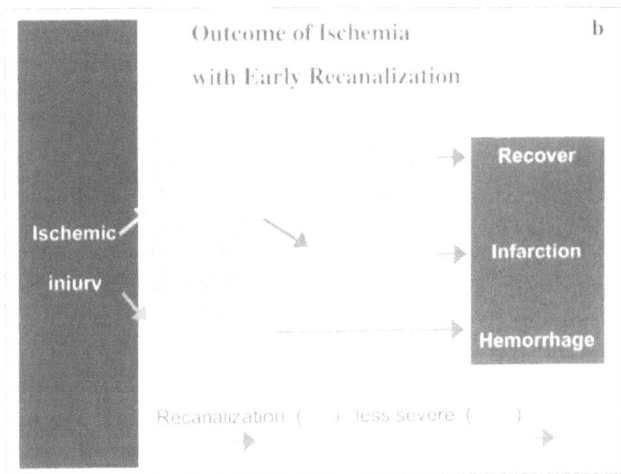

Fig. 2. Definitions and terminology (**a**) related to various ranges of CBF, and their significance (**b**) related to the ischemic injury (viability and reversibility) prior to and after treatment

CBF between the ischemic and infarction thresholds mentioned previously [16, 18-20]. The existence of this ischemic penumbra has been suggested by perfusion and diffusion imaging studies of untreated patients [21-23]. However, without timely successful recanalization, the penumbra eventually progresses to irreversible infarction that cannot be differentiated from core areas of ischemia detected in earlier phases of stroke. Interestingly, although the classic range of CBF for ischemic penumbra is between 10-20 ml × min^{-1} 100 g^{-1} in animal studies (Fig. 1a) [15], clinical studies have shown that this region of potentially reversible ischemia depends on time and anatomic location, and varies in individual patients. This suggests that an absolute measurement of CBF may not be necessary for determining potential viability and reversibility during emergent triage of a stroke patient [11, 24, 25]. This has led our group to apply semiquantitative and relative measurements of residual cerebral blood flow for the purposes of rapid determination of potential salvage ability (reversibility) and risk of hemorrhage (viability) in the setting of acute stroke intervention.

Hemorrhagic complications associated with both spontaneous and therapeutic arterial revascularization in the setting of acute stroke are believed to be related to reperfusion injury within the microvascular bed of nonviable brain tissue (Fig. 2b). Theoretically, ischemic brain that has adequate collateral circulation may remain viable long enough so that revascularization will not result in reperfusion injury and consequent hemorrhagic complication. Ischemic brain that remains viable at the time of revascularization may be salvageable (i.e. reversible) if successful and timely reperfusion is achieved. However, it is also possible that brain tissue that is viable at the time of attempted revascularization may have actually suffered irreversible ischemic injury that progresses to infarction. In this setting, early reperfusion is associated with low risk of hemorrhage despite the progression to infarction.

The concepts of temporal viability and ischemic reversibility can only be properly assessed in a setting of demonstrated early recanalization, such as commonly achieved with intravenous and intra-arterial thrombolysis. Amazingly, most prior studies have only evaluated untreated patients. We have taken the approach of assessing relative differences in residual CBF estimated with Tc99-HMPO single photon emission computed tomography (SPECT). Our preliminary data suggest that in patients who have undergone successful recanalization, the CBF thresholds for viability and reversibility are approximately 35% and 55%, respectively (when compared to normal brain parenchyma) (Fig. 1b) [7]. Our study also demonstrated that most hemorrhages (71%) occurred during early therapeutic intervention (3-5 hours) in patients with low residual CBF (below 35%). These findings suggest that the conventional time window alone cannot differentiate between patients at low and high risk for reperfusion hemorrhage. Instead, it appears that the pretreatment residual CBF may differentiate three categories of treatment outcomes for ischemic lesions. These can be conveniently categorized as: (i) hemorrhage, (ii) infarction, and (iii) reversible ischemia (Fig. 1b). Another interesting observation from our preliminary data is that certain ischemic insults with relatively high residual CBF may be successfully salvaged up to 12 hours after the onset of symptoms. Finally, it should be noted that the viability threshold of CBF reduction found with SPECT is similar what we observed using perfusion magnetic resonance imaging (MRI) in an untreated group of patients with acute stroke [26].

Neuroimaging in Acute Stroke

Neuroimaging techniques have made significant improvements in stroke imaging, particularly for early detection and delineation of acute ischemia. This has been almost exclusively based upon observations of untreated patients [21, 27-42]. Currently, there is no reliable and definitive pretreatment imaging means to identify individuals who are at risk for hemorrhagic complications or those who will potentially benefit by early restoration of CBF [1].

Diffusion-weighted imaging (DWI) has a sensitivity of 88%-100% and a specificity of 95%-100% in the diagnosis of acute stroke [27-36]. DWI may be positive as early as 30 minutes after the onset of symptoms [37]. This capability is essential for the early confirmation and delineation of acute ischemia and to facilitate early therapeutic intervention [21, 37-42]. The efficacy of DWI in the assessment of tissue viability and reversibility, particularly for considering early intervention, has not been established [25, 26, 43-46]. Abnormal diffusion measurements in the setting of acute stroke may consist of early intracellular and extracellular changes in water distribution associated with both reversible and irreversible cerebral ischemia [46]. The ischemic lesion volume and apparent diffusion coefficient (ADC) values measured by diffusion MRI may have predictive value for clinical outcome in untreated patients [47, 48]. However, Baird and Warach [49] have argued that there is no absolute threshold of ADC decrease that predicts evolution to infarction. Furthermore, diffusion abnormalities in the setting of acute stroke may be reversible if early reperfusion occurs [21, 29, 43, 44, 50]. It is likely that DWI only indirectly reflects the severity of hypoperfusion, as supported by the lack of a linear relationship between the magnitude of ADC reduction and degree of ultimate ischemic injury [50, 51]. Furthermore, the apparent threshold of CBF reduction needed to produce abnormalities on DWI is higher than the experimentally defined ischemic and infarction thresholds [52, 53]. Diffusion abnormalities are likely to represent a summation of changes from cellular dysfunction over a period of time [53, 54]. This suggests that DWI is sensitive in detecting ischemia but may not be as specific as perfusion imaging for the assessment of viability and reversibility [43, 44, 55, 56].

Perfusion MRI provides more direct information related to aberrations in regional CBF that may be more reflective of the primary underlying pathophysiology of an acute ischemic insult. Although at present perfusion MRI cannot produce absolute values of CBF, it is capable of making semiquantitative estimates of relative mean transit time (rMTT), relative cerebral blood volume (rCBV), and relative CBF (rCBF) that can be mapped to the cerebral anatomy. These maps can be generated quickly, having already been proven to be feasible and valuable in decision making for acute stroke intervention [26, 45, 57]. Based upon the dynamic contrast enhancement curve, a flow-related map can be generated by various parameters (e.g. mean transit time, peak time) and a blood volume map can be estimated. The relationship between the CBF, MTT and CBV can be expressed as the following:

$$rCBF = rCBV / rMTT$$

The increased signal intensity on the flow-related maps such as the rMTT map is equivalent to an increased vascular resistance as seen in Ohm's law (V=IR), if we consider relative CBF to be equivalent to current (I) and rCBV equivalent to voltage (V). An increase of signal intensity on the rMTT map may not indicate ischemia or infarction, as seen in patients with asymptomatic carotid stenosis or occlusion. Therefore, flow-related maps such as the rMTT map only suggest increased vascular resistance [58-60] and are less ideal than rCBV and rCBF maps in the assessment of ischemic viability and reversibility, as frequently done in the past.

A recent report suggested that the combined use of perfusion imaging and DWI may be beneficial in monitoring the efficacy of thrombolytic therapy [61]. Our group has reported that ischemic tissues with prolonged rMTT and a marked decrease in rCBV tend to suffer irreversible ischemic injuries [62]. A mild decrease in rCBV with prolonged rMTT suggests that it is possible to differentiate between severely ischemic tissue and peri-infarct parenchyma by rCBV maps in hyperacute ischemia [63]. Using the combination of perfusion and diffusion measurements in untreated patients, others have suggested that significant mismatching of perfusion and diffusion abnormalities may serve as a basis for selecting patients who are most likely to benefit from therapeutic revascularization [23, 64]. However, such an approach has certain theoretical limitations that require further evaluation, and also require proper validation when applied to an appropriate patient population. There are several reasons for this. First, the observations of these studies are mostly based upon an untreated population of patients that may not be representative (in terms of demographics, clinical status and, possibly, pathophysiology) of patients being prospectively considered for acute therapeutic intervention. Second, these studies utilized rMTT mapping, which is highly sensitive to any homodynamic compromise that produces a state of hypoperfusion. However, as stated earlier, increased rMTT can be likened to a relative increase in vascular resistance, which can occur in various settings of acute-subacute ischemia or chronic oligemia [62]. Therefore, this type of perfusion mapping cannot differentiate the time of onset of the resistance or functional significance of a given rMTT abnormality, which in our experience is not always indicative of ischemia. Third, the size and magnitude of hyperintensity in rMTT maps are highly dependent upon the proximity and severity of vascular narrowing, respectively, which again does not always translate to actual ischemia. For example, a proximal stenosis of a major cerebral artery is more likely to produce a larger area of abnormal rMTT than an occlusion of a more distal branch within the same territory. Finally, since the CBF reduction threshold for producing positive findings on both diffusion imaging and rMTT maps is likely much higher than the "true" ischemia and infarction thresholds, qualitative assessments alone of DWI and rMTT may overestimate the severity of ischemic injury in a given patient, which would result in denying some patients the potential benefit of thrombolytic therapy [51, 52]. We believe that better patient selection for thrombolytic therapy will eventually be possible by assessing cerebral ischemic viability and reversibility using more quantitative comparisons of diffusion abnormalities with both rMTT and rCBV maps in patients with proof of early and successful recanalization.

Nuclear perfusion imaging of the brain using Tc99m-HMPAO SPECT also has been advocated for the management of acute stroke, particularly in assisting clinical decision making for proper patient selection [5, 65-67]. Relative comparisons of the residual CBF can be made by calculating ratios of activity in normal and affected regions of the brain. Shimosegawa et al. [68] showed that these ratios could be used to estimate the infarction (viability) threshold in an untreated group of patients imaged within 6 hours of symptoms onset; the reported threshold was 0.48 (SD=0.14). In another study, reperfusion occurring within approximately 7 hours after onset of symptoms significantly reduced the development of infarction (reversibility) with a R/CE ratio (the ratio of ischemic regional activity to cerebellar activity) between 0.55 and 0.75 [69]. Others found that so-called moderate ischemia with residual relative CBF ratios between 0.35 and 0.70 was suitable for intra-arterial thrombolysis [70]. Our data show that the pretreatment CBF judged by SPECT in patients with complete recanalization is significantly different among reversible ischemia, infarction, and hemorrhage (Fig. 1b) [7]. The risk of hemorrhagic transformation in acute stroke, when treated within 5 hours with intra-arterial thrombolysis, primarily depended on residual CBF of ischemic tissue judged by pretreatment SPECT (35%). Within 5 hours of symptoms onset, the development of infarction or hemorrhage appeared to depend on both the residual CBF and on the duration of ischemia (Fig. 1b). However, beyond 5 hours from the onset of symptoms, the residual CBF was the only parameter that appeared to be predictive of treatment outcome. It must be stressed that our data also showed that relative reductions in rCBF during an acute stroke correlated with the neurological outcome in the setting of acute therapeutic intervention, supporting the notion that such perfusion measurements can provide important information that could be used for optimizing patient selection. This predictability included both overall neurological outcome and risk of hemorrhagic conversion for a wide spectrum of time intervals from symptoms onset, including some cases that were well beyond the conventional 6-hour therapeutic window used for intra-arterial thrombolysis [7, 71].

Conclusions

The role of acute stroke imaging is evolving from simple detection and delineation of ischemic injury to the more important issue of predicting therapeutic outcome. To achieve this goal, hemorrhage revealed with conventional diagnostic imaging and functional imaging in an untreated population of patients may not always be useful for assessing the true capabilities of various imaging modalities that can be used for predicting therapeutic outcome in acute stroke intervention. Most published studies focused on patients and lesions that neither received treatment nor had demonstrable evidence of reperfusion. The effectiveness of pretreatment imaging or therapy cannot be adequately addressed if a salvaging effort has not been attempted or failed. With the coexisting heterogeneity of disease state among patients or lesions, and the various imaging modalities available for assessing cerebral ischemia, the traditional efforts to obtain absolute measurements of various predictive parameters may detract from the more important goal of finding prompt and practical assessments that can rapidly facilitate triage of the acute stroke patient considered for therapeutic intervention. This need may favor use of somewhat more simplistic and semiquantitative methodologies. Currently, cerebral perfusion imaging using either SPECT or MRI appears to be able to provide this type of prompt and predictive information since it is most closely tied to the primary underlying pathophysiology (i.e. hypoperfusion). Therefore, we believe further efforts need to be made in applying these modalities prospectively for the purpose of improving treatment eligibility (extending therapeutic window) and effectiveness.

Note: This chapter is based on: Imaging helps identify who benefits frome stroke intervention. 1999, Diagn Imaging 19:70-82.

References

1. Furlan AJ, Kanoti G (1997) When is thrombolysis justified in patients with acute ischemic stroke? A bioethical perspective. Stroke 28:214-218
2. The National Institute of Neurological Disorders and Stroke rt-PA Stroke Study Group (1995) Tissue plasminogen activator for acute ischemic stroke. N Engl J Med 333:1581-1587
3. Kwiatkowski TG, Libman RB, Frankel M, Tilley BC, Morgenstern LB, Lu M et al (1999) Effects of tissue plas-

minogen activator for acute ischemic stroke at one year. N Engl J Med 340:1781-1787
4. Kenton EJ (1999) Advocacy and research, making a difference. Stroke Connection Magazine, vol 2
5. Adams H, Brott T, Furlan A, Gomez C. Grotta J, Helgason C, Kwiakowski T, Lyden P, Marler J, Torner J, Feinberg W, Mayberg M, Thies W (1996) Guidelines for thrombolytic therapy for acute stroke: a supplement to the guidelines for the management of patients. Circulation 94:1167-1174
6. Zeumer H, Freitag H, Zanella F, Thie A, Arning C (1993) Local intra-arterial fibrinolytic therapy in patients with stroke: urokinase versus recombinant tissue plasminogen activator (r-TPA). Neuroradiology 35:159-162
7. Ueda T, Sakaki S, Yuh WTC, Nochide I, Ohta S (1999) Outcome in acute stroke with successful intra-arterial thrombolysis and predictive value of initial single-photon emission-computed tomography. J Cereb Blood Flow Metab 19:99-108
8. Ueda T, Sakaki S, Kumon Y, Yuh WTC (1999) Multivariable analysis of long-term outcome in acute stroke patient with intraarterial thrombolysis. In: Proceedings of the Annual Meeting of the American Society of Neuroradiology, 23-28 May 1999, San Diego
9. Ueda T, Sakaki S, Kumon Y, Yuh WTC (1999) Comparison of SPECT values and neurologic scores in pre- and postintraarterial thrombolysis for acute stroke patients. In: Proceedings of the Annual Meeting of the American Society of Neuroradiology, 23-28 May 1999, San Diego
10. Yuh WTC, Ueda T (2003) Perfusion imaging assessment of ischemic viability and reversibility by perfusion imaging and its potential role for the endovascular treatment of acute stroke. Stroke 34:4-1104
11. Furlan MGM, Viader F, Derlon J, Baron J (1996) Spontaneous neurological recovery after stroke and the fate of the ischemic penumbra. Ann Neurol 40:216-226
12. Hacke W, Zeumer H, Ferbert A, Bruchman H, del Zoppo G (1988) Intra-arterial thrombolytic therapy improves outcome in patients with acute vertebrobasilar occlusive disease. Stroke 19:1216-1222
13. Cross DeWitte T III, Moran CJ, Akins PT, Angtuaco EE, Diringer MN (1997) Relationship between clot location and outcome after basilar artery thrombolysis. AJNR Am J Neuroradiol 18:1221-1228
14. Obrenovitch TP (1995) The ischaemic penumbra: twenty years on. Cerebrovasc Brain Metab Rev 7:297-323
15. Jones T, Morawetz R, Crowell R, Marcoux F, FitzGibbon S, DeGirolami U, Ojemann R (1981) Thresholds of focal cerebral ischemia in awake monkeys. J Neurosurg 54:773-782
16. Astrup J, Symon L, Siesj B (1981) Thresholds in cerebral ischemia - the ischemic penumbra. Stroke 12: 723-725
17. Powers WJ, Zivin J (1998) Magnetic resonance imaging in acute stroke: not ready for prime time. Neurology 50:842-843
18. Fisher M, Garcia J (1996) Evolving stroke and the ischemic penumbra. Neurology 47:884-888
19. Symon L, Branston N, Strong A, Hope T (1977) The concept of thresholds of ischaemia in relation to brain structure and function. J Clin Pathol 30[Suppl 11]:149-154
20. Hossmann KA (1994) Viability thresholds and the penumbra of focal ischemia. Ann Neurol 36:557-565
21. Sorensen AG, Buonanno FS, Gonzalez RG et al (1996) Hyperacute stroke: evaluation with combined multisection diffusion-weighted and hemodynamically weighted echo-planar MR imaging. Radiology 199:391-401
22. Kucharczyk J, Mintorovitch J, Asgari HS, Moseley M (1991) Diffusion/perfusion MR imaging of acute cerebral ischemia. Magn Reson Med 19:311-315
23. Sorenson AG, Copen WA, Ostergaard L et al (1999) Hyperacute stroke: simultaneous measurement of relative cerebral blood volume, relative cerebral blood flow, and mean tissue transit time. Radiology 210:519-527

24. Tamura A, Graham D, McCulloch J, Teasdale G (1981) Focal cerebral ischemia in the rat. 2. Regional cerebral blood flow determined by [14C]iodoantipyrine autoradiography following middle cerebral artery occlusion. J Cereb Blood Flow Metab 1:61-69

25. Yuh WTC, Maeda M, Wang AM et al (1995) Fibrinolytic treatment of acute stroke: are we treating reversible cerebral ischemia? AJNR Am J Neuroradiol 16:1994-2000

26. Ueda T, Yuh WTC, Maley JE, Quets JP, Hahn PY, Magnotta VA (1999) Outcome of acute ischemic lesions detected by diffusion and perfusion MR imaging. AJNR Am J Neuroradiol 20:983-989

27. Minematsu K, Li L, Fisher M, Sotak CH, Davis MA, Fiandaca MS (1992) Diffusion-weighted magnetic resonance imaging: rapid and quantitative detection of focal brain ischemia. Neurology 42:235-240

28. Moseley ME, Cohen Y, Mintorovitch J et al (1990) Early detection of regional cerebral ischemia in cats: comparison of diffusion- and T2-weighted MRI and spectroscopy. Magn Reson Med 14:330-346

29. Marks MP, de Crespigny A, Lentz D, Enzmann DR, Albers GW, Moseley ME (1996) Acute and chronic stroke: navigated spin-echo diffusion-weighted MR imaging. Radiology 199:403-408

30. Beauchamp NJ, Barker PB, Wang PY, van Zijl PCM (1999) Imaging of acute cerebral ischemia. Radiology 212:307-324

31. Benveniste H, Hedlund LW, Johnson GA (1992) Mechanisms of detection of acute cerebral ischemia in rats by diffusion-weighted magnetic resonance microscopy. Stroke 23:746-754

32. Norris DG, Niendorf TG, Leibfritz D (1994) Healthy and infarcted brain tissue studies at short diffusion times: the origins of apparent restriction and the reduction in apparent diffusion constant. NMR Biomed 7:304-310

33. Helpern JA, Ordidge RJ, Knight RA (1992) The effect of cell membrane water permeability on the apparent diffusion coefficients of water. In: Society of Magnetic Resonance in Medicine (abstract)

34. Duong TQ, Ackerman JJH, Ying HS, Neil JJ (1998) Evaluation of extra- and intracellular apparent diffusion in normal and globally ischemic rat brains via 19F NMR. Magn Reson Med 40:1-13

35. van der Toorn A, Sykova EDRM, Vorisek I et al (1996) Dynamic changes in water ADC, energy metabolism, extracellular space volume, and tortuosity in neonatal rat brain during global ischemia. Magn Reson Med 36:52-60

36. Matsumoto K, Lo EH, Pierce AR, Wei H, Garrido L, Kowall NW (1995) Role of vasogenic edema and tissue cavitation in ischemic evolution on diffusion-weighted imaging: comparison with multiparameter MR and immunohistochemistry. AJNR Am J Neuroradiol 16:1107-1115

37. Warach S, Gaa J, Siewert B, Wielopolski P, Edelman RR (1995) Acute human stroke studied by whole brain echo planar diffusion-weighted magnetic resonance imaging. Ann Neurol 37:231-241

38. Löblad KO, Laubach HJ, Baird AE et al (1998) Clinical experience with diffusion-weighted MR in patients with acute stroke. AJNR Am J Neuroradiol 19:1061-1066

39. Gonzalez RG, Schaefer PW, Buonanno FS et al (1999) Diffusion-weighted MR imaging: diagnostic accuracy in patients imaged within 6 hours of stroke symptom onset. Radiology 210:155-162

40. Tong DC, Yenari MA, Albers GW, O'Brian M, Marks MP, Moseley ME (1998) Correlation of perfusion- and diffusion-weighted MRI with NIHSS score in acute (<65 hour) ischemic stroke. Neurology 50:864-870

41. Warach S, Dashe JF, Edelman RR (1996) Clinical outcome in ischemic stroke predicted by early diffusion-weighted and perfusion magnetic resonance imaging: a preliminary analysis. J Cereb Blood Flow Metab 16:53-59

42. Singer MB, Chong J, Lu D, Schonewille WJ, Turhim S, Atlas SW (1998) Diffusion-weighted MRI in acute subcortical infarction. Stroke 29:133-136

43. Jahan R, Kidwell SC, Alger JR, Saver JL, Mattiello J, Starkman S, Duckwiler G, Gobin YP, Vinuela F, Kalafut M, Vespa P (1999) Reversibility of abnormal diffusion MR imaging postthrombolysis for acute ischemic stroke. In: Proceedings of the 37th Annual Meeting of American Society of Neuroradiology, San Diego, May 17-21

44. Kidwell CS, Alger JR, Di Salle F, Starkman S, Villablanca P, Bentson J, Saver JL (1999) Diffusion MRI in patients with transient ischemic attacks. Stroke 30:1174-1180

45. Sunshine JL, Tarr RW, Lanzieri CF, Landis DMD, Selman WR, Lewin JS (1999) Hyperacute stroke: ultrafast MR imaging to triage patients prior to therapy. Radiology 212:325-332

46. Bryan RN (1998) Diffusion-weighted imaging: to treat or not to treat? That is the question. AJNR Am J Neuroradiol 19:396-397

47. van Everdingen KJ, van der Grond J, Kappelle LJ, Ramos LMP, Mali WPTM (1998) Diffusion-weighted magnetic resonance imaging in acute stroke. Stroke 29:1783-1790

48. Löblad KO, Baird AE, Schlaug G et al (1997) Ischemic lesion volumes in acute stroke by diffusion-weighted magnetic resonance imaging correlate with clinical outcome. Ann Neurol 42:164-170

49. Baird AE, Warach S (1998) Magnetic resonance imaging of acute stroke. J Cereb Blood Flow Metab 18:583-609

50. Miyabe M, Mori S, van Zijl PCM et al (1996) Correlation of the average water diffusion constant with cerebral blood flow and ischemic damage after transient middle cerebral artery occlusion in cats. J Cereb Blood Flow Metab 16:881-889

51. Busza AL, Allen KL, King MD, van Bruggen N, Williams SR, Gadian DG (1992) Diffusion-weighted imaging studies of cerebral ischemia in gerbils: potential relevance to energy failure. Stroke 23:1602-1612

52. Kohno K, Hoehn-Berlage M, Mies G, Back T, Hossmann KA (1995) Relationship between diffusion-weighted MR images, cerebral blood flow, and energy state in experimental brain infarction. Magn Reson Imaging 13:73-80

53. Baird AE, Benfield A, Schlaug G et al (1997) Enlargement of human cerebral ischemic lesion volumes measured by diffusion-weighted magnetic resonance imaging. Ann Neurol 41:581-589

54. Du C, Hu R, Csernansky CA, Hsu CY, Choi DW (1996) Very delayed infarction after mild focal cerebral ischemia: a role for apoptosis? J Cereb Blood Flow Metab 16:195-201

55. Minematsu K, Li LM, Sotak CH, Davis MA, Fisher M (1992) Reversible focal ischemic injury demonstrated by diffusion-weighted magnetic resonance imaging in rats. Stroke 23:1304-1311

56. Müller TB, Haraldseth O, Jones RA et al (1995) Combined perfusion and diffusion-weighted magnetic resonance imaging in a rat model of reversible middle cerebral artery occlusion. Stroke 26:451-458

57. Maeda M, Yuh WTC, Ueda T et al (1999) Severe occlusive carotid artery disease: Hemodynamic assessment by MR perfusion imaging in symptomatic patients. AJNR Am J Neuroradiol 20:43-51

58. Gückel F, Brix G, Rempp K, Deimling M, Jachim R, Georgi M (1994) Assessment of cerebral blood volume with dynamic susceptibility contrast enhanced gradient-echo imaging. J Comput Assist Tomogr 18:344-351

59. Finelli DA, Hopkins AL, Selman WR, Crumrine RC, Bhatti SU, Lust WD (1992) Evaluation of experimental early acute cerebral ischemia before the development of edema: use of dynamic, contrast-enhanced and diffusion-weighted MR scanning. Magn Reson Med 27:189-197

60. Hamberg LM, Macfarlane R, Tasdemiroglu E et al (1993) Measurement of cerebrovascular changes in cats after transient ischemia using dynamic magnetic resonance imaging. Stroke 24:444-451

61. Jiang Q, Zhang RL, Zhang ZG, Ewing JR, Divine GW, Chopp M (1998) Diffusion-, T2-, and perfusion-weighted nuclear magnetic resonance imaging of middle cerebral artery embolic stroke and recombinant tissue plasminogen activator intervention in the rat. J Cereb Blood Flow Metab 18:758-767

62. Maeda M, Maley J, Crosby D, Quets J, Zhu M, Lee G, Lawler G, Ueda T, Bendixen B, Yuh W (1997) Application of contrast agents in the evaluation of stroke: conventional MR and echoplanar MR imaging. J Magn Reson Imaging 7:23-28

63. Röther J, Gückel F, Neff W (1996) Assessment of regional cerebral blood volume in acute human stroke by use of single-slice dynamic susceptibility contrast-enhanced magnetic resonance imaging. Stroke 27:1088-1093

64. Barber PA, Darby DG, Desmond PM et al (1998) Prediction of stroke outcome with echoplanar perfusion- and diffusion-weighted MRI. Neurology 51:418-426

65. Giubilei F, Lenzi G, Piero V, Pozzilli C, Pantano P, Bastianello S, Argentino C, Fieschi C (1990) Predictive value of brain perfusion single-photon emission computed tomography in acute ischemic stroke. Stroke 21:895-900

66. Hanson S, Grotta J, Rhoades H, Tran H, Lamki L, Barron B, Taylor W (1993) Value of single-photon emission-computed tomography in acute stroke therapeutic trials. Stroke 24:1322-1329

67. Baird A, Donnan G, Austin M, Fitt G, Davis S, McKay W (1994) Reperfusion after thrombolytic therapy in ischemic stroke measured by single-photon emission computed tomography. Stroke 25:79-85

68. Shimosegawa E, Hatazawa J, Inugami A, Fujita H, Ogawa T, Aizawa Y, Kanno I, Okudera T, Uemura K (1994) Cerebral infarction within six hours of onset: prediction of completed infarction with technetium-99m-HMPAO SPECT. J Nucl Med 35:1097-1103

69. Sasaki O, Takeuchi S, Koizumi T, Koike T, Tanaka R (1996) Complete recanalization via fibrinolytic therapy can reduce the number of ischemic territories that progress to infarction. AJNR Am J Neuroradiol 17:1661-1668

70. Ezura M, Takahashi A, Yoshimoto T (1996) Evaluation of regional cerebral blood flow using single photon emission tomography for the selection of patients for local fibrinolytic therapy of acute cerebral embolism. Neurosurg Rev 19:231-236

71. Ueda T, Ohta S, Nochide I, Kohno K, Kumon Y, Sakaki S (1996) Relationship between residual carebral blood flow and neurological outcome in patients with intra-arterial thrombolysis for acute ischemic stroke. In: Taki W (ed) Advances in interventional neuroradiology and intravascular neurosurgery. Amazon, Seattle, pp 487-490

Brain Ischemia

R. von Kummer

Department of Neuroradiology, Universitätsklinikum Carl-Gustav-Carus, Dresden, Germany

Introduction

Acute focal cerebral ischemia, with brain perfusion below 20 ml/min per 100 g tissue, causes an immediate loss of function of the affected brain area and a cascade of pathologic events including tissue water uptake resulting in tissue necrosis if perfusion declines further. Patients with acute cerebral ischemia present with hemiparesis, hemianopia, speech disturbance, or impairment of consciousness. The differential diagnosis includes intracranial hemorrhage, congestive or hypertensive cerebral edema, focal encephalitis, demyelination disorder, metabolic disturbance, or tumor. Brain imaging is absolutely necessary for an exact diagnosis and to assess the acute pathology of the brain. Information provided by computed tomography (CT) and magnetic resonance imaging (MRI) should guide the management of stroke patients and can thus finally influence clinical outcome if the applied treatment is effective.

Imaging can be clinically efficacious on 5 different levels: (1) technical capacity; (2) diagnostic accuracy; (3) diagnostic impact; (4) therapeutic impact; and (5) patient outcome [1]. The technical advantage of CT and MRI in acute stroke is the capability to reproducibly display recognizable images that demonstrate stroke pathology with good intra- and interobserver reliabilities [2]. This paper concentrates on the first level of clinical efficacy in stroke imaging, because there are few prospective data showing that imaging has a proved impact on treatment and outcome.

CT and MRI are capable of detecting intracranial hemorrhage and other diseases that may mimic stroke, the pathology of major brain arteries, brain tissue hypoperfusion, brain swelling, ischemic brain edema, and brain tissue necrosis. Not all information may be crucial to treat the patient properly. Currently, only reperfusion therapy with intravenous recombinant tissue plasminogen activator (rt-PA) or intra-arterial prourokinase within the first 6 hours of stroke onset has been shown to be effective [3-6]. The rationale for reperfusion therapy is a volume of ischemic brain tissue that has chances to regain function. Consequently, imaging should aim to differentiate the following pathological states:

1. Intracranial hemorrhage and other pathologies that cause a stroke-like syndrome, because thrombolytic agents are ineffective or even risky in these diseases.
2. Brain tissue at risk of hypoperfusion, i.e. tissue that cannot survive without enhancement of blood flow, but is still viable at the time of examination for an unknown period. Reperfusion therapy may be beneficial if a considerable volume of such tissue is present [7-8].
3. Irreversibly injured brain tissue, because this tissue cannot recover by definition, even if blood supply is restored immediately after diagnosis. Moreover, reperfusion of damaged brain tissue may increase ischemic edema and the risk of severe hemorrhage [9].

Imaging of Intracranial Hemorrhage

Computed Tomography

After acute intracranial hemorrhage, blood appears on CT as a hyperattenuated, often space-occupying mass and is easily detected within cerebrospinal fluid (CSF) or brain parenchyma. The degree of hyperattenuation depends on the amount of blood, whether it is clotted or not, and whether the blood is intermixed with CSF or brain tissue. Consequently, the assessment of brain hemorrhage can be difficult if blood is only one component of the brain pathology. Sensitivity of CT for detection of parenchymal hemorrhage is considered to be as high, although it was not tested due to a lack of a gold standard. Small hemorrhages in the brain parenchyma or subarachnoid space can be missed. Emergency physicians had an error rate in stroke detection by CT twice that of neurologists and radiologists, and only 17% of emergency physicians, 40% of neurologists and 52% of radiologists recognized all intracranial hemorrhages [10].

Acute hemorrhages usually present as hyperattenuating clots without surrounding edema. If marked edema is present under these circumstances, underlying neoplasm or venous obstruction should be suspected. The location of the hematoma often provides clues about its underlying etiology. Multiple hemorrhagic lesions should make one think about metastatic disease, coagulopathy, or cerebral amyloid angiopathy.

In the subacute and chronic stages, cerebral bleedings become isodense on CT, whereas they display high and low signal intensity on MRI caused by methemoglobin and hemosiderin, which can be detected even years after bleeding [11].

Magnetic Resonance Imaging

On MRI, an acute hemorrhage containing mainly oxyhemoglobin is isointense on T1-weighted images and hyperintense on T2-weighted images. Thus, it is easily missed if located within the CSF space or misinterpreted if located within brain parenchyma (Fig. 1). While MRI has traditionally been considered to be insensitive to hematomas in the clinical setting, it is now quite obvious that MRI can reliably detect acute cerebral hemorrhages. Susceptibility-sensitive gradient echo techniques like T2*-weighted sequences demonstrate acute intracerebral hematomas with low signal intensity due to the susceptibility effect of deoxyhemoglobin. Linfante et al. [12] found that acute hematoma is composed of 3 distinct areas: (1) a center, which has an isointense or hyperintense heterogeneous signal on T2*-weighted and T2-weighted images; (2) a periphery that is hypointense (susceptibility effect) on susceptibility-weighted and T2-weighted images; and (3) a rim that is hypointense on T1-weighted images and hyperintense on T2-weighted images, representing vasogenic edema encasing the hematoma [12].

MRI shows hemorrhage in its different stages, enabling the assessment of bleeding onset, whereas CT is positive only for acute and subacute hemorrhages. In stroke patients, MRI may show cerebral deposits of hemosiderin after clinically silent microbleeds, which may be a risk factor for major cerebral hemorrhages [13, 14]. Moreover, there are hints that MRI can detect acute cerebral bleedings earlier than CT. If this can be proved in larger studies, MRI will become the gold standard for assessing intracerebral hemorrhage and will be required before thrombolytic and antithrombotic therapies.

Regarding the differential diagnosis between ischemic and nonischemic lesions like brain tumors, plaques of multiple sclerosis, encephalitis, metabolic disorders, and venous infarctions, MRI offers a variety of advantages over CT, like better tissue contrast and multiplanar imaging. Systematic studies comparing the technical capacity of both imaging modalities in this regard are however lacking.

Imaging of Tissue at Risk

Three possibilities exist to identify, using CT or MRI, brain tissue at risk of being irreversibly injured by hypoperfusion:

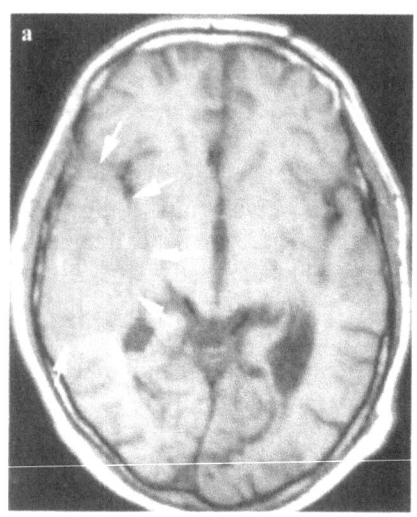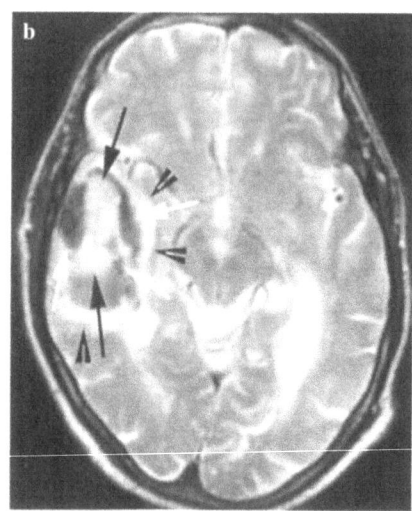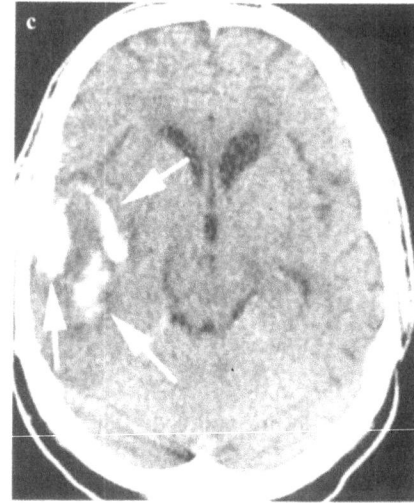

Fig. 1a-c. *A 72-year-old man with sudden onset of memory disturbance, headache and disorientation one day before imaging.* **a** T1-weighted image shows an isointense mass in the right temporal lobe (*arrows*). **b** On T2-weighted image, this mass has hyper- and hypointense portions representing an acute hemorrhage with oxyhemoglobin (hyperintense, *black arrows*) and deoxyhemoglobin (hypointense, *white arrows*). The surrounding hyperintense rim (*arrow heads*) most probably represents edema. **c** CT scan obtained within 1 hour of the MR images. Interestingly, it shows hyperattenuation only in the somewhat older portions of the hemorrhage with deoxyhemoglobin (*arrows*). The other portions of the hemorrhage are still isodense indicating that CT may be insensitive for acute hemorrhage

1. Assessment of arterial occlusion with estimation of the territory supplied by this artery.
2. Assessment of brain tissue swelling due to compensatory arterial vasodilatation.
3. Direct assessment of hypoperfused tissue volume.

These approaches require additional information about the proportion of tissue that is already irreversibly injured.

Arterial Occlusion

The site of arterial occlusion can be detected with cross-sectional CT or MRI, CT or MR angiography, Doppler ultrasound, and digital subtraction angiography (DSA).

CT and CT Angiography

Thromboembolic occlusion of major brain arteries may present on unenhanced CT as a hyperattenuating arterial segment in comparison to other arterial segments. The interobserver agreement on such "hyperdense artery signs" varies between poor (κ=0.20) and moderate (κ=0.63) [15-17].

Computed tomographic angiography (CTA) requires spiral CT techniques and the bolus injection of a contrast agent [18]. Thus, patients with allergic reactions to iodine or renal dysfunction usually cannot be studied with CTA. The CTA examination can be performed immediately after an unenhanced CT scan. Preliminary data suggest that CTA is reliable in visualizing obstruction of major intracranial arteries and veins [18]. CTA is an ex-

cellent technique to find out whether the obstruction of a major artery is the cause of stroke, to differentiate between basilar artery and middle cerebral artery (MCA) occlusion, and to assess whether spontaneous recanalization has occurred.

MRI and MR Angiography

On spin echo sequences, the major brain-supplying arteries display low signal because of high blood flow velocity (signal flow void). High signal or lack of flow void indicates arterial occlusion or low flow (Fig. 2a). In the case illustrated in Fig. 2, the territory of disturbed diffusion (Fig. 2b) does not match that of the distal MCA trunk occlusion. Moreover, the time-to-peak (TTP) parameter image (Fig. 2c) shows increased flow with earlier appearance of the contrast peak within the left basal ganglia. These findings are explained by an initial occlusion of the proximal MCA trunk and distal migration of the thrombus.

Magnetic resonance angiography (MRA) using time-of-flight (TOF) or phase contrast (PC) sequences is a noninvasive test that can image larger extra- and intracranial arteries and veins. After a bolus injection of contrast medium, the brain-supplying arteries can be imaged from the aortic arch up to the circle of Willis within 10 seconds. These contrast-enhanced images are independent of blood flow velocity and turbulence in contrast to TOF and PC techniques. They thus reflect arterial morphology and pathology more reliably than TOF and PC images. Contrast-enhanced MRA may be the method of choice if a quick overview over the extra- and intracranial

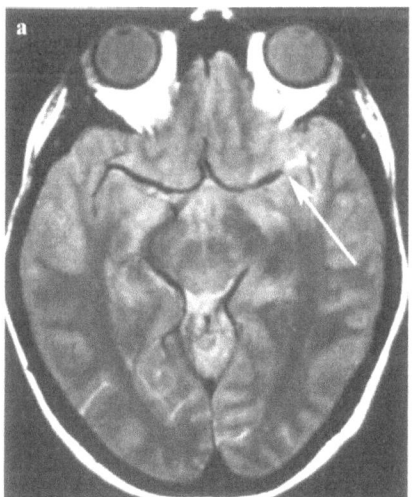 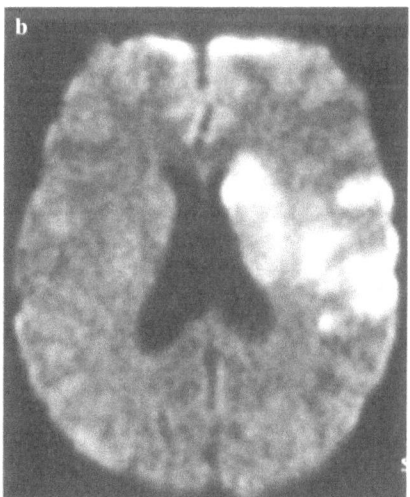 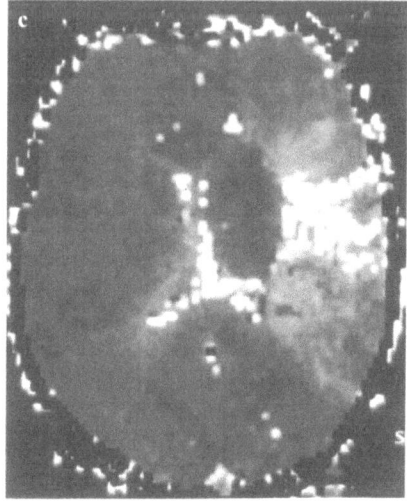

Fig. 2a-c. *A 37-year-old woman with MCA occlusion.* **a** Proton density-weighted MR image shows a lack of flow void in the left distal middle cerebral artery trunk (*arrow*). The occlusion was confirmed by DSA. **B** Diffusion-weighted image (DWI) shows increased signal in the middle portion of the MCA territory and additionally within the left striatum, a territory supplied by the lenticulostriatal arteries that originates proximal to the occlusion site. **c** Time-to-peak (TTP) parameter image shows an area of delayed contrast peak exactly matching the high signal on DWI. Within the striatum, however, blood flow is accelerated. This mismatch can be explained by initial proximal MCA trunk occlusion, followed by a migration of the thrombus into the periphery. In fact, a hyperdense segment of the proximal MCA trunk was visible on the first CT scan obtained 30 minutes after the onset of symptoms

arteries is wanted. Three-dimensional (3D) PC sequences are useful in the diagnosis of venous occlusions. MRA can be performed immediately after brain tissue imaging. The results of TOF or PC MRA should be interpreted with caution because a high-grade stenosis is often overestimated.

Detection of Brain Tissue Swelling and Vasodilatation

The enlargement of anatomical structures such as the cerebral cortex and the effacement of CSF spaces suggest brain tissue swelling and can be detected with CT and MRI. CT may detect brain tissue swelling without hypoattenuation for a short period early after arterial obstruction. Compensatory arterial dilatation due to low perfusion pressure or passive arterial dilatation due to high venous pressure cause this type of swelling [19, 20]. Six neuroradiologists agreed on tissue swelling in 45 CT images of acute stroke patients with a κ of 0.56-0.59 [16]. Compensatory arterial dilatation is associated with a prolongation of the mean transit time. Flow velocity affects the intraluminal signal on MRI so that contrast enhancement becomes visible in vessels with slow flow (Fig. 3a, b). Vascular enhancement is an MRI sign of compromised flow [21].

Perfusion Imaging

Brain perfusion means the volume of blood that flows per minute through a certain amount of brain tissue, usually 100 g. To quantify brain perfusion, clinicians use a contrast agent such as an intra-arterial nondiffusible flow tracer. Both CT and MRI permit clinicians to follow the contrast agent's concentration over time in each tissue voxel and to calculate the mean transit time (MTT), cerebral blood volume (CBV), and cerebral blood flow (CBF) from the concentration curve. True quantification of perfusion requires several conditions that can hardly be achieved [22, 23]. A robust method to image cerebral perfusion without true quantification is the determination of the time from contrast medium entry to peak concentration ("time-to-peak", TTP). A parameter image then displays areas of delayed concentration peaks on CT or MRI. This method is sensitive to detect differences between gray and white matter (Fig. 3c). Perfusion imaging with CT is restricted to 1-4 sections, whereas MRI sequences allow clinicians to image the entire brain. Because CBF often changes over time, it makes sense to repeat perfusion imaging. MRI has then the advantage of avoiding radiation injury.

Imaging of Irreversibly Injured Brain Tissue

Because of its high vulnerability, brain tissue may be already irreversibly injured when the patient presents. Reperfusion treatment is ineffective when a relevant proportion of brain tissue is already dead. Moreover, severely injured brain tissue is prone to malignant edema or clinically relevant bleeding during reperfusion. A reliable assessment of the amount of ischemic damage is, therefore, regarded to be most important for stroke treatment.

The early assessment of irreversibly injured brain tissue is not easy even with histological examination [24].

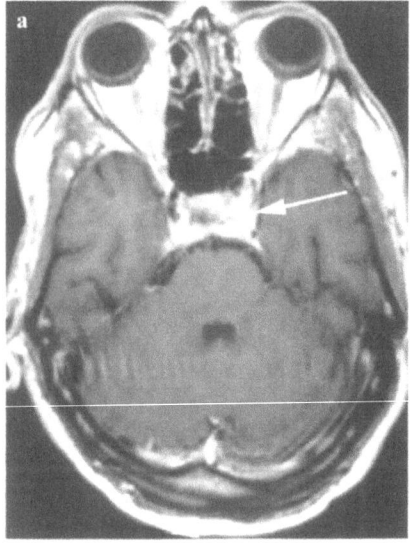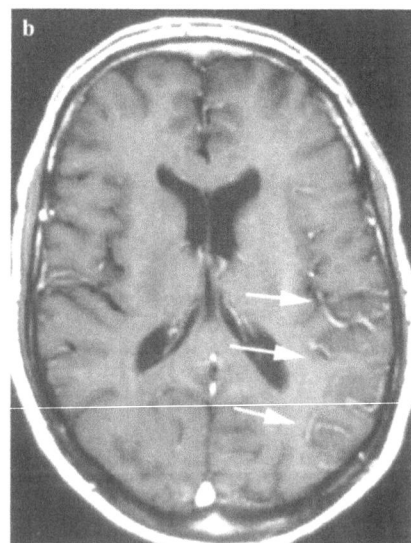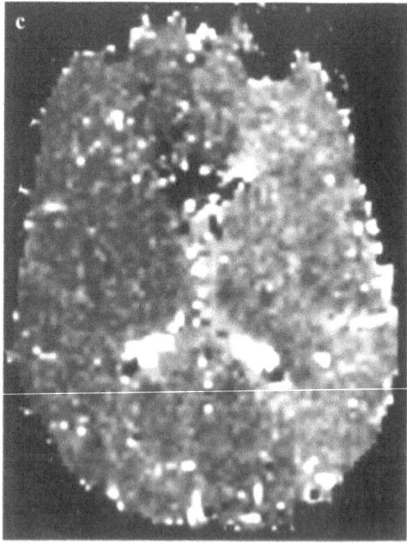

Fig. 3a-c. *A 51-year-old man with attacks of right-sided hemiparesis and remaining weakness of right hand.* **a, b** T1-weighted MR images after contrast medium injection of show (**a**) lack of flow void in the left carotid siphon (*arrow*) and (**b**) marked intra-arterial contrast enhancement on the distal branches of the left middle cerebral artery indicating low flow and hemodynamic compromise (*arrows*). **c** Time-to-peak parameter image shows a delay of contrast medium peaks in the left middle cerebral artery territory

Cerebral blood flow (CBF) of 8-12 ml/min per 100 g is accepted to be the flow threshold for structural integrity [25]. A sudden decrease in cerebral perfusion below 8 ml/min per 100 g causes the gray matter to immediately take up water [26-28]. The amount of water accumulating during ischemia was significantly correlates with the duration of ischemia [29]. Significant resolution of brain edema is possible only if ischemia has lasted less than 15 minutes. This early type of ischemic edema occurs in tissue that was exposed to perfusion below the threshold for maintaining structural integrity. Imaging ischemic edema may be useful to identify the proportion of ischemic brain tissue that is irreversibly damaged [30].

Computed Tomography

X-ray attenuation is linearly proportional to specific gravity and thus allows monitoring tissue water content [31]. An increase of tissue water content by 1% causes a decrease of X-ray attenuation by 2.6 HU in gels [32] and by 2.1 HU in experimental, cryogenically induced brain edema. Coregistration of CT attenuation and CBF revealed that hypoattenuation develops only in areas of critically hypoperfused brain tissue [33]. The mean CBF in the affected MCA territory of patients with hypoattenuating basal ganglia (7 ml x min^{-1} 100 g^{-1}) was significantly lower than that of patients who did not have these findings (17 ml x min^{-1} 100 g^{-1}) [34]. A decline in cerebral blood volume (CBV) may add to the decrease in X-ray attenuation.

Using a CT window width of 80 HU, the minimal visible contrast is at 3-4 HU, which corresponds to an increase in brain tissue water content of about 1.5%. This suggests that the first and potentially reversible stage of the developing ischemic edema cannot be seen on CT because the decline of attenuation has not reached the contrast resolution of 4 IIU. In other words, a normal CT examination in a patient with stroke excludes hemorrhage and other disease, but cannot exclude ischemic edema in an early stage. This insensitivity of CT for the first stage of ischemic edema has, however, a clear advantage by the increased specificity of the finding: CT depicts ischemic edema only at its irreversible stage. Hypoattenuating brain parenchyma on CT after arterial occlusion indicates severe ischemia under the critical level of structural integrity for 1-3 hours. Under clinical conditions, hypoattenuation may appear already 22 minutes after the onset of symptoms [30]. It is not yet known, however, whether hypoattenuation of ischemic brain tissue can disappear if the tissue is reperfused within less than 30-60 minutes and to what extent changes in CBV contribute to changes in CT attenuation.

Because of its subtlety, early ischemic edema (Fig. 4) is recognized with only moderate interobserver reliability [16, 17, 35]. The National Institute of Neurological Disorders and Stroke rt-PA Stroke Trialists and others demonstrated that training in CT reading considerably affects the sensitivity of detecting ischemic edema [35, 36].

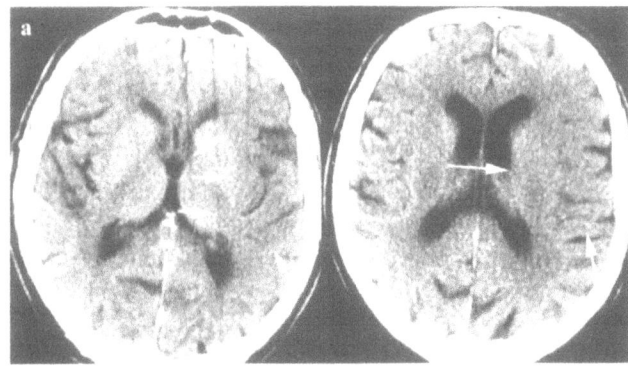

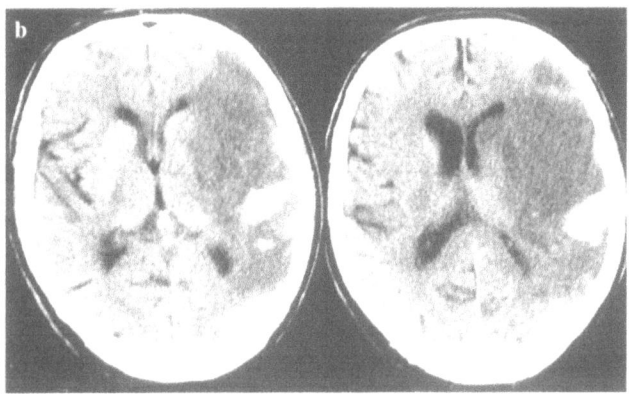

Fig. 4a, b. *Patient with severe right-sided hemiparesis.* **a** The early CT image (1 hour after onset of symptoms) shows subtle hypoattenuation of the left insular, frontal, and temporal cortices (*arrows*). **b** Twenty-four hours later, this area became clearly hypodense, shows a space-occupying effect, and contains a small hematoma

Attempts were made to improve the capability of CT in detecting ischemic edema by performing a density-difference analysis between both cerebral hemispheres, by varying window width and center level, and by using a quantitative score [37-39].

Magnetic Resonance Imaging

MRI has more than one possibility to image ischemic brain tissue changes. It is generally accepted that signal changes that appear relatively late after focal ischemia represent irreversible damage. The increase in signal on T2-weighted spin echo sequences and the corresponding decrease on T1-weighted sequences mainly represent tissue water uptake and may indicate ischemic edema or, later, ischemic necrosis. These signal changes appear hours after stroke onset and are, therefore, irrelevant for acute stroke treatment. However, MR images that have been specifically sensitized to the translational diffusion of water (diffusion-weighted images, DWI) can reveal tissue contrast based on properties essentially very different from those exploited by standard sequences [40, 41]. In ischemic brain areas with CBF values of 30 ml/min per 100 g and less, the extracellular fluid compartment is reduced because of a shift of water from the extracellular space into the cells [27]. At the same ischemic threshold, proton diffusion becomes impaired [42, 43].

Within 15-30 minutes after onset of focal ischemia below that threshold, the apparent diffusion coefficient (ADC) decreases by 30%-50%, while T1- and T2-weighted MR images remain normal [40]. This time course is consistent with the complete loss of tissue adenosine triphosphate, loss of sodium and potassium membrane pump activities, and consequent cellular edema in severely ischemic brain tissue [44]. Increased signal on DWI precisely indicates the areas with ATP depletion. Induction of cellular edema by means other than focal ischemia also reduces ADC [45].

It is clear from these observations in experimental animals that DWI is highly sensitive in detecting brain areas with ATP depletion and consequently high risk for irreversible injury. Moreover, its negative predictive value for ischemic damage must be high. In stroke patients, brain tissue with high signal on DWI or with low ADC is either going to die or may recover with reperfusion [46-48].

Conclusions

The differentiation of the stroke syndrome and the assessment of acute brain pathology are the main conditions for a carefully directed and successful treatment. CT and MRI have the technical capacity to reproducibly display recognizable images that demonstrate pathology of acute stroke, brain-supplying vessels, and diseases that mimic stroke. MRI is superior to CT in detecting acute and chronic states of brain hemorrhage. DWI is highly sensitive in detecting ischemic brain regions with depletion of ATP and high risk of irreversible tissue damage. If DWI is negative in an acute stroke patient or shows only small areas of disturbed diffusion, the patient has a good prognosis if cerebral blood flow is quickly restored. Hypoattenuating brain tissue on CT is difficult to recognize in the very early stage of ischemic brain edema, but is a highly specific finding representing irreversibly injury. If a volume of hypoattenuating brain tissue is detected, the extent of damaged tissue determines the patient's prognosis and response to treatment.

References

1. Kent D, Larson E (1992) Disease, level of impact, and quality of research methods; three dimensions of clinical efficacy assessment applied to magnetic resonance imaging. Invest Radiol 27:245-254
2. Powers W (2000) Testing a test. A report card for DWI in acute stroke. Neurology 54:1549-1551
3. NINDS Stroke Study Group (1995) Tissue plasminogen activator for acute ischemic stroke. N Engl J Med 333:1581-1587
4. Hacke W, Kaste M, Fieschi C, Toni D, Lesaffre E, von Kummer R, Boysen G, Bluhmki E, Höxter G, Mahagne M, Hennerici M (1995) Intravenous thrombolysis with recombinant tissue plasminogen activator for acute hemispheric stroke. The European Cooperative Acute Stroke Study (ECASS). JAMA 274:1017-1025
5. Hacke W, Kaste M, Fieschi C, von Kummer R, Davalos A, Meier D, Larrue V, Bluhmki E, Davis S, Donnan G, Schneider D, Diez-Tejedor E, Trouillas P (1998) Randomised double-blind placebo-controlled trial of thrombolytic therapy with intravenous alteplase in acute ischaemic stroke (ECASS II). Lancet 352:1245-1251
6. Furlan A, Higashida R, Wechsler L, Gent M, Rowley H, Kase C, Pessin M, Ahuja A, Callahan F, Clark W, Silver F, Rivera F (1999) Intra-arterial prourokinase for acute ischemic stroke. JAMA 282:2003-2011
7. Jansen O, Schellinger P, Fiebach J, Hacke W, Sartor K (1999) Early recanalisation in acute ischaemic stroke saves tissue at risk defined by MRI. Lancet 353:2036-2037
8. Parsons M, Barber A, Chalk J, Darby D, Rose S, Desmond P, Gerraty R, Tress B, Wright P, Donnan G, Davis S (2002) Diffusion- and perfusion-weighted MRI response to thrombolysis in stroke. Ann Neurol 51:28-37
9. Dzialowski I, Weber J, Dörfler A, Forsting M, von Kummer R (2002) CT monitoring of ischemic edema during reperfusion after transient middle cerebral artery occlusion. Stroke 33:408
10. Schriger D, Kalafut M, Starkman S, Krueger M, Daver J (1998) Cranial computed tomographic interpretation in acute stroke. Physician accuracy in determining eligibility for thrombolytic therapy. JAMA 279:1293-1297
11. Wardlaw J, Statham P (2000) How often is haemosiderin not visible on routine MRI following traumatic intracerebral haemorrhage? Neuroradiology 42:81-84
12. Linfante I, Llinas R, Caplan L, Warach S (1999) MRI features of intracerebral hemorrhage within 2 hours from symptom onset. Stroke 30:2263-2267
13. Kidwell C, Saver J, Villablance J, Duckwiler G, Fredieu A, Gough K, Leary M, Starkman S, Gobin Y, Jahan R, Vespa P, Liebeskind D, Alger I, Vinuela F (2002) Magnetic resonance imaging detection of microbleeds before thrombolysis: an emerging application. Stroke 33:95-98
14. Nighoghossian N, Hermier M, Adeleine P, Blanc-Laserre K, Derex I, Honnorat J, Phillipeau F, Dugor J, Froment J, Trouillas P (2002) Old microbleeds are a potential risk factor for cerebral bleeding after ischemic stroke. A gradient-echo T2*-weighted brain MRI study. Stroke 33:735-742
15. Tomsick T, Brott T, Chambers A, Fox A, Gaskill M, Lukin R, Pleatman C, Wiot J, Bourekas E (1990) Hyperdense middle artery sign on CT: efficacy in detecting middle cerebral artery thrombosis. AJNR Am J Neuroradiol 11:473-477
16. von Kummer R, Holle R, Grzyska U, Hofmann E, Jansen O, Petersen D, Schumacher M, Sartor, K (1996) Interobserver agreement in assessing early CT signs of middle cerebral artery infarction. AJNR Am J Neuroradiol 17:1743-1748
17. Marks M, Holmgren E, Fox A, Patel S, von Kummer R, Froehlich J (1999) Evaluation of early computed tomographic findings in acute ischemic stroke. Stroke 30:389-392
18. Knauth M, von Kummer R, Jansen O, Hähnel S, Dörfler A, Sartor K (1997) Potential of CT angiography in acute ischemic stroke. AJNR Am J Neuroradiol 18:1001-1010
19. Gibbs J, Wise R, Leenders K, Jones T (1984) Evaluation of cerebral perfusion reserve in patients with carotid-artery occlusion. Lancet 8372:310-314
20. Yuh W, Simonson T, Wang A, Koci T, Tali E, Fisher D, Simon J, Jinkins J, Tsai F (1999) Venous sinus occlusive disease: MR findings. AJNR Am J Neuroradiol 15:309-316
21. Essig M, von Kummer R, Egelhof T, Winter R, Sartor K (1996) Magnetic resonance imaging of vascular contrast enhancement in cerebrovascular disease. AJNR Am J Neuroradiol 17: 887-894
22. Rempp K, Brix G, Wenz F, Becker C, Gückel F, Lorenz W (1994) Quantification of regional cerebral blood flow and volume with dynamic susceptibility contrast-enhanced MR imaging. Radiology 193:637-641

23. Koenig M. Klotw e, Luka B, Venderink D, Spittler J, Heuser L (1998) perfusion CT of the brain: diagnostic approach for early detection of ischeic stroke. Radiology 209:85-93
24. Garcia J, Liu KF, Ho KL (1995) Neuronal necrosis after middle cerebral artery occlusion in Wistar rats progresses at different time intervals in the caudoputamen and the cortex. Stroke 26:636-643
25. Hossmann KA (1994) Viability thresholds and the penumbra of focal ischemia. Ann Neurol 36:557-565
26. Watanabe O, West CR, Bremer A (1977) Experimental regional cerebral ischemia in the middle cerebral artery territory in primates. Part 2: Effects on brain water and electrolytes in the early phase of MCA stroke. Stroke 8:71-76
27. Schuier FJ, Hossmann KA (1980) Experimental brain infarcts in cats. II. Ischemic brain edema. Stroke 11:593-601
28. Todd N, Picozzi P, Crockard,A, Ross Russel R (1986) Duration of ischemia influences the development and resolution of ischemic brain edema. Stroke 17:466-471
29. Todd N, Picozzi P, Crockard A, Ross Russel R (1986) Reperfusion after cerebral ischemia: Influence of duration of ischemia. Stroke 17:460-465
30. von Kummer R, Bourquain H, Bastianello S, Bozzao L, Manelfe C, Meier D, Hacke W (2001) Early prediction of irreversible brain damage after ischemic stroke by computed tomography. Radiology 219:95-100
31. Rieth KG, Fujiwara K, Di Chiro G, Klatzo I, Brooks RA, Johnston GS, O'Connor CM, Mitchell LG (1980) Serial measurements of CT attenuation and specific gravity in experimental cerebral edema. Radiology 135:343-348
32. Unger E, Littlefield J, Gado M (1988) Water content and water structure in CT and MR signal changes: possible influence in detection of early stroke. AJNR Am J Neuroradiol 9:687-691
33. Grond M, von Kummer R, Sobesky J, Schmülling S, Heiss WD (1997) Early computed tomography abnormalities in acute stroke. Lancet 350:1595-1596
34. Firlik A, Kaufmann A, Wechsler L, Firlik K, Fukui M, Yonas H (1997) Quantitative cerebral blood flow determinations in acute ischemic stroke. Relationship to computed tomography and angiography. Stroke 28:2208-2213
35. Grotta J, Chiu D, Lu M, Patel S, Levine S, Tilley B, Brott T, Haley E, Lyden P, Kothari R, Frankel, M, Lewandowski C, Libman R, Kwiatkowski T, Broderick J, Marler J, Corrigan J, Huff S, Mitsias P, Talati S, Tanne D (1999) Agreement and variability in the interpretation of early CT changes in stroke patients qualifying for intravenous rtPA therapy. Stroke 30:1528-1533
36. von Kummer R (1998) Effect of training in reading CT scans on patient selection for ECASS II. Neurology 51[Suppl 3]:S50-S52
37. Bendszus, M, Urbach H, Meyer B, Schultheiß R, Solymosi L (1997) Improved CT diagnosis of acute middle cerebral artery territory infarcts with density-difference analysis. Neuroradiology 39:127-131
38. Lev M, Farkas J, Gemmete J, Hossain S, Hunter G, Koroshetz W, Gonzalez R (1999) Acute stroke: improved nonenhanced CT detection - Benefits of soft-copy interpretation by using variable window width and center level settings. Radiology 213:150-155
39. Barber P, Demchuk A, Zhang J, Buchan A (2000) Validity and reliability of a quantitative computed tomography score in predicting outcome of hyperacute stroke before thrombolytic therapy. Lancet 355:1670-1674
40. Moseley M, Cohen Y, Mintorovitch J, Chileuitt L, Shimizu H, Kucharczyk J, Wendland M, Weinstein P (1990) Early detection of regional cerebral ischemia in cats: comparison of diffusion- and T2-weighted MRI and spectroscopy. Magn Reson Med 14:330-346
41. Kuroiwa T, Nagaoka T, Ueki M, Yamada I, Miyasaki N, Akimoto H (1998) Different apparent diffusion coefficient. Water content correlations of gray and white matter during early ischemia. Stroke 29:859-865
42. Busza A, Allen K, King M, van Bruggen N, Williams S, Gadian D (1992) Diffusion-weighted imaging studies of cerebral ischemia in gerbils. Potential relevance to energy failure. Stroke 23:1602-1612
43. Wang Y, Hu W, Perez-Trepichio A, Ng T, Furlan A, Majors A Jones S (2000) Brain tissue sodium is a ticking clock telling time after arterial occlusion in rat focal cerebral ischemia. Stroke 31:1386-1392
44. Mintorovitch J, Yang G, Shimizu H, Kucharczyk J, Chan P, Weinstein P (1994) Diffusion-weighted magnetic resonance imaging of acute focal cerebral ischemia: comparison of signal intensity with changes in brain water and Na+, K+ -ATPase activity. J Cereb Blood Flow Metab 14:332-336
45. Back T, Hoehn-Berlage M, Kohno K, Hossmann K (1994) Diffusion NMR imaging in experimental stroke: correlation with cerebral metabolites. Stroke 25:494-500
46. Lövblad K, Laubach H, Baird A, Curtin F, Schlaug G, Edelman R, Warach S (1998) Clinical experience with diffusion-weighted MR in patients with acute stroke. AJNR Am J Neuroradiol 19: 1061-1066
47. Kidwell C, Alger J, Di Salle F, Starkman S, Villablanca P, Bentson J, Saver J (1999) Diffusion MRI in patients with transient ischemic attacks. Stroke 30:1174-1180
48. Kidwell C, Saver J, Mattielloo J, Starkman S, Vinuela F, Duckwiler G, Gobin Y (2000) Thrombolytic reversal of acute human cerebral ischemic injury shown by diffusion/perfusion magnetic resonance imaging. Ann Neurol 47:462-469

Haemorrhagic Cerebral Vascular Disease

J. Byrne

Department of Neuroradiology, Radcliffe Infirmary, University of Oxford, Oxford, UK

Introduction

This paper outlines a logical strategy for managing the imaging investigation of patients presenting with spontaneous intracranial haemorrhage. Details of the patient's acute and past medical histories may point to the cause of intracranial bleeding but in most instances it is imaging that distinguishes the victims of haemorrhagic from those with ischemic stroke. This crucial distinction triggers completely different diagnostic and therapeutic management paths.

In the following paragraphs, I describe my protocols for identifying underlying structural lesions that require interventions to prevent rebleeding or progression. These lesions are most commonly vascular and, in some circumstances, emergency interventions may be life-saving. It is therefore important for investigations to be appropriate and timely.

How Should the Patient with Haemorrhagic Stroke be Investigated?

The first step is to triage patients (Fig. 1) into those likely to have an underlying structural lesion carrying a risk of rebleeding, those likely to have a 'non-structural' cause

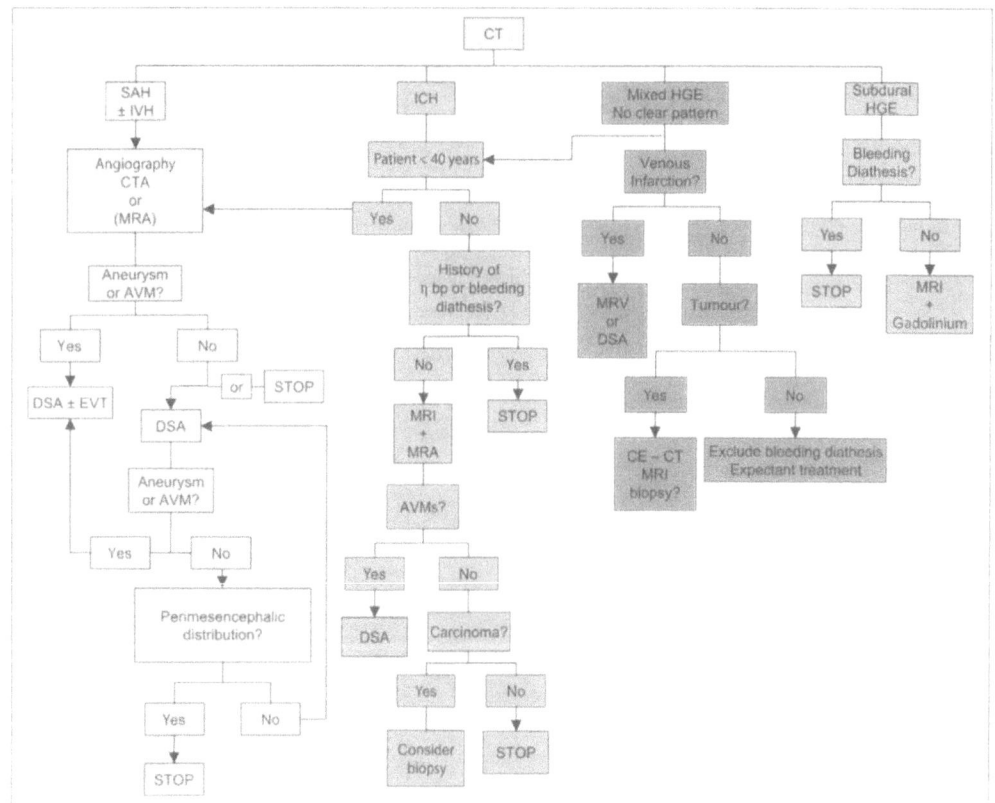

Fig. 1. Flow diagram showing CT based diagnostic triage routes for patients with spontaneous intracranial haemorrhage

that requires urgent diagnosis and treatment, and those unlikely to have an underlying lesion and therefore not requiring urgent interventions.

Causes of Subarachnoid Haemorrhage

Common causes of subarachnoid haemorrhage are:
- Saccular aneurysm
- Arterial dissection
- Angiogram-negative perimesencephalic haemorrhage

Rarer causes are:
- Brain or spinal arteriovenous malformations (AVMs) or arteriovenous fistulae (AVFs)
- Dural AVFs
- Pitituary apoplexy
- Infectious aneurysms
- Drug abuse (e.g. cocaine)
- Sickle cell disease (in children)
- Bleeding diathesis (e.g. excessive anticoagulation)

Causes of Spontaneous Intracranial Haemorrhage

Common causes of spontaneous intracranial haemorrhage in the basal ganglia and thalamus are:
- AVMs, including cavernous malformations and cryptic AVMs
- Lipohyalinosis
- Moyamoya syndrome
- Tumour
- Bleeding diathesis

In the lobar region, causes are:
- AVMs, including cavernous malformations and cryptic AVMs
- Saccular aneurysms
- Venous thrombosis
- Amyloid angiopathy
- Tumour
- Amphetamine and cocaine abuse

- Infectious endocarditis
- Bleeding diathesis

Finally, in the cerebellum and brain stem, causes are:
- AVMs, including cavernous malformations and cryptic AVMs
- Lipohyalinosis
- Tumour
- Amyloid angiopathy
- Bleeding diathesis

Causes of Spontaneous Subdural Haemorrhage

Typical causes of spontaneous subdural haemorrhage are:
- Saccular aneurysm
- Rupture of small pial vessels
- Moyamoya syndrome
- Dural AVFs
- Dural metastases
- Coagulation defects

Conclusions

This presentation discusses the role of computed tomography (CT), magnetic resonance imaging (MRI), and digital subtraction angiography (DSA) in the diagnosis of these pathologies, with illustrative examples. The crucial role of CT as the primary imaging tool is emphasised and the student will be taught to distinguish predominantly lobar, subarachnoid, intraventricular and subdural locations of haemorrhage. Students will be taught features of the evolving cerebral haemorrhage over time and the resulting effect on the imaging appearances of haematomas.

Suggested Reading

Davis S, Fisher M, Warach S (eds) (2003) Magnetic resonance imaging in stroke. Cambridge University, Cambridge
Warlow CP et al (eds) (1996) Stroke: a practical guide to management. Blackwell Science, Oxford

Hemorrhagic Vascular Pathology

M. Forsting, I. Wanke

Department of Radiology and Neuroradiology, Institute of Diagnostic and Interventional Radiology, University of Essen, Essen, Germany

Imaging Intracranial Hemorrhage

Intracranial hemorrhage (ICH) is a frequent indication for emergent neuroimaging. To understand the appearance of clots on computed tomography (CT) and magnetic resonance imaging (MRI), it is mandatory to know some details of clot formation.

Initially, an intracerebral hematoma is composed of 95%-98% oxygen-saturated hemoglobin, mainly containing erythrocytes. Over the first 4-6 hours, the protein clot retracts, still containing intact biconcave red blood cells (RBCs) with oxygenated hemoglobin. During the next 48 hours, the RBCs shrink and hemoglobin desaturates. During this period, the hematoma contains predominantly deoxygenated intracellular hemoglobin (remember, the RBCs are still intact). In the early subacute phase (a few days after the initial hemorrhage), oxidative denaturation of the hemoglobin progresses and deoxyhemoglobin is gradually converted to methemoglobin (MetHb). These changes first occur around the periphery of the hematoma and then progress centrally. RBCs continuously lyse and release MetHb into the extracellular space. Afterwards, the hematoma starts to shrink to finally form a slit-like cavity containing a fluid similar to cerebrospinal fluid (CSF) and, as a long-standing marker of bleeding, ferritin- and hemosiderin-laden macrophages.

Computed Tomography

Fresh intracerebral blood typically appears hyperdense on CT due to the high protein concentration and high mass density. However, acute intracerebral hematoma occasionally appears isodense or even hypodense on CT. This occurs with extreme anemia, i.e. when the hemoglobin concentration drops to 8 g/dl. Another reason for primary isodense clots on CT is a coagulation disorder. Failure of clot retraction results in a relatively isodense, acute ICH.

Within 1-6 weeks, hemorrhage becomes virtually isodense with adjacent brain. Due the breakdown of the blood-brain barrier, hemorrhage can mimic an abscess on contrast-enhanced studies.

Magnetic Resonance Imaging

MRI of intracerebral hemorrhage is complex and requires much knowledge on the pathophysiology of blood degradation. The signal is mainly influenced by the oxidation state of hemoglobin (Hb) and by the protein concentration. Extrinsic factors are the pulse sequences and the field strength of the MRI system. Generally speaking, deoxy-Hb appears isointense with brain on T1-weighted images and hypointense on T2-weighted images; extracellular MetHb (subacute clots) appears bright on T1- and T2-weighted images; and hemosiderin (chronic state) is dark on T1- and T2-weighted images. However, this is only a rough summary. We strongly recommend further study of hemoglobin degradation and its relationship to the MRI signal. This allows one to recognize intratumoral hemorrhages because the oxygen content within a tumor is lower and, therefore, the time course of signal changes is delayed.

Hemorrhagic Diseases

The three most common hemorrhagic diseases are hypertension, aneurysms and vascular malformations. Hypertensive hemorrhage is the most common cause of intracranial hemorrhage and has a predilection for areas supplied by penetrating branches of the middle cerebral and basilar arteries. Two thirds of these bleedings are located in the basal ganglia; in 50% of these, there is also associated intraventricular hemorrhage. Other relatively common sites of hypertensive ICH are the cerebellum and pons. In addition to the location of the bleeding, findings of lacunar stroke or white matter disease may further enhance the suspicion of a hypertensive cause.

Patients usually undergo CT first. If in doubt about the hypertensive character of the hematoma, MRI is a second step. Finally, the majority of these patients needs angiography, especially if younger than 70 years and with bleeding in a so-called atypical location.

If the hemorrhage is not hypertensive (i.e. the patient has no specific history and the hematoma is atypically located), a vascular malformation or an intracranial aneurysm is the most likely cause of ICH. The purpose of this summary is not to fully cover the large field of these diseases, but to give a short overview of pathology, clinical presentation, imaging findings and treatment options. The seminar itself provides numerous illustrations to enhance knowledge in this field.

Intracranial Aneurysms

Usually, intracranial aneurysms are divided into three basic types: saccular, fusiform and dissecting. They can arise as solitary (70%-75%) or multiple (25%-30%) vascular lesions, usually located at the circle of Willis. The vast majority of aneurysms (85%) are located in the anterior circulation and only 15% are in the posterior circulation. Most saccular aneurysms are not considered to be congenital, but develop during life. The most common location (30%-35%) is the anterior communicating artery. However, many of these so-called AcomA aneurysms do have their origin at the A1-A2 junction of the anterior cerebral artery and do not involve the anterior communicating artery. Internal carotid and posterior communicating artery aneurysms account for 30% and middle cerebral artery (MCA) bifurcational aneurysms account for 20%. Approximately 10% of intracranial aneurysms arise at the vertebrobasilar circulation: half develops at the basilar tip (with various levels of involvement of the P1 segments) and the other half is from other posterior fossa vessels. Extremely rare are aneurysms of the anterior inferior cerebellar artery (AICA) and of the vertebral artery (VA) without involvement of the VA-PICA junction or the vertebrobasilar union.

Most intracranial aneurysms remain undetected until the time of rupture. Subarachnoid hemorrhage (SAH), a medical emergency, is by far the most common initial clinical presentation. A history of abrupt onset of a severe headache of atypical quality ("the worst headache in my life") is typical of SAH. Headache onset may or may not be associated with brief loss of consciousness, nausea and vomiting, focal neurologic deficits, or meningism. Despite the characteristic history, SAH is frequently misdiagnosed. Nearly half of patients presents with milder symptoms caused by a warning leak before full rupture of the aneurysm.

Although the pathogenesis and etiology of cerebral aneurysms have been studied extensively, both are still poorly understood. Endogenous factors such as elevated blood pressure, the special anatomy of the circle of Willis or the effect of hemodynamic factors, particularly originating at vessel bifurcations, are all known to be involved in the growth and rupture of an aneurysm. Arteriosclerosis and inflammatory reactions, however, may also have an impact. Exogenous factors such as cigarette smoking, heavy alcohol consumption and certain medications are thought to be risk factors in the pathogenesis of aneurysm or to at least increase the risk of rupture.

Furthermore, a genetic component is discussed. First-degree relatives of patients with an aneurysmal SAH have a significantly higher risk of harboring a cerebral aneurysm compared to the normal population.

The annual incidence of SAH in the Western world is around 6-10 per 100 000 persons, peaking in the sixth decade, with risk for SAH increasing linearly with age. The annual incidence in other countries like Finland or Japan is higher – about 15 per 100 000 persons. SAH accounts for one-quarter of cerebrovascular deaths. Aneurysms increase in frequency with age beyond the third decade, are approximately 1.6-times more common in women, and are associated with a number of genetic conditions.

Hydrocephalus, rebleeding from aneurysmal rerupture, and cerebral vasospasm with ischemia are the three major complications following SAH. Intracerebral hematoma occurs in up to 30% of patients with aneurysmal rupture. The outcome is clearly worse than with SAH alone. If a space-occupying hematoma compressing neural structures is present, immediate evacuation of the hematoma is mandatory, eventually in combination with clipping of the aneurysm, if it can be identified. In this setting, CT angiography is a valuable and fast imaging modality to disclose the aneurysm prior to surgical intervention. Immediate surgical evacuation is also indicated in acute subdural hematoma, which is usually associated with recurrent aneurysmal rupture. However, this can also occur with the initial SAH or can be the only extravascular space involved after aneurysmal rupture.

Vasospasm is a major cause of morbidity and mortality in patients after SAH and is often associated with delayed cerebral ischemia. However, many patients are asymptomatic despite various degrees of angiographically visible vasospasm. Although vasospasm is noted angiographically after SAH in 70% of cases, it becomes symptomatic only in about one-half of these patients.

If SAH is suspected clinically, CT of the brain is the initial diagnostic imaging modality of choice and clearly the gold standard to identify, localize and quantify subarachnoid hemorrhage. Typically, the subarachnoid blood appears hyperdense on an unenhanced CT image. The pattern of SAH can suggest the location of the underlying aneurysm. Intraparenchymal hemorrhage occurs with aneurysms of the posterior communicating artery and middle cerebral artery more frequently than with other locations. Interhemispheric or intraventricular hemorrhage, occurring in about 50% of patients in autopsy studies, is characteristic of anterior communicating artery or distal anterior cerebral artery aneurysms. Ruptured posterior inferior cerebellar artery (PICA) aneurysms almost always coexist with hydrocephalus and intraventricular hemorrhage in the fourth ventricle, which can also be seen on CT. Intracerebral hemorrhage is also more common in patients who rebleed, since the first bleeding may lead to fibrosis of the surrounding subarachnoid space and adhesion of the aneurysm to the brain.

Subdural hematoma occurs in about 5% of patients, but is rarely the only location of bleeding.

Small amounts of SAH may be overlooked, thus CT images should be carefully read. However, even if the CT scan is really normal (no reading fault), aneurysmal SAH cannot be ruled out. The sensitivity of CT for detecting SAH depends on the volume of the extravasated blood, the hematocrit, and the time elapsed after the acute event. Using modern scanners and performing the analysis within 24 hours after ictus, CT detects SAH in up to 95% of cases. However, due to dilution by CSF, the density of the hematoma decreases rapidly over time; thus after only a few days it may be impossible to demonstrate subarachnoid blood on CT. Sensitivity of CT thus decreases to 80% at day 3, 70% at day 5, 50% at one week, and 30% at 2 weeks.

However, if CT is negative despite a convincing history of sudden headache, lumbar puncture is still the next diagnostic step to rule out SAH, if there is no contraindication such as a bleeding disorder or space-occupying intracranial lesion. Lumbar puncture should not be performed before 6 hours after onset of headache; preferably 12 hours should elapse between onset of headache and spinal tap. After this interval, sufficient lysis of erythrocytes has occurred to form bilirubin and oxyhemoglobin. These pigments give the CSF the "typical" xanthochrome yellowish tinge after centrifugation, an essential feature in the differentiation from traumatic SAH. This xanthochromia is invariably detectable for at least 2 weeks, usually 3 (in 70% of patients) to 7 weeks after SAH.

Identification of factors predictive of outcome or specific complications is important in the management of SAH. The risk of a given patient to suffer from vasospasm can be estimated by the location, thickness, and density of subarachnoid blood on CT. In 1980, Fisher and colleagues described 47 patients in whom the amount and distribution of subarachnoid blood after aneurysmal rupture on the initial CT correlated with the subsequent occurrence of vasospasm demonstrated by angiography. Two (11%) of 18 patients developed vasospasm when no or diffuse thin SAH was present on CT, whereas none did with only intraventricular or intracerebral hemorrhage. Of 24 patients with diffuse, thick SAH, 23 (96%) developed severe symptomatic vasospasm. Since then, the CT-based Fisher classification (Table 1) of quantifying local amounts of subarachnoid blood as a powerful predictor for the occurrence of vasospasm and delayed cerebral is-

chemia has been confirmed by several clinical and experimental studies. However, the predictive value of the Fisher grading system is not perfect. Never be too sure that a patient with a low Fisher score will not develop vasospasm. All patients with SAH have to be carefully monitored during the first two weeks after ictus, regardless of the initial Fisher score.

Sensitivity of single-slice CT angiography (CTA) in the investigation of intracranial aneurysms has been reported to range from 67% to 100%, with an accuracy of approximately 90% and an interobserver agreement ranging from 75% to 84%. Nevertheless, this technique has limited sensitivity for aneurysms smaller than 3 mm (25%-64% compared with 92%-100% for aneurysms >3 mm). Moreover, CTA has pitfalls if the aneurysm is located in a site where adjacent bone or considerable vessel overlap exist, such as the paraclinoid and terminal segments of the internal carotid artery (ICA) or at the MCA bifurcation.

The implementation of multidetector row technology led to a major step forward in the field of CTA, notably for small vessels and intracranial aneurysms. This technique reduces acquisition time despite the use of pitch values inferior to unity. Improvements in image quality and spatial resolution give better diagnostic results for intracranial aneurysms. Multirow CT technology will clearly facilitate work in emergency departments. Patients with a never-experienced-before headache and a negative unenhanced CT scan will get a quick and reliable CTA examination. To optimize treatment planning and work-flow, CTA may also be used to stratify patients into endovascular and surgical treatment groups. However, whether CTA really will allow us to decide which therapeutic modality is best still has to be determined. In our opinion, there are drawbacks when describing the anatomy of the neck and the true relationship of tiny vessels originating near the entrance of the aneurysm or adjacent to the aneurysmal dome. However, CTA clearly plays a role in the pretherapeutic phase in large or giant aneurysms. In these patients, it is often more difficult to visualize the exact anatomy of the neck and the relationship to adjacent bony structures, such as in the paraophthalmic region, than with conventional digital subtraction angiography (DSA) alone. Moreover, CTA is helpful in the pretherapeutic planning of partially calcified and thrombosed aneurysms, and may help to determine the best treatment modality. In patients with large, space-occupying hematomas, CTA is clearly enough to rule out an underlying aneurysm. In this specific situation, DSA is probably no longer indicated.

MRI and MR angiography (MRA) are increasingly used in the diagnostic work-up of patients with cerebral aneurysms. However, MRI is less suitable than CT in patients with acute SAH because they are often restless and need extensive monitoring. MRI is used in patients with a negative angiogram to detect other causes of SAH, such as a thrombosed aneurysm or spinal vascular malforma-

Table 1. Fisher's grading scale for subarachnoid hemorrhage (SAH)

Group	Subarachnoid blood	Risk of vasospasm
1	No blood	Low
2	Diffuse or vertical layers <1 mm	Only moderate
3	Localized clot or vertical layer >1 mm	High
4	Intracerebral or intraventricular clot with only diffuse or no SAH	

tion, and it will increasingly be used in screening programs and as a follow-up tool after endovascular therapy.

Conventional MRI sequences are less sensitive than CT to SAH. Since SAH is mostly arterial in origin, the predominant form of hemoglobin is oxy-Hb. Immediately after the extravasation of blood into the subarachnoid space, there is a shortening in T1 due to the increase in hydration layer water owing to the higher protein content of CSF. This results in an increased signal on T1-weighted and proton-density images. Fluid-attenuation inversion recovery (FLAIR) sequences are highly sensitive. The signal from CSF is almost completely reduced while producing a heavy T2-weighting. On FLAIR images, SAH appears hyperintense compared to CSF and the surrounding brain. Currently, it is widely accepted that even subtle amounts of subarachnoid blood can be detected by MRI when using FLAIR or proton-density weighted sequences. False-positive FLAIR results may be caused by flow-related enhancement within the CSF. Even hyperacute SAH can be detected with MRI. Compared with CSF, hyperacute blood has slightly lower signal intensity on T2*-weighted gradient echo images and increased signal intensity on T2-weighted spin echo images. Aneurysm size is a crucial factor for the sensitivity. MRA studies consistently indicate sensitivity rates of more than 95% for aneurysms larger than 6 mm, but much less for smaller aneurysms. For aneurysms smaller than 5 mm, which constitute as many as one-third of aneurysms in asymptomatic patients, detection rates of 56% and less have been reported. However, these aneurysms should not be ignored even if their rupture risk is low. In our experience, in most patients, MRA can detect aneurysms as small as 3 mm; the problem to detect lesions below this size is well known. This should be taken into account for all screening programs, but also for those follow-up examinations (after coiling) when the initial size of the aneurysm was around 3 mm.

Present indications for MR angiography in the evaluation of cerebral aneurysms include:
- Incidental findings on CT or MRI suspicious for an aneurysm
- Evaluation of specific clinical symptoms (e.g. third cranial nerve palsy) or non-specific symptoms in patients in whom an aneurysm may explain the clinical presentation (e.g. those with thunderclap-headache).
- Contraindications for conventional angiography
- Noninvasive follow-up of patients with known aneurysms or endovascularly treated aneurysms
- Screening in high risk patients (e.g. first-degree relatives of patients with SAH or multiple aneurysms, patients with polycystic kidney disease or with connective tissue disease)

Owing to its excellent spatial resolution, conventional cerebral angiography is still the gold standard for the detection of a cerebral aneurysm. Currently, this is performed during the first available moment after presentation of the patient in hospital. Considering that the risk of hemorrhage is highest in the first 24 hours (4%), an early angiogram is crucial for any therapeutic decision and for the patient's outcome.

Cerebral angiography can localize the lesion, reveal its shape and geometry, determine the presence of multiple aneurysms, define the vascular anatomy and collateral situation, and assess the presence and degree of vasospasm. Due to the frequency of multiple aneurysms, a complete four-vessel angiography examination is essential. However, in case of a space-occupying hematoma, angiography of the most likely affected vessel is sufficient. Anteroposterior, lateral, and oblique views are systematically performed with cross-compression to demonstrate the anterior communicating artery, if necessary. Additional views may be necessary to optimize demonstration of the aneurysmal neck. If no aneurysm is found, selective catheterization of both external carotid arteries is performed to exclude a dural arteriovenous fistula. The potential for collateral circulation from the vertebrobasilar system may be evaluated when the vertebral artery is injected during carotid artery compression (Allcock's test), demonstrating the patency, size and collateral potential of the P1 segment of the posterior cerebral artery (PCA) and the posterior communicating artery ipsilateral to the compressed carotid artery.

As a prerequisite to angiography, survey of renal function and coagulation factors is required in all patients. DSA is necessary; biplanar angiography facilitates the diagnostic work-up and is useful for safe and fast therapeutic interventions. It shortens examination time and increases the safety during aneurysm obliteration. High-quality fluoroscopy and roadmapping are essential to perform intracranial interventions.

The primary treatment goal of cerebral aneurysms is prevention of rupture. Surgical clipping has been the treatment modality of choice for both ruptured and unruptured cerebral aneurysms for decades. Twenty years ago, endovascular treatment was mainly restricted to those patients with aneurysms unsuitable for clipping due to the size or location, or in whom surgical clipping was contraindicated because of the general medical condition. Since the introduction of controlled detachable coils for packing of aneurysms, endovascular embolization is increasingly used. Numerous observational studies have published complications rates, occlusion rates and short-term follow-up results. These have been summarized up to March 1997 in a systematic review of 48 eligible studies of 1383 patients with ruptured and unruptured aneurysms. Permanent procedural complications occurred in 3.7% of 1256 patients. More than 90% occlusion of the aneurysm was achieved in around 90% of patients. The most frequent procedural complication was cerebral ischemia and the second most frequent complication was aneurysm perforation, which occurred in about 2% of patients. Rerupture of angiographically successful coiled aneurysms may occur; long-term rates of rebleeding after endovascular coiling still need to be established. In 2002, the results of the International Subarachnoid Aneurysm Trial (ISAT) were published; the clear benefits of endovascular coiling will definitely change treatment strategies for patients with intracranial aneurysms. The endovascular approach will become the first-line treatment option, wherever it is available. New devices like selfexpandable stents for intracranial use now allow surgeons to treat even broad-based aneurysms. As a rule of thumb, around 70%-80% of intracranial aneurysms can nowadays be treated via the endovascular approach.

Cavernomas

Cavernomas, also called cerebral cavernous malformations or cavernous angiomas, are characterized by endothelium-lined, sinusoidal blood cavities without other features of normal blood vessels like muscular and adventitial layers. No brain tissue is present between the blood cavities, which are embedded in connective tissue. This is, from a pathological viewpoint, the major difference between cavernoma and capillary telangiectasia. In the latter, there is intervening brain parenchyma between the vascular channels. During follow-up, growth of cavernomas can occur, but this is exclusively related to osmotic changes or differences (like in chronic subdural hematoma) and never related to infiltration or any active growth. The sinusoidal walls may be locally thickened or hyalinized with spots of calcification. Cavernomas may occur sporadically or after radiation therapy, and may also be hereditary following an autosomal dominant trait.

No reliable study gives exact rates of incidence and prevalence of cavernomas, but some data are available. The prevalence, estimated on the basis of autopsy and MRI studies, is 0.5%-0.7%. The incidence has been estimated to be 0.4%-0.9%. Cavernomas account for 8%-15% of all intracranial vascular malformations. During the last two decades, incidence data have been confirmed by MRI-based retrospective studies. There is no gender preponderance, and up to 25% of all cavernomas are found in the pediatric population. Multiple cavernomas occur in up to 90% of familial cases and in around 25% of sporadic cases. Therefore, whenever you see a single cavernoma on the MR scan of a patient, make sure that this is the only one.

Patients with cavernomas present with a variety of symptoms. Seizures are the most common symptom, accounting for 38%-55% of complaints. Other symptoms include focal neurologic deficits in 12%-45% of patients, recurrent hemorrhage in 4%-32%, and chronic headaches in 5%-52%. Brain stem cavernomas nearly never cause seizures. Most of these patients have typical brain stem symptoms such as diplopia, face or body sensory disturbances, and ataxia. Without imaging, it is difficult to distinguish on clinical grounds alone this subgroup of patients with intratentorial cavernomas from those with multiple sclerosis.

The majority of patients becomes symptomatic between the third and fifth decades, and there is no definite association between symptoms and gender. The frequency of asymptomatic cavernomas is not precisely known, but according to the literature, it seems to be around 40%.

The central clinical problem in patients with cavernomas is the question of hemorrhage. On a first view, this should be a simple question with a simple answer. However, both are wrong. The problem starts with the definition of hemorrhage and ends with rather individual answers for individual patients.

On one side, hemorrhage can be defined clinically: first or sudden onset of new neurologic symptoms in a patient with a cavernoma is usually related to a new or first hemorrhagic event. However, the literature contains an amazing number of definitions and terms to describe cavernoma-related hemorrhage: overt hemorrhage, symptomatic hemorrhage, gross hemorrhage, microhemorrhage, intralesional or perilesional ooze or diapedesis, clinically significant hemorrhage, subclinical hemorrhage and others. The reason for this variety of descriptions is that sometimes only clinical events were used to define hemorrhage and in other studies different imaging modalities (mainly MRI) had a major impact on the definition of hemorrhage. We suggest using the established Zabramski classification scheme in order to compare different patient groups and studies. However, the problem in defining a hemorrhage is a major reason for the still ongoing debate about the risk of hemorrhage and bleeding rates in patients with cavernomas.

Most estimates assume that cavernomas are present since birth; risk of hemorrhage and bleeding rates are mainly based on that assumption. In 1991, Del Curling et al. and Robinson et al. were the first to calculate the annual hemorrhage rate and found that it is between 0.25% and 0.7% per patient. Aiba et al. (1995) analyzed patients based on the initial finding: if bleeding was the initial symptom, the annual hemorrhage rate was 22.9%; if seizure was the first symptom, the annual bleeding rate was 0.39% per patient. Kondziolka (1995) also stratified his patient group into those who had previously experienced a hemorrhage and those who had not. Patients with one previous hemorrhage had a 4.5% yearly risk of hemorrhage, whereas those without a previous hemorrhage had a 0.6% yearly risk. An analysis of the symptomatic bleeding risk in untreated patients who had experienced two or more hemorrhages found the rate to be approximately 30% per year. Other authors, usually not differentiating between initial symptoms, published hemorrhage rates between 1.1% and 3.1%. Porter et al. reported in 1999 that brain stem cavernomas may have a significantly increased risk of hemorrhage and calculated it at 5% per person annually. Contrarily, Kupersmith and coworkers found a bleeding rate of 2.46% in brain stem cavernomas. However, the rebleeding rate – and this is quite well supported by other data – was beyond 5% in brain stem cavernomas. All studies suggest that the occurrence of rebleeding is an indication of a higher bleeding probability of a given cavernoma. The risk of a symptomatic rebleed at least doubles in comparison to asymptomatic cavernomas. These findings clearly should impact upon therapeutic decisions. The bleeding incidence is higher in patients with the inherited form of cavernomatosis, however, not for a single given cavernoma, but in terms of patient-years.

Patients younger than 35 years experienced more bleeding episodes, and the same was true for those with cavernomas of at least 10 mm. A number of studies addressed the increased bleeding risk in women; the majority, however, did not find any gender difference in bleeding risks.

The main problem in all these studies is a substantial selection bias and the definition of hemorrhage. Another, but probably more important aspect for patients when discussing bleeding risks is the clinical significance of hemorrhage and the probability of a good recovery. The probability of a fatal hemorrhage is rather low and many patients do have complete or nearly complete recovery after the initial bleeding. In general, bleeding rates given by surgical groups tend to be higher than those observed by others.

Finally, when discussing the risks of cavernoma with patients, it is important to consider that the majority of studies calculated an annual risk of 0.5%-1%, much lower than that for true arteriovenous malformations (AVMs), and a low risk of fatal hemorrhage. In the majority of patients, specifically those older than 35 years, harboring a single cavernoma less than 10 mm in diameter and with seizures as the initial symptom, a wait-and-see strategy is reasonable. In patients presenting with an initial hemorrhage, the repeat hemorrhage risk is much higher, especially if already more than one bleeding event has happened.

As mentioned previously, the majority of patients with cavernomas presents with seizures as the initial symptom. It is important to know that in the vast majority of patients, these seizures are not related to acute bleeding events, but to hemosiderin deposition adjacent to neurons. Hemosiderin and ferritin are well-known epileptogenic agents (at least in animal experiments). If surgical removal of the cavernoma is considered, understanding the relationship between seizures and hemosiderin deposition is especially important because of pharmacological not treatable seizures. It is of utmost importance not only to remove those parts of the cavernoma with blood flow, but also to remove the hemosiderin ring around the cavernoma within the adjacent brain tissue. This part of the malformation is responsible for the seizure.

Due to the slow blood flow, cavernomas are angiographically occult vascular malformations. If the lesion has hemorrhaged, an avascular area with moderate mass effect can sometimes be identified. Occasionally (less than 10%) a faint blush on the late capillary or early venous phase of high-resolution angiograms can be seen. Angiography is rarely necessary in typical cavernomas. If associated with a developmental venous angioma (DVA), presurgical DSA may be indicated to analyze the venous drainage pattern. The same is true for those cavernomas that do not have the typical MRI appearance. In some of these, DSA can increase the diagnostic confidence. On CT and, even more, on MRI, imaging features are more or less pathognomonic.

The CT appearance of a cavernoma depends on the amount of internal thrombosis, hemorrhage and calcification. The lesions appear hyperdense compared to the adjacent brain parenchyma, but can have variable attenuation values. Because the density of blood on CT depends on clot formation, the attenuation of a thrombosed cavernoma changes with time. Calcifications do not change that much, however, cavernomas tend to calcify only partially. In patients with a recent hemorrhage, the cavernoma may be suspected on CT mainly by taking into account the site of hemorrhage and the patient's history, and thus by excluding other typical causes of intracerebral bleeding. Differential diagnosis must cover calcified brain tumor, mainly oligodendroglioma, which has a high tendency of intratumoral bleeding. Contrast enhancement can be observed on CT, but usually requires a substantial delay between contrast agent injection and scanning. Even with a standardized 10-15 minute delay between contrast agent injection and scanning, the enhancement of a cavernoma varies from none or minimal to striking.

The imaging modality of choice is MRI. Typically, cavernomas have a popcorn-like appearance with a well-delineated complex reticulated core of mixed signal intensities representing hemorrhage in different stages of evolution or blood flow at different velocities. Typical is a low-signal hemosiderin rim that completely surrounds the lesion. The dark signal "blooms" on T2-weighted images, and is best visible on gradient echo T2*-weighted studies. Brunereau and colleagues studied the sensitivity of T2-weighted MRI versus gradient echo (GRE) sequences in patients with the familial form of cavernomas. The mean numbers of lesions detected on SE images and on GRE images were significantly different (7.2 vs. 20.2 in symptomatic subjects). Owing to the blood stagnation phenomenon or to the presence of true chronic microhemorrhages, cavernous angiomas contain deoxyhemoglobin or hemosiderin, which generates susceptibility effects and decreases signal intensity. This loss of signal intensity is much better demonstrated with T2*-weighted GRE sequences. This sequence should be part of the imaging protocol in all patients with a positive family history of cavernoma, a suspicion of focal or generalized seizures, or venous angiomas (there is a significant coincidence between occurrence of venous angiomas and cavernoma). However, turbo spin echo sequences using a long echo train, i.e. all FLAIR sequences, are insensitive to this susceptibility effect. Furthermore, even large lesions may not have a visible hemosiderin ring if there were no relevant, associated bleeding episodes.

Arteriovenous Malformations

Arteriovenous malformations of the brain (brain AVMs) correspond to congenital cerebrovascular anomalies, also known as intracerebral or pial AVMs. These are not neo-plastic lesions; therefore they are not "angiomas", which is obviously an inappropriate term although it is a commonly used.

Because of the rarity of the disease and the existence of asymptomatic patients, establishing a true prevalence rate is difficult, and probably not feasible. When considering unselected populations, Al-Shahi et al., in a retrospective study in a region of Scotland, found a prevalence of 15 per 100 000 living adults over 16 years of age. In this series, prevalence was obviously underestimated, since it did not consider asymptomatic AVMs. Only large post-mortem studies in the general population can give an accurate estimate of the prevalence of both symptomatic and clinically silent AVMs. However, such a series does not exist. Even though brain AVMs are considered to be a congenital disorder, nonsystemic familial AVMs are extremely rare and only few familial cases have been reported. No genetic predisposition was found and occurrence of brain AVMs in two members of the same family could have been a fortuitous event. Autopsy data showed that only 12% of AVMs are symptomatic while the patient is alive and that intracranial hemorrhage was the most common clinical presentation.

Regarding macroscopic pathology, brain AVMs are composed of: (1) clustered and abnormally muscularized feeding arteries, which may also show changes such as duplication or destruction of the elastica, fibrosis of the media and focal thinning of the wall; (2) arterialized veins of varying size and wall thickness; (3) structurally ambiguous vessels formed solely of fibrous tissue or displaying both arterial and venous characteristics; and (4) intervening gliotic neural parenchyma. Brain AVMs anastomose with normal cerebral vessels. Intracranial hemorrhage is the most frequent clinical presentation of brain AVM, with a frequency comprised between 30% and 82% (Mast, 1995). Overall, the percentages are relatively close between the different series, with annual rates of bleeding between 2% and 4%.

The occurrence of a first hemorrhage seems to be associated with an increased risk of subsequent hemorrhage. In the series of Graf et al., patients with ruptured AVMs had a 6% risk of rebleeding in the first year after hemorrhage and 2% thereafter. On the basis of retrospective analysis, the rupture of brain AVMs is estimated to be less severe than that of intracranial aneurysms, with a death rate between 10% and 15% and an overall morbidity rate less than 50% (The Arteriovenous Malformation Study Group, 1999). Hemorrhage of brain AVMs can be subarachnoid (30%), parenchymal (23%), intraventricular (16%) or combined (31%). Parenchymal hemorrhages were most likely to result in neurological deficit (52%). Overall, in the series of Hartmann (1998), 47% of patients had a good outcome after bleeding and an additional 37% were independent in daily living. In patients with a sudden onset of neurological deficit, CT is usually the first imaging modality used, mainly to rule out hemorrhage. CT is able to show early parenchymal, sub-

arachnoid and intraventricular bleeding. The diagnosis of brain AVM should be discussed when the patient is young, if the parenchymal hematoma has a lobar topography, and if calcifications or spontaneously hyperdense serpiginous structures are visible.

In case of unruptured AVM, unenhanced CT scans can be normal. However, in some patients slightly hyperdense serpiginous structures can be seen. Parenchymatous calcifications are observed in 20% of cases related to intravascular thrombosis or evolution of an old hematoma. Contrast agent injection is absolutely mandatory to depict brain AVM on CT. Abnormalities of the parenchymal density are visible in approximately 25% of cases, related to the presence of gliosis or old hematoma. Abnormalities of the ventricular system can be observed: focal dilatation in case of associated parenchymal atrophy; and compression of the ventricular system in case of mass effect caused by the AVM. Hydrocephalus can be observed in cases of previous hemorrhage or if the ventricular system is compressed by enlarged draining veins of the AVM. MRI is currently used in cases of unruptured AVM or to find the underlying lesion in cases of lobar hematoma, generally days or weeks after bleeding.

Given the different sequences available, MRI permits three levels of analysis of an AVM:
– Anatomical analysis using conventional sequences,
– Vascular analysis using MR angiography, and
– Functional analysis using fMRI.

Despite recent developments, CTA and MRA are currently not sufficient to obtain a precise description of the AVM from an anatomical and hemodynamical point of view. Selective angiography is still always necessary to make a decision regarding the treatment. In summary, the diagnosis of an AVM nowadays is usually based on CT or MRI, while the exact and therapeutically relevant anatomical and functional information still has to be obtained by angiography.

Technically, selective angiography has to be performed with a rigorous protocol. To assess as precisely as possible the anatomical components of the AVM, it is important to performed selective injection of internal and external carotid arteries and vertebral arteries. Arterial feeders, nidus, and venous drainage are analyzed by performing multiple projections (anteroposterior, lateral and oblique). Three-dimensional angiography may be helpful.

However, even excellent angiograms are often inadequate for correct therapeutic decisions. The exact anatomy of large feeding arteries may be obscure with selective injections. Small feeding arteries are sometimes not visible on selective angiograms. Although the size of the nidus is generally well evaluated by selective angiography, intranidal aneurysms and direct intranidal arteriovenous fistulas are often misdiagnosed. The venous drainage of the AVM is generally well studied by selective angiography, but the compartments of the AVM and their venous drainage are often not depicted, because the AVM is injected as a whole.

For these reasons, superselective angiography often gives a more detailed analysis of the AVM and may become more important in the diagnosis decision. Superselective angiography is performed by manual injection of each separate arterial feeder. It is usually the first step of embolization.

Suggested Reading

Forsting M (ed) (1994) Intracranial vascular malformations and aneurysms: from diagnostic work-up to endovascular therapy. Springer, Berlin Heidelberg New York

Molyneux A, Kerr R, Stratton I, Sandercock P, Clarke M, Shrimpton J, Holman R (2002) International Subarachnoid Aneurysm Trial (ISAT) of neurosurgical clipping versus endovascular coiling in 2143 patients with ruptured intracranial aneurysms: a randomised trial. Lancet 360:1267-1274

Ondra SL, Troupp H, George ED et al (1990) The natural history of symptomatic arteriovenous malformations of the brain: a 24-year follow-up assessment. J Neurosurg 73:387-391

Pollock BE, Flickinger JC, Lunsford LD et al (1996) Factors that predict the bleeding risk of cerebral arteriovenous maformations. Stroke 27:1-6

Porter RW, Detwiler PW, Spetzler RF, Lawton MT, Baskin JJ, Derksen PT et al (1999) Cavernous malformations of the brainstem: experience with 100 patients. J Neurosurg 90(1):50-58

Rigamonti D, Hadley MN, Drayer BP, Johnson PC, Hoenig-Rigamonti K, Knight JT, Spetzler RF (1988) Cerebral cavernous malformations. Incidence and familial occurence. N Engl J Med 319:343-347

Robinson JR, Awad IA, Little JR (1991) Natural history of the cavernous angioma. J Neurosurg 75:709-714

Spetzler RF, Martin NA (1986) A proposed grading system for arteriovenous maformations. J Neurosurg 65:476-483

Wiebers DO, Whisnant JP, Huston J 3rd, Meissner I, Brown RD Jr, Piepgras DG, Forbes GS, Thielen K, Nichols D, O'Fallon WM, Peacock J, Jaeger L, Kassell NF, Kongable-Beckman GL, Torner JC (2003) Unruptured intracranial aneurysms: natural history, clinical outcome, and risks of surgical and endovascular treatment. Lancet 362:103-110

White PM, Wardlaw JM, Easton V (2000) Can noninvasive imaging accurately depict intracranial aneurysms? A systematic review. Radiology 217:361-370

Demyelinating Diseases

K.K. Koeller[1], R.G. Ramsey[2]

[1] Department of Radiologic Pathology, Armed Forces Institute of Pathology, Washington, DC, USA
[2] Premier Health Imaging, Chicago, IL, USA

Introduction

The spectrum of white matter diseases is broad, with conditions ranging from the relatively benign to the progressively debilitating to the rapidly fulminant and fatal. While a specific diagnosis based on the imaging appearance alone is often not possible because of considerable overlap among the diseases, magnetic resonance imaging (MRI) remains ideal for the detection of many of these diseases because of its sensitivity in identifying free water within the normally myelinated white matter.

The oligodendrocyte, located predominantly within the white matter, is the cell responsible for the production of myelin and is also the least common of the three major cells (after neurons and astrocytes) that compose the brain parenchyma. Demyelinating diseases are not characterized by neoplastic growth. Rather, the attack on the oligodendrocyte leads to a loss of myelin. Consequently, the hallmark imaging manifestation of a demyelinating process is a white matter lesion with T2 hyperintensity that produces little mass effect for the size of the lesion. This brief review focuses on the classic demyelinating process, multiple sclerosis, and other demyelinating conditions arising from viral infection, chronic toxic conditions, iatrogenic causes, vascular disease, and inherited metabolic white matter disease.

Primary Demyelination

The prototypical white matter disease is multiple sclerosis (MS). Despite the more than 160 years since the first clinical features of the disease were recognized in 1837 by Carswell and Cruveilhier, much of this demyelinating process is not well understood. Although many etiologies, including trauma and viral infection, have been proposed, many authorities now believe that the disease is primarily autoimmune in nature and modulated by genetic factors (chromosome 6). This hypothesis is supported by the frequent association of MS with many other autoimmune conditions (e.g. Graves' disease, myasthenia gravis, Crohn's disease, systemic lupus erythematosus).

The incidence of MS varies with geography, with increased frequency of the disease in cooler climates. In the United States and countries of northern Europe, the incidence is about 1 per 1000. MS is primarily a disease of young and middle-aged adults (95% of cases occur in patients between the ages of 18 and 50 years) and it is the second most common disabling disease of young adults, with only acquired immune deficiency syndrome (AIDS) being more common. Most (60%) patients with the disease are female [1].

Typical clinical presenting symptoms include paresthesia, numbness, diplopia, weakness, gait disturbance, and burning sensations. About 7% of patients present with symptoms reflecting myelitis in which hemiparesis, constipation, urinary retention, or incontinence are typical features. Seizure activity occurs in about 5% of cases. Uthoff's phenomenon gained prominence decades ago as a provocative test for MS, based on the observation that patients with MS have a worsening of their symptoms when they are exposed to warm temperatures. The test was abandoned when it was noted that some patients would not return to their neurologic baseline. MS is rarely seen in children, especially before the age of puberty. Clinical exacerbations in women are common in the first 6 months of the post-partum period. Detection of oligoclonal gammopathy on cerebrospinal fluid examination is an important laboratory finding but may not always be present [2].

The phenomenon of optic neuritis, characterized clinically by retrobulbar pain, a central monocular loss of vision, and an afferent papillary defect (Marcus Gunn pupil) is especially useful as a clinical hallmark for MS. The likelihood of a female patient with optic neuritis having MS, either at the time of presentation or sometime in the future, is 74%. While the diagnosis is best substantiated by clinical inspection, magnetic resonance imaging remains valuable in directing therapy. When 2 or more MS-like lesions are noted, intravenous corticosteroid therapy is advocated and may slow the development of full-blown MS [3].

The clinical criteria required to establish the diagnosis are complex and require strict implementation to be effective [4]. In general, two distinctly different clinical "attacks" from two different lesions in the central nervous system are required to make the diagnosis, although many variations on this theme are possible with adjunctive laboratory and imaging findings. Three forms of the disease are recognized: relapsing-remitting, progressive, and monosymptomatic [5]. The majority (70%) of patients with MS present clinically with the relapsing-remitting form of the disease. Typical symptoms include numbness, dysesthesia, and burning sensations. A patient must have at least 2 clinical attacks from two clinically distinct lesions. The episodes must be for at least 24 hours duration and be at least 30 days apart [4]. Partial or complete remission for months or years is expected for patients with this form.

The second most common form of MS is the progressive form, affecting about 20% of patients, and it is further subdivided into primary and secondary subtypes. In the primary progressive form of the disease, the clinical presentation is marked by a slow onset without the distinct attacks that are typical for the relapsing-remitting form. In the secondary progressive form, the patient presents initially in the relapsing-remitting form with later transformation into progressively worsening disability in addition to individual clinical relapses.

The most controversial form is the "monosymptomatic demyelinating" form occurring in about 10% of MS patients. Patients with this form have one or two episodes of characteristic symptoms, followed by complete recovery to their neurologic baseline. By its very nature, it is clearly an unusual form of MS and some authorities question whether it is truly part of the MS family but may instead be an entirely distinct clinicopathologic disease.

Several variant types of MS have been identified. An especially aggressive form, known as acute fulminant MS of the Marburg type, manifests with a rapidly progressive neurologic deterioration from severe axonal loss, leading to death within a few months [6]. Another variant, neuromyelitis optica (Devic's disease), is characterized by both visual and myelopathic symptoms because of involvement of the optic nerve and spinal cord. Baló concentric sclerosis is a variant form characterized by alternating concentric bands of demyelination and normal myelination. These features are not only noted histologically but are also well seen on cross-sectional imaging studies [7].

Pathologically, MS is an inflammatory process with focal hypercellularity from microglial infiltration combined with perivascular cuffing of lymphocytes marking the acute phase of a *sclerose en plaque* or MS plaque. In this phase, the oligodendrocyte – the cell responsible for the production of myelin – is most affected by these changes and results in the overall loss of myelin. The plaque, which has a predilection for the periventricular zone, may be either active, characterized by inflammatory changes with breakdown of the blood-brain barrier, or inactive, characterized by gliosis and complete loss of myelin. Later on, destruction of axons leads to parenchymal loss and cerebral atrophy.

Magnetic resonance imaging (MRI) is the modality of choice for the evaluation of patients suspected of having MS and is an essential tool in assessing the natural course of the disease and effects of treatment. MRI frequently identifies many lesions that are not suspected from clinical examination [8]. Small focal hyperintense lesions, particularly in a periventricular distribution, with relatively less mass effect for the size of the lesion characterize the disease on T2-weighted images [9]. Many MS lesions are ovoid in shape with their long axis perpendicular to the ventricular wall, corresponding to the pathway of periventricular white matter vessels, and corroborate a pathologic feature, known as Dawson's finger [10]. An especially important location for MS plaques is the corpus callosum-septum pellucidum interface. The detection of lesions at this site carries increased specificity for the diagnosis of MS [11]. Fluid-attenuated inversion recovery (FLAIR) imaging is particularly helpful in identifying periventricular lesions, although lesions of the brain stem and cerebellum may be less obvious with this technique because of susceptibility effects [12].

On initial inspection, the imaging appearance of some large plaques may mimic that of a brain tumor. Closer evaluation reveals the relative lack of mass effect for the size of these "tumefactive" MS plaques and provides a valuable clue to the correct diagnosis [13]. Distinction between plaques in the active phase and plaques in the chronic phase can be made with contrast-enhanced MRI as active plaques enhance while chronic plaques do not [9, 14]. The enhancement correlates with the presence of inflammatory cells and signifies the loss of a normal blood-brain barrier [9].

In the advanced stages of the disease, cerebral atrophy is noted on MRI studies with prominent ventriculomegaly and sulcal enlargement and appears to be more common in patients with the secondary progressive form of the disease than in patients with the relapsing-remitting form [15]. The presence of cerebral atrophy, as evidenced by thinning of the corpus callosum and enlargement of the third ventricle width, or by using computer-aided techniques, correlates better with clinical disability than the number of lesions on T2-weighted images [15, 16]. Advanced MRI techniques are providing even more information about the nature of the MS plaque and hold the promise of better assessment of the effects of therapy. Magnetization transfer imaging reveals differences in magnetization transfer between MS plaques and other white matter lesions, such as senescent white matter lesions [17]. On MR spectroscopy, a decreased peak of *N*-acetylaspartate (NAA), decreased NAA:creatine ratio, and an increased choline:creatine ratio have been seen in both active and chronic plaques, although the incidence varies among the different clinical types of the disease. Increased amounts of choline, lipids, lactic acid, and inositol have also been variably reported and highlight the dynamic nature of the MS plaque [18, 19]. Recently, MR perfusion studies have shown regions of decreased perfusion, believed to represent areas of hemodynamic and microvascular abnormality, in patients with MS even though no abnormal T2 hyperintensity was noted on other MR sequences. This supports the belief that MS is truly a diffuse white matter disease, with more involvement beyond readily identifiable plaques.

About 7% of all MS cases involve the spinal cord. MS plaques in this territory tend to involve 2 or more vertebral body segments, compared to transverse myelitis, which is usually limited to one vertebral body segment. MS myelitis also tends to involve the dorsal columns. Most (60%) patients with spinal cord MS plaques have cerebral plaques as well.

Despite all of these imaging features, it is important to emphasize two "truths" about MS. First, the MS plaque is a dynamic entity, not only fluctuating between an active phase and a chronic phase but also showing remyelination, inflammatory changes, gliosis, and demyelination at any given time. Second, the diagnosis of MS is still only established with clinical correlation. None of the imaging presentations, either alone or in combination, described previously is pathognomonic. The diagnosis of MS carries a tremendous emotional undercurrent for the patient. With this in mind, the radiologist should strictly avoid labeling a patient as "having MS" in a radiological report in the absence of clinical confirmation.

White Matter Disease from Viral Infection

Acute Disseminated Encephalomyelitis

Acute disseminated encephalomyelitis (ADEM) is a demyelinating disease that is typically seen 1-3 weeks after patients are vaccinated or have a viral infection. Neurologic symptoms in ADEM vary from mild (headache and meningeal signs) to severe (neurologic deficits and coma). In contrast to MS, ADEM is a monophasic illness and children are more commonly affected. Since ADEM is a diagnosis of exclusion, long-term follow-up is required to completely exclude MS. Most (80%) patients have a good prognosis but 10%-20% have a persistent neurologic deficit. Rarely, the disease can result in death. It is believed that ADEM represents an autoimmune response that triggers perivenous demyelination in immunocompetent patients. No virus or bacterium has been isolated in any patient with ADEM on autopsy examination. A rare hyperacute aggressive form, acute hemorrhagic leukoencephalitis, may occur in children and is usually fatal, secondary to herniation.

On computed tomography (CT), ADEM may not be detected or it may have an ill-defined non-specific hypoattenuation. On MRI, the lesions of ADEM are frequently asymmetric, varying in size and number, with little or no mass effect, a hallmark feature of a demyelinating process. Variable enhancement is seen on contrast-enhanced studies. Similar to MS, lesions may occasionally involve the optic nerve or spinal cord [20].

Progressive Multifocal Leukoencephalopathy

Progressive multifocal leukoencephalopathy (PML) is overwhelmingly a disease of the immunocompromised patient population and most (55%-85%) cases are related to AIDS. There is a wide age range of involvement, with the peak age of presentation in the sixth decade. The disease is caused by reactivation of a papovavirus (JC virus) that selectively attacks the oligodendrocyte, leading to demyelination. In contrast to patients with ADEM, patients with PML have an extremely poor prognosis, with death common in the first 6 months following establishment of the diagnosis.

Like ADEM, the lesions of PML display little mass effect or enhancement. Rarely, some lesions may be large enough to be associated with some mass effect and, in these circumstances, it may be difficult to differentiate them from true neoplasms. Most lesions involve the subcortical white matter and deep cortical layers of the parieto-occipital or frontal white matter, although gray matter and posterior fossa lesions may occur in up to 50% of cases. PML lesions tend to be more confluent in their appearance than ADEM lesions. Scalloping of the lateral margin of the lesion at the gray-white matter junction is common. Occasionally, the lesions contain hemorrhage [21].

Human Immunodeficiency Virus Encephalopathy

Human immunodeficiency virus (HIV) encephalopathy results from direct infection of the brain by the virus itself. Most patients are severely immunocompromised at the time of onset and exhibit psychomotor slowing, impaired mental status, and memory difficulties. Histologically, demyelination and vacuolation with axonal loss are noted, along with occasional microglial nodules. Mild cerebral atrophy is the first and sometimes only imaging feature of the disease, which is also known as AIDS dementia complex, HIV dementia, and HIV-associated dementia complex. Involvement of the central white matter, basal ganglia, and thalamus is characteristic. Typically, bilaterally symmetric areas of abnormal hyperintensity in the basal ganglia and small focal areas in the periventricular regions are noted on T2-weighted MR images. Regression of these findings has been seen following institution of antiretroviral therapy [22].

White Matter Disease from Toxic Imbalance

Chronic Alcohol Ingestion and its Consequences

Chronic alcohol ingestion predominantly causes atrophy that involves the entire cerebral hemisphere and the superior cerebellar vermis. Two diseases – Marchiafava-Bignami disease and Wernicke's encephalopathy – involve necrosis of distinct locations and are important consequences of chronic alcoholism. Selective demyelination and necrosis of the corpus callosum is the hallmark of Marchiafava-Bignami disease. Originally described by two Italian physicians who documented the disease in a series of poorly nourished patients who died from the effects of excessive consumption of Italian red wine, Marchiafava-Bignami disease can occur in any population and from any alcoholic agent. It has even been reported in poorly nourished non-drinkers. The necrotic zones are especially well seen as abnormal hyperintense foci on sagittal T2-weighted images. If the patient survives, atrophy of the corpus callosum is seen [23].

Wernicke's encephalopathy causes necrosis in the medial thalamic nuclei and mamillary bodies, which results from thiamine deficiency. Patients with the disease typically present with ophthalmoplegia, ataxia, and confusion. The disease is uniformly fatal unless replacement thiamine therapy is instituted within 24-72 hours of presentation. Abnormal T2 hyperintensity within the medial portions of the thalami is the hallmark imaging feature of this disease. While the thalamic changes are potentially reversible, atrophy of the mamillary bodies is permanent.

Osmotic Myelinolysis

Formerly called "central pontine myelinolysis", the term "osmotic myelinolysis" was proposed a few years ago to emphasize the nature of this disease: rapid intravascular osmotic change causes endothelial injury in the regions where the gray and white matters are most closely apposed, i.e. in the central portion of the pons. The end result of this endothelial injury is demyelination. Clinical symptoms usually include acute mental status changes, lethargy, dysphagia, and progressive quadriparesis. Once thought to be uniformly fatal, it is now known that this is not necessarily true and a return to a normal imaging appearance and clinical status may be seen over a variable period of time. The classic imaging appearance of osmotic myelinolysis is hypoattenuation on CT and T1 and T2 prolongation on MRI within the center of the pons. Distinctive sparing of the pons periphery is noted. Extrapontine involvement may be noted in about 10% of cases and usually involves the basal ganglia and others locations within the brain [24].

White Matter Disease Associated with Radiation Therapy and Chemotherapy

Radiation Injury and Necrosis

The spectrum of radiation injury to the brain is broad. Three distinct categories of disease are noted: acute radiation injury, early delayed radiation injury, and late radiation injury. In acute radiation injury, mild transient encephalopathic symptoms present very shortly after initiation of radiation. No CT or MRI findings are seen with this form of injury. Early delayed radiation injury produces demyelination within the white matter at least 2 months after the start of radiation therapy. Lesions predominate in

the white matter, basal ganglia, and cerebral peduncles. Late radiation injury has 3 different forms: focal radiation necrosis, diffuse radiation injury, and necrotizing leukoencephalopathy. While the first two generally occur at least one year after the start of therapy, the last entity may manifest as early as 3 months after onset of therapy [25]. Distinguishing radiation necrosis from recurrent malignant brain tumor, such as glioblastoma multiforme, is frequently impossible using conventional MRI. Both lesions may have mass effect and surrounding vasogenic edema, and may enhance on contrast-enhanced studies. Metabolic imaging (e.g. positron emission tomography) or MR spectroscopy (MRS) may facilitate differentiating between the two possibilities. Radiation necrosis is iso- to hypometabolic on metabolic imaging studies and has a characteristic lactic acid peak and near-normal peaks for N-acetylaspartate (NAA) and choline on MRS. In contrast, recurrent high-grade gliomas are hypermetabolic and typically show elevated choline levels compared to NAA without or with elevated lactic acid levels.

Diffuse radiation injury is characterized by white matter changes that are "geographic" in nature, i.e. the areas of abnormal signal intensity or attenuation are limited to the regions of the brain that correspond to the radiation portal. This can produce striking differences between the involved zones and the spared surrounding white matter. The involved territories are often symmetric and do not enhance on post-contrast studies.

While originally reported in children with leukemia, diffuse necrotizing leukoencephalopathy has also been observed following treatment for many other malignancies in both children and adults. The disease may occur following chemotherapy alone but the incidence of disease is highest when chemotherapy is combined with radiation therapy. Both the histologic findings and imaging features bear resemblance to radiation necrosis. Axonal swelling, demyelination, coagulation necrosis, and gliosis dominate the histologic picture. Diffuse white matter changes, with hypoattenuation on CT and T1 and T2 prolongation on MRI, are common and often involve an entire hemisphere [26].

Mineralizing Microangiopathy

Usually seen in children with cancer who have been treated with chemotherapy alone or in combination with radiation therapy, mineralizing microangiopathy results from deposits of calcium in and around small penetrating blood vessels of the deep brain leading to local areas of necrosis. This is the most common neuroradiologic abnormality noted in this group of patients. The disease has a predilection for the basal ganglia, especially the putamen, and, more rarely, the cerebral cortex. On CT and MRI, evidence of cortical atrophy, abnormal attenuation and signal intensity changes within the white matter are typically noted. Of all chemotherapeutic agents, methotrexate is the one classically associated with mineralizing microangiopathy. Patients younger than 5 years of age who have meningeal leukemia and have received high-dose methotrexate therapy are at greatest risk for developing this complication of therapy [27].

Vascular Causes of White Matter Disease

Posterior Reversible Encephalopathy Syndrome

Under normal circumstances, cerebral perfusion pressure is maintained at a relatively constant level by autoregulation, a physiologic mechanism that compensates for wide changes in systemic blood pressure. Hypertensive encephalopathy is believed to result from loss of normal autoregulation, with competing regions of vasodilatation and vasoconstriction as a result. Current theory espouses that the vessels of the posterior cerebral circulation, having less sympathetic innervation compared to those of the anterior circulation, are unable to vasoconstrict in a normal manner and therefore bear the brunt of these vascular changes. Accordingly, visual field deficits are common, as are headaches, somnolence, and an overall impaired mental status. Since this hypertensive encephalopathy is also reversible if treated promptly, it has been referred to as posterior reversible encephalopathy syndrome (PRES). The disease is also associated with renal failure, preeclampsia, eclampsia, and the use of immunosuppressive agents such as cyclosporin A and FK506.

On MRI studies, abnormal T2 hyperintensity is most commonly seen in the distribution of the posterior circulation, although other sites including the frontal lobes and corpus callosum may be noted as well. Frequently, the lesions are bilaterally symmetric. Diffusion-weighted imaging may be normal or show restricted water diffusion while perfusion studies indicate normal to increased perfusion in these zones. When biopsy of these regions is performed, white matter edema is seen histologically. Following treatment or removal of the offending immunosuppressive agent, the lesions resolve and the involved sites return to normal signal intensity [28].

Ischemia and Vascular Disease

Small focal lesions of T2 hyperintensity are quite common in the white matter of adult patients. They are not associated with mass effect, do not enhance, and are typically isointense compared to normal white matter on T1-weighted images. When these lesions have been biopsied, histologic examination reveals a wide range of findings including gliosis, loss of myelination, and areas of ischemia. Senescent white matter lesions tend to be located in the periventricular white matter (although not immediately adjacent to the ventricular margin), centrum semiovale, and optic radiation. In contrast to MS lesions, they do not involve the corpus callosum, an important distinguishing feature. Since the lesions are so ubiquitous and appear to be a part of "normal" aging, various terms have been proposed: senescent white matter changes or

disease, deep white matter ischemia, etc. In general, the more lesions present, the more likely it is that the patient will have cognitive problems or difficulties with neuropsychologic testing. However, it is not possible to predict a particular patient's status simply based on the imaging appearance alone. Hence, the diagnosis of Binswanger's dementia should be avoided unless substantiated with clinical evidence.

The presence of periventricular and subcortical lesions in an adult 30-50 years of age, with a family history of similarly affected relatives, should raise the possibility of cerebral autosomal dominant arteriopathy with subcortical infarcts and leukoencephalopathy (CADASIL). A defect on the long arm of chromosome 19 has been identified and apparently evokes an angiopathy affecting small and medium-sized vessels. Most lesions occur in the frontal and temporal lobes. Less commonly, the thalamus, basal ganglia, internal and external capsules, and brain stem may be involved [29].

Many other conditions and diseases are associated with small vessel injuries that commonly involve the white matter as small, focal areas of abnormal T2 hyperintensity. These include autoimmune disease, particularly systemic lupus erythematosus, Behçet's disease, and giant cell arteritis, as well as arteritis associated with drug use (e.g. metamphetamine and heroin), radiation injury, and malignancy.

Dysmyelinating and Metabolic Diseases

The number and understanding of inherited metabolic white matter diseases have exponentially increased in the last 50 years and continue to expand yearly. Most will manifest in childhood, especially during infancy, and many are transmitted in an autosomal recessive fashion. Imaging features in these diseases are rarely pathognomonic and practically all require biochemical analysis of blood, urine, and skin to establish the diagnosis. From a pathophysiologic basis, these disorders are categorized based on the cellular organelle in which the altered metabolism is located. Lysosomal disorders, or "storage disorders", are a clinically heterogeneous group caused by an enzyme deficiency that results in the accumulation of phospholipids, glycolipids, mucopolysaccharides, or glycoproteins, all of which interfere with myelin production. Peroxisomal disorders are caused by an enzyme deficiency within peroxisomes, an organelle that is particularly common in oligodendrocytes, and alter normal lipid metabolism with the accumulation of very long-chain fatty acids. The mitochondrial disorders are a clinically heterogeneous group of diseases that result in spongy degeneration of myelin in various locations and also frequently involve muscles. Amino and organic acid disorders are rare and the clinical presentation is dependent on which acid is involved. Special types of leukodystrophies compose the last group. These represent those that are associated with macrocrania (Canavan's disease, Alexander's disease) or sudanophilic deposits noted on histologic examination (Cockayne's disease, Pelizaeus-Merzbacher disease) [30].

Diseases that tend to involve the "central" white matter first include Krabbe's disease, X-linked adrenoleukodystrophy and other peroxisomal disorders, metachromatic leukodystrophy, and Pelizaeus-Merzbacher disease. Diseases that tend to involve the peripheral white matter first include Alexander's disease, Canavan's disease, and Cockayne's disease. Diseases that involve gray matter in addition to the white matter involvement include mitochondrial disorders and the mucopolysaccharidoses. If hemorrhage is seen within a white matter lesion on an imaging study, it should provoke consideration of a diagnosis other than an inherited metabolic disorder.

References

1. Hauser SL (1994) Multiple sclerosis and other demyelinating disease. In: Isselbacher KJ, Graunwald E, Wilson JD, Martin JD, Fauci AS, Kasper DL (eds) Harrison's principle of internal medicine. McGraw-Hill, New York, pp 2287-2295
2. Farlow MR, Bonine JM (1993) Clinical and neuropathological features of multiple sclerosis. Neuroradiol Clin N Am 3:213-228
3. Trobe JD (1994) High-dose corticosteroid regimen retards development of multiple sclerosis in optic neuritis treatment trial. Arch Ophthalmol 112:35-36
4. McDonald WI, Compston A, Edan G, Goodkin D, Hartung H-P, Lublin FD et al (2001) Recommended diagnostic criteria for multiple sclerosis: guidelines from the International Panel on the Diagnosis of Multiple Sclerosis. Ann Neurol 50:121-127
5. Grossman RI, McGowan JC (1998) Perspective of multiple sclerosis. AJNR Am J Neuroradiol 19:1251-1265
6. Niebler G, Harris T, Davis T, Roos K (1992) Fulminant multiple sclerosis. AJNR Am J Neuroradiol 13:1547-1551
7. Gharagozloo AM, Poe LB, Collins GH (1994) Antemortem diagnosis of Balo concentric sclerosis: correlative MR imaging and pathologic features. Radiology 191:817-819
8. Barkhof F, Scheltens P, Frequin STFM, Nauta JJP, Tas MW, Valk J et al (1992) Relapsing-remitting multiple sclerosis: sequential enhanced MR imaging vs. clinical findings in determining disease activity. AJR Am J Roentgenol 159:1041-1047
9. Nesbit GM, Forbes GS, Scheithauer BW, Okazaki H, Rodrigucz M (1991) Multiplc sclcrosis: histopathologic and MR and/or CT correlation in 37 cases at biopsy and three cases at autopsy. Radiology 180:467-474
10. Horowitz AL, Kaplan RD, Grewe G, White RT, Salberg LM (1989) The ovoid lesion: a new MR observation in patients with multiple sclerosis. AJNR Am J Neuroradiol 10:303-305
11. Gean-Marton AD, Vezina LG, Marton KI, Stimac GK, Peyster RG, Taveras JM et al (1991) Abnormal corpus callosum: a sensitive and specific indicator of multiple sclerosis. Radiology 180:215-221
12. Hashemi RH, Bradley WG Jr, Chen DY, Jordan JE, Queralt JA, Cheng AE et al (1995) Suspected multiple sclerosis: MR imaging with a thin-section fast FLAIR pulse sequence. Radiology 196:505-510
13. Dagher AP, Smirniotopoulous JG (1996) Tumefactive demyelinating lesions. Neuroradiology 38:560-565
14. Grossman RI, Gonzalez-Scarano F, Atlas SW, Galetta S, Silberberg DH (1986) Multiple sclerosis: gadolinium enhancement in MR imaging. Radiology 161:721-725
15. Ge Y, Grossman RI, Udupa JK, Wei L, Mannon LJ, Polansky M et al (2000) Brain atrophy in relapsing-remitting multiple sclerosis and secondary progressive multiple sclerosis: longitudinal quantitative analysis. Radiology 214:665-670
16. Dietemann JL, Beigelman C, Rumbach L, Vogue M, Tajahmady T, Faubert C et al (1988) Multiple sclerosis and corpus callosum atrophy: relationship of MRI findings to clinical data. Neuroradiology 30:478-480
17. Mehta RC, Pike GB, Enzmann DR (1996) Measure of magnetization transfer in multiple sclerosis demyelinating plaques, white matter ischemic lesions, and edema. AJNR Am J Neuroradiol 17:1051-1055
18. Grossman RI, Lenkinski RE, Ramer KN, Gonzalez-Scarano F, Cohen JA (1992) MR proton spectroscopy in multiple sclerosis. AJNR Am J Neuroradiol 13:1535-1543
19. Falini A, Calabrese G, Filippi M, Origgi D, Lipari S, Colombo B et al (1998) Benign versus secondary-progressive multiple sclerosis: the potential role of proton-MR spectroscopy in defining the nature of disability. AJNR Am J Neuroradiol 19:223-229
20. Singh S, Alexander M, Korah IP (1999) Acute disseminated encephalomyelitis: MR imaging features. AJR Am J Roentgenol 173:1101-1107
21. Whiteman M, Post MJD, Berger JR, Tate LG, Bell MD, Limonte LP (1993) Progressive multifocal leukoencephalopathy in 47 HIV-seropositive patients: neuroimaging with clinical and pathologic correlation. Radiology 187:233-240
22. McArthur JC, Sacktor N, Seines O (1999) Human immunodeficiency virus-associated dementia. Semin Neurol 19:105-111
23. Izquierdo G, Quesada MA, Chacon J, Martel J (1992) Neuroradiologic abnormalities in Marchiafava-Bignami disease of benign evolution. Eur J Radiol 15:71-74
24. Miller GM, Baker HL, Okazaki H, Whisnant JP (1988) Central pontine myelinolysis and its imitators: MR findings. Radiology 168:795-802
25. Valk PE, Dillon WP (1991) Radiation injury of the brain. AJNR Am J Neuroradiol 12:45-62
26. Chan Y, Leung S, King AD, Choi PH, Metreweli C (1999) Late radiation injury to the temporal lobes: morphologic evaluation at MR imaging. Radiology 213:800-807
27. Davis P, Hoffman JJ, Pearl G, Braun I (1986) CT evaluation of effects of cranial radiation therapy in children. AJR Am J Roentgenol 147:587-592
28. Post JD, Beauchamp NJ (1998) Reversible intracerebral pathologic entities mediated by vascular autoregulatory dysfunction. Radiographics 18:353-367
29. Yousry TA, Seelos K, Mayer M, Bruning R, Uttner I, Dichgans M et al (1999) Characteristic MR lesion pattern and correlation of T1 and T2 lesion volume with neurologic and neuropsychological findings in cerebral autosomal dominant arteriopathy with subcortical infarcts and leukoencephalopathy (CADASIL). AJNR Am J Neuroradiol 20:91-100
30. Kendall BE (1992) Disorders of lysosomes, peroxisomes, and mitochondria. AJNR Am J Neuroradiol 13:621-653

Brain Degeneration and Aging

M.A. van Buchem

Department of Radiology, Leiden University Medical Center, Leiden, The Netherlands

Introduction

Many diseases result in degeneration of the nervous system. To name a few: infection, multiple sclerosis, and tumors destroy neuronal tissue. However, the term neurodegenerative disorders refers to a group of diseases that share the characteristic of death of subsets of specific classes of neurons. Another common feature of the class of neurodegenerative disorders is the fact that they are idiopathic, the etiology of these diseases is not completely understood. With increasing knowledge of the pathogenesis of these diseases, disorders that are presently classified as neurodegenerative will be grouped among diseases with a known pathogenesis, and consequently, the list of degenerative disorders will decrease. This paper discusses the neuroradiological aspects of a number of disorders that are presently considered to be neurodegenerative.

Normal Aging

The most common neurodegenerative disorder is aging. Aging is associated with degenerative changes of the brain. With increasing life expectancy of the population, the number of elderly persons increases in industrialized societies. Therefore, radiologists in such societies will increasingly be confronted with age-related changes in the brain. Knowledge of these changes is thus essential for every radiologist.

Before describing the abnormalities that occur with aging, it is important to be aware of a few facts. First, age-related abnormalities do not occur in all elderly persons. Some elderly individuals have a perfectly normal brain that is indistinguishable from that of a young person. This observation is in line with the concept of subdividing human aging in *successful aging* and *usual aging*. Successful aging is defined as minimal physiologic loss, even when compared with younger individuals, while usual aging is the presence of disturbance of physiologic functions (such as systolic hypertension, abnormal glucose tolerance) without overt neurologic symptoms. Elderly individuals with a normal appearance of the brain on imaging may be representatives of the group of successfully aging human beings.

Second, age-related changes that are apparent on radiological examinations do not always have functional consequences. An impressive load of brain lesions may be an incidental finding in an elderly individual who has no neurological or intellectual complaints whatsoever and who, apparently, is capable of having a normal, independent life.

Third, normal aging and neurodegenerative disorders may be difficult to distinguish. One reason is the similarity of the abnormalities that are associated with these conditions. In several neurodegenerative disorders, the abnormalities only differ in pattern from those occurring in normal aging. In other neurodegenerative disorders, the abnormalities really are similar, also in pattern, and the amount of abnormalities in relation to a patient's age is the only factor that permits distinction from normal aging. Another phenomenon that complicates distinguishing normal aging from other neurodegenerative disorders is the fact that due to the high prevalence of the latter, these conditions often coexist in the elderly with changes that are due to normal aging. In such circumstances it may be impossible to separate the abnormalities in terms of their origin.

An important task for radiologists, when confronted with a brain study in an elderly patient, is to screen for the presence of neurodegenerative disorders. In this process, changes should not be attributed too easily to normal aging. In order to be able to separate usual aging and other neurodegenerative disorders, a radiologist should be familiar with the changes that occur in normal aging. In the following section such changes are described.

Atrophy

With normal aging, mild to moderate atrophy of the brain occurs. This is mainly due to a gradual loss of white matter, based on loss of myelinated fibers and thinning of capillary walls. Since, the cerebrospinal fluid (CSF) compensates for the decreasing volume that the brain occupies in the skull, the CSF space directly reflects brain atrophy. CSF spaces that are to be evaluated when screening for signs of atrophy are the pericerebral and pericerebellar spaces, the caliber of the ventricles, and the presence and size of Virchow-Robin spaces (VRS).

In both radiologic and pathologic studies it has been demonstrated that progressive enlargement of the ventricles, cerebral sulci, and cerebellar CSF space occurs with aging. From 10 to 50 years of age, the CSF-to-brain ratio remains constant. In the fifth decade the contribution of CSF to the intracranial volume starts increasing. However, this increase is highly variable, and in 30%-50% of the elderly the CSF space remains in the range of those of young adults. Furthermore, in a large community-living, elderly population, sex differences have been demonstrated for the association of age and atrophy. In elderly men, atrophy is more pronounced than in elderly women.

In general, the increase of CSF space that is associated with normal aging occurs diffusely. However, in specific locations atrophy is more pronounced on imaging studies. An early finding may be third ventricular enlargement, due to atrophy of the median nuclei of the thalamus. The temporal horns of the lateral ventricles enlarge only mildly with normal aging. Widening of the cortical sulci occurs first in the frontal and parietal parasagittal regions, whereas the sulci in the central, precentral, post-central, and superior frontal gyri widen later in life. The frontal interhemispheric fissure and the CSF space around the cerebellar vermis are often widened clearly in normal elderly. The anterior portion of the sylvian fissure widens earlier than the posterior part. Moreover, in all age groups, the left sylvian fissure and left lateral ventricle are generally wider than their equivalents on the right side.

Another reflection of atrophy in the elderly is increased visibility of VRS. VRS are an extension of the subarachnoid space around perforating vessels that extent up to the level of the capillaries. Consequently, these perivascular spaces are filled with CSF. Local dilatations of VRS occur in all age groups, and are considered a normal anatomical variant. Such dilatations may render them visible on computed tomography (CT) and magnetic resonance imaging (MRI). On cross-sectional images, VRS appear as sharply delineated round, oval, or curvilinear structures that have no mass effect. The content of VRS follows the characteristics of CSF on CT and on all pulse sequences of MRI. VRS have sites of predilection: in the basal ganglia at the level of the anterior commissure, in the convexity, in the subinsular cortex, and in the midbrain. At these sites VRS often occur bilaterally and symmetrically. With advancing age, the number and size of VRS that are visible on cross-sectional imaging increase, in particular at the convexity and less so in the basal ganglia. État criblé is an extreme form of dilated VRS that may occur in aging. Age-related widening of VRS has been considered a manifestation of atrophy of the brain, similar to the increased pericerebral CSF space enlarge-

ment. In addition, it has been attributed to increased tortuosity of penetrating arteries and arterioles that is associated with aging.

Since atrophy often is a global process, it may be difficult to assess qualitatively on cross-sectional images whether atrophy of the brain is present or not. Evaluation of the volume of the corpus callosum on a mid-sagittal image is easier. Since the corpus callosum generally reflects brain volume and thus atrophy, looking at the corpus callosum may help detecting atrophy.

Gray Matter Hypointensities

On MRI, the signal intensity of the deep gray matter nuclei changes with age. These changes comprise lowering of the signal intensity on T2-weighted images. It has been postulated that the substrate for these changes is an increasing deposition of ferritin, a storage form of non-heme iron. The visibility of these changes depends on field strength and specifications of the MRI sequence used.

In the first 10 years of life, the signal intensity of the deep gray matter nuclei on T2-weighted images is similar to that of the cerebral cortex. By age 25 years, the signal intensities at 1.5 tesla of the globus pallidus, red nucleus and pars reticulata of the substantia nigra become hypointense to the cortical gray matter and white matter. At that age, the dentate nucleus has low signal intensity in only one-third of cases. With aging, the hypointensity is relatively constant in the red nucleus, substantia nigra, and dentate nucleus. However, the volume of hypointensity in the globus pallidus increases with aging. In the putamen, hypointensity is only found in the elderly population (older than 60 years of age), and may equal that in the globus pallidus in the eighth decade. In the healthy elderly, hypointensity on T2-weighted images is never found in the caudate nucleus and thalamus. Hypointensity in these structures in elderly suggests disease.

White Matter Hyperintensities

With age the prevalence of focal lesions in white matter increases. These lesions can be subdivided in dilated VRS, infarct-like lesions, and aspecific white matter lesions. VRS have been discussed earlier in this document, and are characterized by a signal intensity that follows that of CSF on all pulse sequences. Infarct-like lesions have been defined as focal, non-mass areas; they are hyperintense to gray matter on proton density-weighted and T2-weighted images and have signal intensities that approximate that of CSF on T1-weighted images. Aspecific white matter lesions are those non-mass lesions with high signal intensity on proton density-weighted-images and T2-weighted images that do not follow the previous definitions. With aging, the prevalence of all these lesions increases, however, in this section, the latter group is discussed. They will be referred to as white matter hyperintensities (WMH).

In most studies, WMH are subdivided in periventricular WMH and subcortical WMH. Postulated causes for WMH are subependymal gliosis and atrophic perivascular demyelination. The prevalence and severity of WMH increase with aging. The reported prevalence in the elderly varies, and depends among other things on the definition of WMH that is used. In the Cardiovascular Health Study, a prevalence of more than 60% was found in a population aged 65 years and older. WMH occur more frequently and more extensively in women than in men, and more white matter change occurs in black individuals than in non-blacks. Furthermore, WMH correlate with ventricular size but not with sulcal size, which suggests that ventricular size reflects white matter atrophy rather than cortical gray matter atrophy. Apart from age, elevated systolic blood pressure, diabetes mellitus, and aortic atherosclerosis have been identified as risk factors for WMH. WMH often are found in individuals who function normally, however in large populations, impaired cognitive and lower extremity functions are associated with WMH. Periventricular WMH are related to late-onset depression, whereas WMH in the deep white matter are associated with cognitive decline.

Abnormal Aging

Classifying the diseases that are discussed in this section is arbitrary. I chose to subdivide the diseases according to their most striking radiological feature: atrophy or WMH. The diseases that are listed in a given category do not only have the feature they are listed under, but may have other features too. Furthermore, in each description an effort is made to describe the difference with normal aging. However, making this difference may often not be possible, since changes due to normal aging and those that are the consequence of a disease may coexist, and also because several neurodegenerative disorders may coexist.

Atrophy

Disorders that are characterized by cerebral atrophy are often associated with dementia. Imaging serves three purposes in dementia: (1) provide criteria for the diagnosis, (2) stage disease severity in Alzheimer's disease (AD), and (3) monitor disease progression. The diagnostic role of imaging in dementia can again be subdivided into: (a) ruling out treatable disorders such as subdural hematoma, hydrocephalus, or intracranial tumor; and (b) providing information that suggests a diagnosis. In the appropriate clinical setting, imaging can contribute to the diagnosis of AD, frontotemporal dementia, vascular dementia, and sporadic and variant forms of Creutzfeldt-Jakob disease.

Alzheimer's Disease

Alzheimer's disease (AD) is the most common cause of dementia, affecting 60%-90% of the elderly with progressive memory loss. Symptoms in AD may occur in patients as young as 30-40 years of age. In such cases, AD often runs in the family and is based on the transmission of an autosomal dominant mutation in the amyloid precursor protein gene, the presenilin-1 or -2 gene. However, in more than 90% of cases, AD is sporadic and becomes symptomatic after age 65 years. Histologic findings in AD are diffuse cerebral atrophy, particularly affecting the gray matter, decreased synaptic density, neuron loss, and the presence of neuritic plaques and neurofibrillary tangles in the cortex. These changes begin in the transentorhinal area and spread gradually via the hippocampus, limbic areas in the medial temporal lobe, neocortical association areas to primary sensory and motor areas. On cross-sectional imaging, AD is characterized by supratentorial atrophy. Atrophy occurs diffusely, but particularly affects the temporal lobes. Manifestations of diffuse atrophy are enlarged sulci and widened lateral and third ventricles. In the temporal lobe, atrophy affects the entorhinal cortex and hippocampus in particular, and this is apparent on cross-sectional images as widening of the temporal horn of the lateral ventricle, the choroidal-hippocampal fissure, suprasellar cistern, and sylvian fissure. This may occur symmetrically, asymmetrically, or focally. Hippocampal and entorhinal atrophy is best defined on coronal images. WMH are frequently found in AD patients. However, in the absence of cardiovascular risk factors, WMH are not significantly more frequent in AD patients compared to normally aging individuals.

Although AD patients share several characteristics with normally aging individuals, on cross-sectional imaging there are several differences. As compared to normal elderly, general cerebral atrophy occurs earlier and increases faster in AD patients, and significantly more atrophy occurs in the entorhinal cortex and hippocampus.

Pick's Disease

Pick's disease is a much less common cause of dementia. Contrary to AD patients, memory functions are initially spared in patients with Pick's disease. However, these patients have prominent behavioral and personality changes. The age at onset is similar to that of AD. Histologically, Pick's disease is characterized by neuronal swelling, neuronal loss, atrophy and gliosis in the cortex and subcortical white matter. On cross-sectional imaging, the most striking characteristic of Pick's disease is severe focal atrophy, apparent as widened sulci with shriveled, sharp gyri and widening of the lateral ventricles. This characteristically occurs in the inferior frontal and anterior temporal lobes and in the frontoparietal region. These atrophic areas contrast sharply with the relatively normal posterior temporal lobe, occipital lobes, pre- and postcentral gyri, and parietal lobes. The left hemisphere is more frequently involved than the right. Atrophy may also be found in the caudate nucleus. On T2-weighted images, increased signal intensity may be found in the cortex and subcortical white matter of the affected areas.

Parkinson's Disease

Clinically, idiopathic Parkinson's disease is characterized by the presence of tremor, rigidity, akinesia, and postural difficulties. Parkinson's disease may coexist with AD. The histological hallmark of the disease is loss of dopaminergic cells and gliosis in the pars compacta of the substantia nigra. On cross-sectional imaging, Parkinson's disease is characterized by non-specific supratentorial atrophy, apparent as widening of sulci and ventricles. More subtle and specific changes that may occur in Parkinson's disease are: diminished width of the pars compacta, hyperintense foci on T2-weighted images in the substantia nigra, and an increase of the signal intensity of the dorsal lateral substantia nigra (which normally is hypointense on T2-weighted images) to isointensity to brain parenchyma without iron.

Huntington's Disease

Huntington's disease (HD) is an autosomal dominant disorder that gives rise to the clinical picture of choreoathetosis, rigidity, and dementia. The disease is expressed in young adulthood. Histologically, HD is characterized by neuronal loss, demyelination, gliosis, and iron accumulation in the striatum. On cross-sectional imaging, the most striking feature of HD is atrophy of the caudate nucleus and putamen. This is apparent as the loss of the usual bulge of the inferolateral borders of the frontal horns of the lateral ventricles. Coexisting abnormalities may be diffuse cerebral atrophy, and hyper- and hypointensity of the striatum on T2-weighted images.

Normal Pressure Hydrocephalus

Normal pressure hydrocephalus (NPH) is clinically characterized by a triad of gait apraxia, dementia, and urinary incontinence. NPH is uncommon under the age of 60 years, and increases in frequency thereafter. The etiology of NPH remains unclear. It has been suggested that inadequate absorption of CSF underlies the disease, but the hypothesis has also been put forward that NPH results primarily from periventricular white matter damage. Whatever the cause is, in a number of patients with NPH the clinical symptoms reverse with shunting, whereas the symptoms would progress without shunting. Since dementia is a horrible disorder, and since NPH is one of the few treatable causes of dementia, it is important to assess on brain scans of every single elderly patient whether NPH could be the underlying disease.

Making the diagnosis of NPH on cross-sectional images is a challenge. The most striking characteristic of NPH is atrophy. In these patients, both ventricles and sulci are widened. However, typically, there is a discrepancy in the amount of widening of the ventricles and that of the sulci, in that the ventricles are wider than would be expected from the caliber of the sulci if both phenomena would just be the consequence of general atrophy. In other words, dilatation of the ventricles is more striking than widening of the sulci. On sagittal MR images, uniform, smooth thinning and elevation of the corpus callosum and dilatation of the optic and infundibular recesses are apparent. Furthermore, there often is a smooth periventricular area of increased signal intensity on T2-weighted images, presumably due to increased transependymal migration of CSF. Lastly, a pronounced flow void may be seen in the aqueduct, due to increased CSF hydrodynamics.

White Matter Hyperintensities

Vascular Dementia

Vascular disease may be the cause of dementia in several ways. It may be due to multiple large vessel infarcts, a single "strategic" infarct, lacunar disease in the basal ganglia, and diffuse white matter disease, or leukoaraiosis.

Whether leukoaraiosis and Binswanger's disease (BD) are the same thing, and whether BD is a symptom or a disease, are still matters of debate. BD refers to a condition characterized by the presence of abnormalities of the white matter on cross-sectional imaging. These areas are hypodense on CT, have increased signal intensity on T2-weighted images, and sometimes have decreased signal intensity on T1-weighted images. Typically, these areas start in the periventricular white matter, and they may spread to the surface of the brain, with sparing of the subcortical U-fibers and cortex. This condition may be associated with widening of the ventricles and with the presence of lacunar disease. Histologically, incomplete infarction is found in the abnormal periventricular white matter areas. It has been suggested that BD is a small vessel disease. BD is found in asymptomatic individuals over 60 years of age as well as in cognitively impaired patients. Still, the extent of the lesions is associated with cognitive decline and gait problems. BD probably shares its pathogenesis with the periventricular changes that occur in normal aging. On cross-sectional images, BD differs from normal aging only by the extent of the white matter abnormalities.

Suggested Reading

Aoki S, Okada Y, Nishimura K et al (1989) Normal deposition of brain iron in childhood and adolescence: MR imaging at 1.5 T. Radiology 172:381-385

Bryan RN, Wells SW, Miller TJ et al (1997) Infarctlike lesions in the brain: prevalence and anatomic characteristics at MR imaging of the elderly - data from the Cardiovascular Health Study. Radiology 202:47-54

Caplan LR (1995) Binswanger's disease - revisited. Neurology 45:626-633

Drayer BP (1988) Imaging of the aging brain. Part I. Normal findings. Radiology 166:785-796

Drayer BP (1988) Imaging of the aging brain. Part II. Pathologic conditions. Radiology 166:797-806

Esiri MM, Hyman BT, Beyreuther K, Masters CL (1997) Ageing and dementia. In: Graham DI, Lantos PL (eds) Greenfield's neuropathology, vol. 2. Arnold, London, pp 153-233

Grossman RI, Yousem DM (2003) Neuroradiology – the requisites, 2nd edn. Mosby, St. Louis.

Guttmann CRG, Jolesz FA, Kikinis R et al (1998) White matter changes with normal aging. Neurology 50:972-978

Jack CR, Lexa FJ, Trojanowski JQ, Braffman BH, Atlas SW (2003) Normal aging, dementia, and neurodegenerative disease. In: Atlas SW (ed) Magnetic resonance imaging of the brain and spine, 3rd edn. Lippincott Williams Wilkins, Philadelphia, pp 1177-1240

Lechner H, Schmidt R, Fazekas F et al (1994) White matter lesions on magnetic resonance imaging in a healthy elderly population: correlations to vascular risk factors and carotid atherosclerosis. J Stroke Cerebrovasc Dis 4:224-228

Milton WJ, Atlas SW, Lexa FJ, Mozley PD, Gur RE (1991) Deep gray matter hypointensity patterns with aging in healthy adults: MR imaging at 1.5 T. Radiology 181:715-719

Nagata K, Basugi N, Fukushima T et al (1987) A quantitative study of physiological cerebral atrophy with aging: a statistical analysis of the normal range. Neuroradiology 29:327-332

Pantoni L, Garcia JH (1995) The significance of cerebral white matter abnormalities 100 years after Binswanger's report - a review. Stroke 26:1293-1301

Roman GC (1996) From UBOs to Binswanger's disease - impact of MRI on vascular dementia research. Stroke 27:1269-1273

Roman GC, Tatemichi TK, Erkinjuntti T et al (1993) Vascular dementia: diagnostic criteria for research studies. Report of the NINDS-AIREN International Workshop. Neurology 43:250-260

Rowe JW, Kahn RL (1987) Human aging: usual and successful. Science 237:143-149

Valk J, Barkhof F, Scheltens P (2002) Magnetic resonance in dementia. Springer, Berlin Heidelberg New York

Ylikoski A, Erkinjuntti T, Raininko R, Sarna S, Sulkava R, Tilvis R (1995) White matter hyperintensities on MRI in the neurologically nondiseased elderly - analysis of cohorts of consecutive subjects aged 55 to 85 years living at home. Stroke 26:1171-1177

Imaging the Effects of Systemic Metabolic Diseases on the Brain

M. Castillo

Department of Neuroradiology, University of North Carolina, Chapel Hill, NC, USA

Introduction

Brain function depends on a consistent supply of oxygen and glucose. Many systemic disorders that interfere with the metabolism of these two substances result in neurological dysfunction. The brain is commonly affected by disorders primarily involving the heart, liver, kidneys, blood, and endocrine organs. Most cardiac disorders result in ischemic brain damage and are not addressed here. The most common liver disorders to affect the brain are those resulting in acute and chronic hepatic failure. The central nervous system (CNS) is also affected by disorders of the metabolism of elemental substances such as salts and metals. The most common disorders in this category involve those related to copper, sodium, and iron metabolism. CNS injuries may also result from extraneous substances, either toxic or those used as medications. Substances toxic to the CNS include carbon monoxide, glycol, lead, methanol, mercury, and toluene. In this paper, I also address miscellaneous disorders including hypoglycemia, anorexia nervosa, chronic fatigue syndrome, porphyria and amyloidosis and their effects on the CNS. CNS disorders may also be associated with gastrointestinal disorders.

Liver Failure and Parenteral Nutrition

Hepatic insufficiency leads to abnormalities on magnetic resonance imaging (MRI) of the brain. T1-weighted images show increased signal in the caudate nucleus, tectum (particularly the inferior colliculi), globus pallidus, putamen, subthalamic nucleus, red nucleus, adenohypophysis, and substantia nigra. Abnormalities are bilateral, symmetrical, and of homogenous signal intensity. There no corresponding abnormalities on T2-weighted images, and computed tomography (CT) results are normal. MRI findings are due to increased amounts of manganese (Mn) and other factors leading to shortening of relaxation time. Increased plasma levels of Mn are found in patients with chronic liver failure and occupational toxicity, and in those receiving long-term parenteral nutrition.

Approximately 95% of Mn is excreted in bile. Mn is involved in enzymatic cycles involving superoxide dismutase and glutamine synthetase. Mn reaches the brain by way of erythrocytes and plasma. Transferrin and albumin are its carriers in plasma. The half-life of blood Mn is 10-42 days but when it reaches the brain it may remain there for prolonged periods of time. Astrocytes have specific transport systems for Mn. Mn is neurotoxic and results in striatal dopamine depletion, NMDA excitotoxicity, and oxidative stress. Mn plays a role in development of hepatic encephalopathy, clinically characterized by pyramidal and extrapyramidal dysfunctions, brisk tendon reflexes, and tremors. The concentration of Mn in the pallidus of cirrhotic patients is 3-fold higher compared to controls. The frequency of MRI abnormalities in cirrhotic patients is about 73%.

Alper's syndrome is a rare childhood disorder characterized by progressive neuronal degeneration with liver disease. These patients develop seizures and liver failure. There is necrosis of deep gray nuclei and cortex. MRI shows high T2 signal in basal ganglia and thalamus. There is atrophy and high T2 signal in the cortex, predominantly occipital. The abnormalities are bilateral and asymmetrical. The abnormalities may reflect mitochondrial dysfunction.

Long-term total parenteral nutrition results in high T1 signal in the same regions. These solutions are rich in Mn and produce neurological symptoms. Once the parenteral nutrition is discontinued, the MRI abnormalities reverse to normal. The amount of time required for these abnormalities to resolve is not clear but most do one year after cessation of parenteral nutrition. In one case, T1 hyperintensity developed in the adenohypophysis and dorsal brain stem 3 months after total parenteral nutrition and reverted to normal 4 months after treatment. Similar findings have been noted in patients following liver transplantation. Although the clinical and imaging abnormalities are reversible in adults, its effects on the child's brain are not known. Repeated episodes of hepatic failure lead to the development of acquired (non-wilsonian) hepatocerebral degeneration. The clinical symptoms are permanent and death follows. By MRI, these patients do not show T1 hyperintensities in basal ganglia as described previously for chronic hepatic encephalopathy. Patients with acquired hepatocerebral degeneration show high T2 signal in the middle cerebral peduncles. These zones correspond to spongiform myelinolytic changes.

Bilirubin Encephalopathy

Kernicterus is now a rare disorder. Most cases result from isoimmunization to Rh factor or from ABO blood group incompatibility. It is almost always a disease of neonates. Later in life, most cases are due to genetic hematologic or liver diseases (e.g. defects of glucose-6-phosphate dehydrogenase, Crigler-Najjar disease, Gilbert's disease) or are secondary to breast-feeding or severe sepsis. In kernicterus, the liver is unable to conjugate bilirubin. The enzyme uridine-diphosphate glucoronyl transferase does not function well and albumin-bound (insoluble) bilirubin cannot be deconjugated into bilirubin diglucoronide or "water soluble" bilirubin. Initially there is hypotonia, then hypertonia and after one week, hypotonia returns. There is yellow staining of the globi pallidi, mamillary bodies, subthalamic nuclei, and indusium griseum. In the brain stem, the substantia nigra and cranial nerve nuclei are involved. In the chronic stage, there is high T2 signal in the globi pallidi and cerebellar dentate nuclei. These structures are atrophic. Acutely, there is high T1 signal in basal ganglia without corresponding abnormalities on T2-weighted images. This finding is probably related to acute hepatic insufficiency.

Wilson's Disease

Wilson's disease (WD) is a genetic disorder of copper metabolism characterized by failure to incorporate copper into ceruloplasmin in the liver, failure to excrete copper by the liver into bile, and accumulation of copper. Its defect is mapped to chromosome 13. Most children present with hepatic failure and adults present with neurological symptoms. Accumulation of copper within Descemet's membrane results in Kayser-Fleischer rings. Copper in the lens results in "sunflower" cataracts. There is cell loss and cavitation in the lentiform nucleus. Other regions involved include thalami, subthalami, red nuclei, substantia nigra, dentate nuclei and brain stem. These regions contain large cells with small nuclei (termed Opalski cells) which are typical of WD. MRI shows abnormalities even in absence of symptoms. Paramagnetic effects of copper are visible by MRI in untreated patients. Basal ganglia lesions are bilateral and symmetrical. The putamina show high T2 signal. Thalamic involvement spares the dorsomedial nuclei. The dentatothalamic, corticospinal and pontocerebellar tracts are involved. The claustrum shows high T2 signal.

The midbrain is T2 bright with relative sparing of its deep nuclei (Panda sign). The high copper concentrations are not responsible for the MRI findings. Copper results in T1 and T2 shortening, thus the MRI findings are probably due to spongy degeneration, cavitation, neuronal loss and gliosis. The abnormal striatum correlates with pseudoparkinsonism, an abnormal dentatothalamic tract with cerebellar signs and an abnormal pontocerebellar tract with pseudoparkinsonism. The presence of portosystemic shunting correlates with abnormalities seen in the globi pallidi. The abnormal T2 signal improves after copper-trapping therapy. Contrast enhancement is rare but may be seen when patients receive treatment with penicillamine.

Carbon Monoxide

Carbon monoxide (CO) results in nearly 6000 accidental and suicidal deaths in the US. Common causes of high CO levels are burning of gasoline, kerosene, wood, coal and propane. Individuals working in enclosed spaces are prone to acute CO intoxication ("warehouse workers headache"). Hemoglobin has 200- to 250-times more affinity for CO than for carbon dioxide. CO affects the cytochrome oxidase system, impairs release of oxygen in tissues and results in lipid peroxidation. Symptoms occur early, but their severity has no correlation with blood levels of CO. Early symptoms include headache, impaired vigilance and abnormal audition and vision. Severe symptoms are nausea, vomiting, seizures, syncope, coma and death. Classic findings, such as "cherry red" mucosa, are rare.

CO has two effects in the brain. First, it binds to regions having high oxygen demand such as the globi pallidi. Second, CO binds to normal iron-containing structures such as the substantia nigra. Systemic hypotension contributes to brain lesions. MRI and CT show lesions mostly in the globi pallidi. The lesions are of low density and high T2 signal and contain no hemorrhage.

Glycol-related Products

Ethylene glycol found in automobile antifreeze, hydraulic fluid and industrial solvents is a common cause of poisoning and suicide. Diethylene glycol and propylene glycol are also toxic and are used to contaminate medications such as acetaminophen. After the ingestion of ethylene glycol, metabolic acidosis ensues and results in kidney damage due to accumulation of calcium and oxalate crystals in urine. Blindness is typical of ethylene glycol poisoning. MRI shows high T2 signal in the putamina, globi pallidi, caudate nuclei and thalami. Symptoms of intoxication with diethylene glycol and propylene glycol include fever, vomiting, diarrhea, cough, abdominal pain, altered mentation, dyspnea and acute renal failure.

Lead

Acute lead (Pb) poisoning is rare. Most lead poisoning occurs in children due to ingestion of peeling paint chips. Since 1978, lead-based paint has not been used in the United States. Acute lead poisoning results in encephalopathy and cerebral edema. Gross examination of the brain shows congestion, petechial hemorrhages, thrombosis and demyelination. In adults, most lead poisoning is chronic. Chronic lead intoxication is a consequence of gasoline sniffing, inhalation of automobile exhaust fumes, lead smelting, consumption of "moonshine" whiskey, battery manufacturing and lead glazing of pottery. Chronic exposure to lead results in intracranial calcifications particularly in the cerebellum. These calcifications are dystrophic and due to vascular damage. CT shows widening of cranial sutures in cases of chronic lead poisoning and hypodensity in the subinsular regions, or may be normal.

Methanol

Methanol (methyl alcohol) is used for production of antifreeze solution, illegal drinks and poor-quality cologne. After ingestion of methanol, there is a latent period varying from 1 to 72 hours. Thereafter, metabolic acidosis and cortical blindness ensue. Other symptoms are parkinsonism, inebriation, headache, dizziness, seizures and coma. Methanol and its byproducts (formaldehyde and formic acid) are toxic to the CNS. Putaminal hemorrhagic necrosis is typical. The putamina are swollen, of low density, and contain small hemorrhages. MRI shows these regions to have either low or high T1 signal and hyperintensity on T2-weighted images. Other patients also show cortical necrosis particularly in the paramedian frontal lobes reflected by high T2 signal. Optic atrophy is seen but the signal in these structures remains normal. The white matter may be edematous.

Mercury

Mercury (Hg) poisoning is rare and occurs after the ingestion of organic or inorganic mercury. Organic mercury intoxication results from eating contaminated fish or pork (due to used of Hg-based fungicides). Symptoms include ataxia, neuropathy, choreoathetosis, visual loss, confusion and coma. Chronic ingestion of Hg-laden fish, first described in Japan (Minamata disease), is now being found in other parts of the world. MRI shows atrophy of the calcarine and post-central cortices and cerebellar vermis. These areas are slightly hypointense on T1-weighted images and of high T2 signal. These findings reflect spongiosis and are correlated with visual field deficits, sensory abnormalities and ataxia.

Inhalant Abuse

Inhaling solvents, volatile substances and glue vapors induces a transient euphoric state. Inhalant abuse occurs in teenagers. Fumes are inhaled directly or by placing the substance in a bag or on a rag. After an initial euphoric state, drowsiness and sleep ensue. These compounds have a great affinity for the lipid-laden brain. Suffocation, aspiration and dangerous behavior are causes of death in subjects who use inhalants.

Chronic abuse of toluene results in cognitive impairment, cerebellar ataxia, tremor, and anosmia. MRI shows cerebral, cerebellar and brain stem atrophy. T2-weighted images show abnormal high signal in white matter due to gliosis. Hypointensity in basal ganglia and thalami is the result of iron deposition. Other MRI findings in toluene abuse are loss of cerebral and cerebellar gray-white matter discrimination, scattered foci of abnormal signal in white matter, a thin corpus callosum and atrophy.

Disorders of Ethanol Abuse

Chronic alcohol consumption results in ataxia and lower limb inco-ordination due to cerebellar atrophy. Cerebellar atrophy is present in over 60% of alcoholics. There is shrinkage of folia particularly in the superior vermis reflecting loss of Purkinje cells. Alcoholic myelopathy and peripheral neuropathy are related to deficiency of thiamine. Acute symptoms of Wernicke-Korsakoff (WK) syndrome include lethargy, confusion, altered memory, nystagmus, ophthalmoplegia and ataxia. WK syndrome is mostly seen in alcoholics but may be due to anorexia, protracted vomiting, digitalis toxicity, gastric plication, starvation and acquired immune deficiency syndrome (AIDS).

A common underlying factor in all these conditions is thiamine (vitamin B1) deficiency. B1 metabolism plays roles in brain glucose oxidation and membrane permeability. After treatment, patients develop chronic memory problems (Korsakoff's psychosis). Glutamate is found in high concentrations in B1-depleted brains. Cerebral lactic acidosis occurs early. Acutely there is vascular dilatation and endothelial swelling involving small arteries followed by neuronal damage and astrocytoma swelling. This leads to ischemia of the mamillary bodies, the dorsomedial thalamic nuclei, pulvinars, walls of the third ventricle, periaqueductal gray matter, colliculi, third cranial nerve nuclei, inferior olives and superior cerebellar vermis. On T2-weighted images, these regions show high signal intensity. Contrast enhancement of the mamillary bodies is pathognomonic of this condition. Hemorrhage is found in 20% of cases. In chronic stages, there is brain atrophy more prominent in the fornices and mamillary bodies.

Marchiafava-Bignami (MB) disease is seen mostly in chronic alcoholics. It was initially described in drinkers of Italian red wine but may be seen in persons ingesting other types of alcoholic beverages. There is cystic necrosis of the corpus callosum, particularly the genu and body. Similar lesions are seen in the optic chiasm, anterior commissure, centrum semiovale and brachium pontis. There is demyelination with axonal preservation. MRI shows the anterior corpus callosum to be of low T1 signal and high T2 signal. Areas of high T2 signal are also seen in the centrum semiovale.

Alcohol is most common teratogenic agent to which human beings are exposed. The fetal-alcohol syndrome (FAS) was first described in the United States and in France but is now prevalent in other countries such as Russia. It is clinically characterized by mental retardation, anomalies of the CNS, dysmorphic facial features, and skeletal, cardiac, and urogenital abnormalities. Unfortunately, the mental deficits are permanent and do not improve with age. The most common brain abnormalities observed in FAS are microcephaly, dysgenesis (and agenesis) of the corpus callosum, dysgenesis of the cerebellum and the brain stem, occipital meningoencephalocele, myelomeningocele, and holoprosencephaly. Facial anomalies include thin lips, small mandible and maxilla, and cleft lip and palate. Alcohol or its metabolites have adverse effects in the gastrulation stage of embryonic development by causing a reduction in the number of cells in the early neural plate and increased cell death (apoptosis) at the margins of the anterior neural folds. This mechanism explains the coexistence of brain and facial anomalies in FAS. Other common teratogens include carbamazepine, valproic acid, retinoin, phenytoin, toluene, trimethadione, warfarin, cocaine, and probably benzodiazepine.

Sodium (Na) imbalance results in a diffuse injury (hyponatremic encephalopathy) or focal lesions (osmotic myelinolysis). Hyponatremia results from excess water and urinary loss of Na cations. Abnormal secretion of antidiuretic hormone (ADH) results in hypervolemia. When plasma osmolality falls, cellular equilibrium is maintained by excretion of intracellular solutes and dilution of the intracellular compartment by influx of water into cells. Cellular damage occurs as a consequence of water influx. In acute hyponatremic encephalopathy, death results from swelling and herniation. Most patients with hyponatremic encephalopathy have one or more of the following conditions: postoperative state, polydipsia-hyponatremia syndrome, congestive heart failure and AIDS. In addition to damage induced by low Na, most patients are hypoxic.

A common demyelinating lesion associated with correction of hyponatremia is central pontine myelinolysis (CPM). Conditions leading to CPM are alcoholism, extensive burns, sepsis, Hodgkin's disease and other tumors. Myelinolysis is not the sequela of hyponatremia but is secondary to its correction. Rapid correction of hyponatremia increases the risk of developing myelinolysis. CPM ensues 2-3 days after a hyponatremic event. Over 85% of patients suspected to have CPM show no imaging abnormalities. Microscopically, CPM consists

in destruction of myelin and relative preservation of axons. The lesion is symmetrical and located in basis pontis. The cerebellar cortex is also affected. About 10% of patients with CPM have other lesions, mostly supratentorial. Myelinolysis often involves the deep gray structures. The thalamus is affected but the cortex and subcortical regions may also be involved. CPM has low T1 signal and high T2 signal. On axial views, the lesion is round or triangular. On coronal views, it has a "Batman" sign configuration. Contrast enhancement is rare. Prognosis is variable: some patients die while others survive. Survivors may improve slowly or not at all.

Hallervorden-Spatz Disease

This disease is related to iron (Fe) overload and degeneration. Little is known about the biochemical abnormalities of Hallervorden-Spatz (HS) disease, although it is linked to an abnormality on chromosome 20p12.3-p13. Iron is deposited in the globi pallidi and pars reticulata of the substantia nigra. Iron deposition leads to axonal swelling and decreased myelin content and production. Microscopy demonstrates abnormal, spherical bodies containing superoxide dismutase. Eventually, these regions are destroyed. Patients demonstrate dystonia, muscle rigidity, hyperreflexia and choreoathetosis. Mental retardation is variable and death occurs 1-2 years after diagnosis. Initially, MRI shows T2 hypointensity in the globi pallidi. When gliosis ensues, the globi pallidi become bright on T2-weighted images and surrounded by hypointensity. This is the "eye of the tiger" sign.

Hypoglycemia and Hyperglycemia

Most cerebral insults due to hypoglycemia occur in young children. Oxygen and glucose are major substrates needed for normal brain metabolism, and absence of either leads to significant injury. The neonatal brain is fairly resistant to hypoglycemia. Acute symptoms of hypoglycemia are jitteriness, seizures and vomiting. Hypoglycemia is diagnosed when whole blood glucose concentration falls below 20 mg/dl in preterm babies, 30 mg/dl in term babies and 45 mg/dl in adults. Sequelae of hypoglycemia are mental retardation, spasticity, visual abnormalities and microcephaly. In neonates, hypoglycemia leads to edema and infarctions. The occipital regions are affected more severely but the basal ganglia are also involved. Chronically, the occipital cortex becomes thin, malacia develops and these findings correlate with visual abnormalities. In adults, hypoglycemia also induces occipital infarctions in addition to infarctions elsewhere (which are generally multiple) and laminar necrosis.

Hyperglycemia may increase cerebral lactic acid and damage the brain primarily or worsen the outcome of patients with underlying infarctions. A typical manifestation is hemichorea-hemiballismus (HH). Symptoms of HH are random and fast jerking motions in the distal extremities (chorea) and violent flinging and kicking mainly in the proximal joints (ballismus). CT shows high density in one lentiform nucleus and head of the ipsilateral caudate nucleus. These regions are of high T1 signal while T2-weighted images are normal. Occasionally, the ipsilateral cerebral peduncle may show T1 hyperintensity in its anteromedial region. Findings are thought to be due to the presence of gemistocytes.

Neuroradiological Diagnosis of Craniocerebral and Spinal Trauma: Current Concepts

P.M. Parizel[1], C.D. Phillips[2]

[1] Department of Radiology, University of Antwerp, Antwerp, Belgium

[2] Department of Radiology, University of Virginia Health System, Charlottesville, VA, USA

Imaging Techniques

Traditionally, X-ray films of the skull have been used to detect skull fractures, intracranial mass effect ("pineal shift"), air-fluid levels and foreign objects (e.g. metal, glass, projectile fragments). However, the diagnostic yield of plain X-ray films is low because there is poor correlation between skull fractures and intracranial injury. When computed tomography is available, plain skull films contribute little or no additional information in the clinical management of the acute trauma patient.

Computed tomography (CT) is the initial imaging study of choice in acute craniocerebral trauma. It is a rapid and accurate technique. The availability of CT has dramatically improved the survival of patients with epidural and subdural hematomas. Critically injured patients can be monitored within the scanner with relative ease. CT is used for the detection of:

- Hemorrhage (intra-axial and extra-axial, including subarachnoid blood),
- Mass effect, edema and brain herniations,
- Fractures and displaced bone fragments (using bone window settings), and
- Foreign bodies.

The CT examination should start with a lateral scout image, which can be used as a digital radiograph to detect fractures. The non-contrast scan is performed with contiguous axial sections (slice thickness, 5 mm) from the base of the skull to the vertex; alternatively, a spiral technique can be used. CT images of the head should be obtained using 3 window settings:

- Brain parenchyma window (level, 40 HU; width, 80-120 HU);
- Bone window (level, 500 HU; width, 2000-4000 HU); recalculation of raw image data with a bone or edge algorithm is useful;
- Subdural window (level, 70-100 HU; width, 150-300 HU) for the detection of a thin layer of blood against the dense calvarium.

If the patient is clinically unstable or rapidly deteriorating, the CT procedure needs to be foreshortened (e.g. single mid-ventricular image). When fractures of the temporal bone, orbit, or maxillofacial structures are suspected, additional thin slices in different orientations should be obtained. Spiral CT with coronal reformatting can be used as an alternative to direct coronal views when the patient cannot tolerate hyperextension of the neck. Multidetector CT (MDCT) is now used in major trauma centers for rapid screening of the skull, spine, and their contents. The MDCT data set can be used for high-resolution three-dimensional (3D) surface reconstructions (Fig. 1).

Magnetic resonance imaging (MRI) is the preferred technique in the evaluation of subacute and chronic brain injury. MRI has the highest sensitivity for parenchymal lesion detection, and is especially useful in evaluating lesions in the

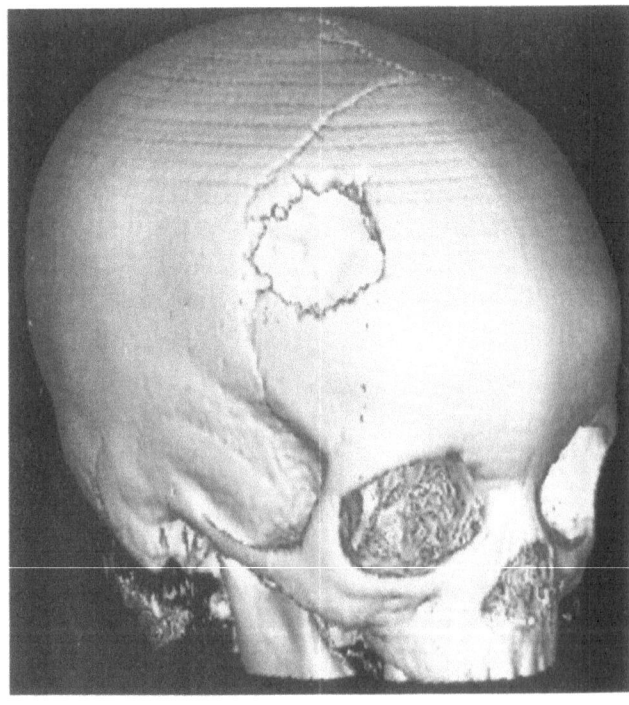

Fig. 1. Depressed skull fracture. Surface shaded display (SSD), obtained from a 3D multidetector CT data set, reveals the irregular, jagged edges of a right frontal depressed skull fracture

posterior fossa or near the skull base (difficult to see on CT due to beam hardening artifacts), diffuse axonal injury due to shearing stresses, and cortical contusions. Important limitations include the relative insensitivity for the detection of subarachnoid hemorrhage, cortical bone injury and small bone fragments. Our standard imaging protocol consists of:

1. Axial fast spin echo (FSE) T2-weighted imaging;
2. Axial fluid attenuated inversion recovery (FLAIR) T2-weighted imaging for the detection of gliosis and encephalomalacia;
3. Axial or coronal gradient echo fast low angle shot (FLASH) imaging with dual echo times (TE, 15 and 35 ms) for the detection of hemorrhagic foci (e.g. in diffuse axonal injury);
4. Sagittal spin echo (SE) or gradient echo T1-weighted imaging for the detection of cortical contusions or post-traumatic encephalomalacia in the anterior and inferior parts of the frontal lobes, and in the anterior temporal lobes;
5. Diffusion-weighted echo planar imaging (EPI) in the acute phase.

Scalp and Skull Lesions

Scalp and skull lesions are commonly observed in head trauma. *Scalp lacerations* occur when the scalp is crushed and split against the underlying bone. These lesions heal well because of the generous blood supply (this also explains why scalp wounds bleed profusely). Scalp wounds must be carefully examined to exclude foreign bodies or depressed bone fragments. CT is the preferred imaging technique for showing soft tissue swelling of the scalp. When the integrity of the skin is disrupted, a scalp hematoma may contain small amounts of air. CT shows not only the scalp lesions, but also the associated osseous and intracranial abnormalities. Multidetector CT allows rapid visualization of the entire cranium, with 3D rendering of the skull bones (Fig. 1).

Caput succedaneum, subgaleal hematoma, subgaleal hygroma, and cephalohematoma are commonly confused (Fig. 2). Table 1 provides a comparative summary of the distinct features of these entities.

Maxillofacial Injuries

Maxillofacial injuries are not uncommon accompaniments to central nervous system (CNS) trauma. The facial skeleton is commonly injured during head trauma. Head trauma may result in intracranial injuries which are often the critical injuries in the immediate trauma setting. However, major facial trauma may be a serious cause of morbidity and mortality. Respiratory problems may accompany major facial trauma. Major morbidity in this patient group may result from facial injuries in the subacute period. The injuries which lead to considerable patient morbidity include: orbital trauma; central skull base and temporal bone fractures, with resulting injury to a number of cranial nerves,

vascular structures and adjacent soft tissue structures; and obvious deformity and loss of function.

The era of fast CT with multidetector units has led to a significant alteration in the acute imaging of patients with maxillofacial injuries. Quite simply, the rapidity of CT – with thin sections and multiplanar reconstruction (MPR)

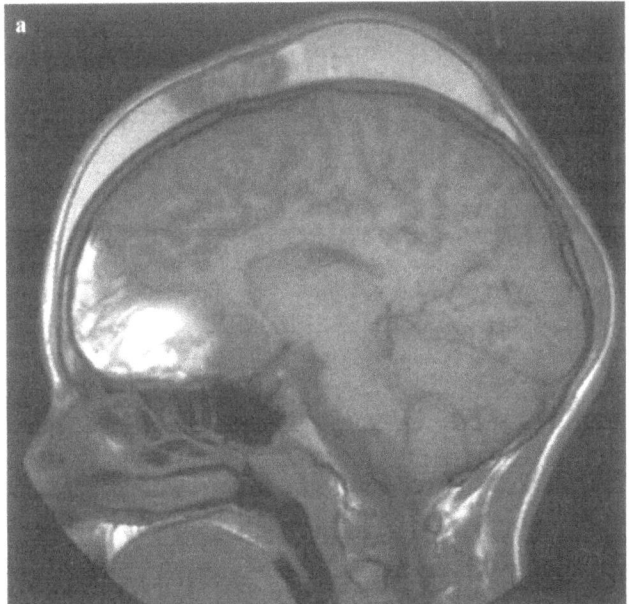

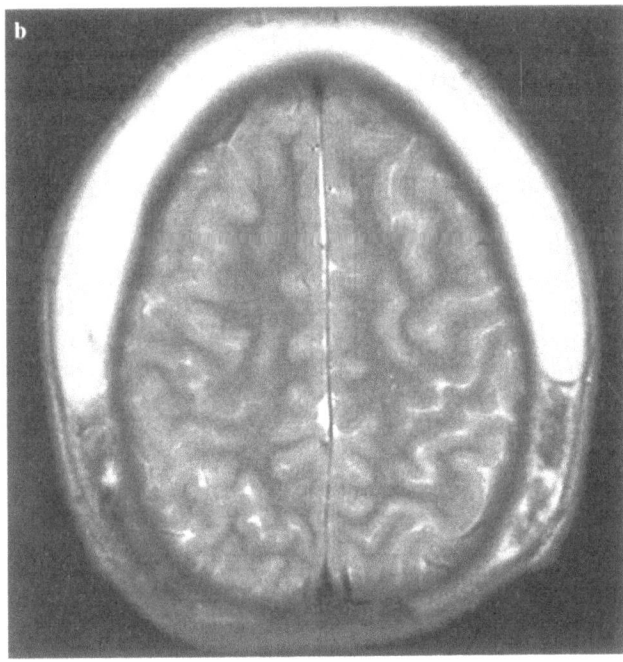

Fig. 2a, b. *Hemorrhagic cerebral contusions and subgaleal hematoma in a 13-year-old boy injured in a motor vehicle accident.* **a** Sagittal SE T1-weighted image. **b** Axial TSE T2-weighted image. Intracranially, there are hemorrhagic cerebral contusions in the right frontal and anterior temporal lobes. Extracranially, there is marked bilateral swelling of the subcutaneous soft tissues due to a massive subgaleal hematoma which extends from the frontal to the posterior parietal region

Table 1. Overview of scalp lesions

	Caput succedaneum	Subgaleal hematoma[a]	Subgaleal hygroma	Cephalohematoma[b]
Occurrence	Normal vaginal delivery	Head trauma (or after birth)	Birth trauma (forceps delivery)	Birth trauma (skull fracture during birth)
Location	Above of the galea aponeurotica	Beneath the galea aponeurotica	Beneath the galea aponeurotica	Subperiosteal (flat flat skull skull bones)
Composition	Edema (with with microscopic hemorrhages)	Venous blood	Cerebrospinal fluid	Subperiosteal hemorrhage
Clinical presentation	Pitting edema	Diffusely spreading, firm, fluctuating mass	Fluctuating collection	Well defined, focal, firm mass
Skull fracture	No ·	Yes or no	Yes	Yes
Crosses suture lines?	Yes	Yes	Yes	No

[a] Extracranial subdural hematoma
[b] Extracranial epidural hematoma

that rival the quality of directly acquired images in the sagittal and coronal planes – has led many services to perform the entire evaluation of a trauma patient (CNS, abdomen, pelvis, spine, and the detailed evaluation of facial trauma) in one setting. We have adopted a series of trauma protocols for patient evaluation, which simplifies the technologists' plan for imaging in this patient group. The initial exam is unenhanced CT of the brain, with the scan simply begun at the level of the midface or mandible (depending on the injuries noted), followed quickly by the requested trauma abdominal, chest, or pelvic examination as required by the trauma service. In the setting of major trauma, the examination then addresses the cervical spine or other affected spinal segments. Cervical spine CT may accompany the initial head and face CT exam. When the patient has significant injuries and there is minimal time to spend in the CT suite, it is possible to obtain good quality examinations of the lumbar or thoracic spine from reformatted data from the abdominal, chest, or pelvic CT study.

We prefer to initially categorize injuries to the facial skeleton by the presence or absence of involvement of the pterygoid plates. Fracture of the pterygoid plates results in dissociation of the facial skeleton and the skull. These fractures were first examined in detail by the French surgeon LeFort. His rather gruesome investigation involved blunt trauma to the midface of cadavers, with subsequent investigation of the patterns of fracture. LeFort categorized three different levels of fracture, a system still utilized to large extent to this day. LeFort I injuries result in a "floating palate", with the fracture plane below the level of the orbital rim, which allows mobility of the inferior maxilla in relation to the remainder of the midface. LeFort II injuries result in dissociation of the palate and the inferior orbital rim on the involved side. The fracture involves the medial and lateral maxilla but will permit displacement of the inferior orbital rim if traction is applied to the palate. LeFort III fractures result in dissociation of the entire midface in relation to the skull, and the superior fracture plane involves the root of the nasal bone. We have found that axial, coronal, and particularly sagittal CT images allow excellent assessment of these

fractures. There are other fairly common patterns of facial injury, easily characterized by CT examination. The "tripod", or trimalar fracture (Fig. 3) accompanies an angular

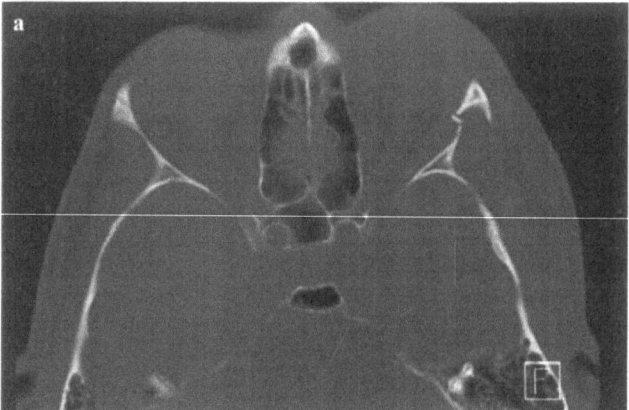

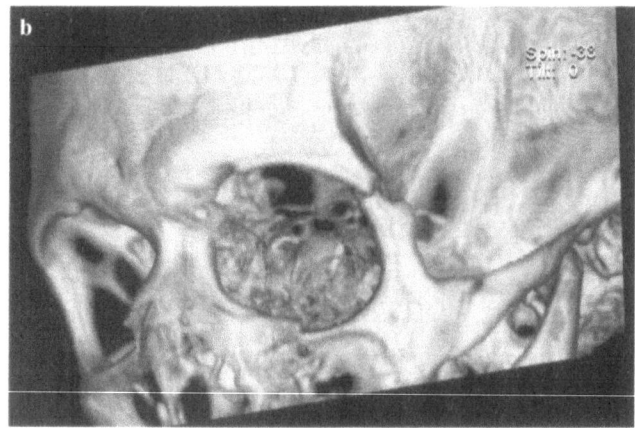

Fig. 3a, b. *Tripod fracture.* **a** Axial CT slice through the orbits. **b** Surface shaded display (SSD), obtained from a 3D multidetector CT data set. These images reveal the typical features of a left-sided tripod injury: there are fractures of the zygomatic arch, the anterior wall of the maxilla, and the posterolateral wall of the maxilla. This type of injury is caused by an angular blow to the midface, typically in proximity to the zygomaticomaxillary suture

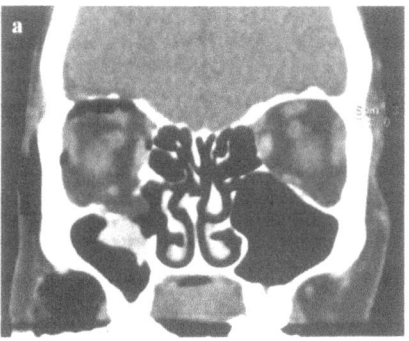 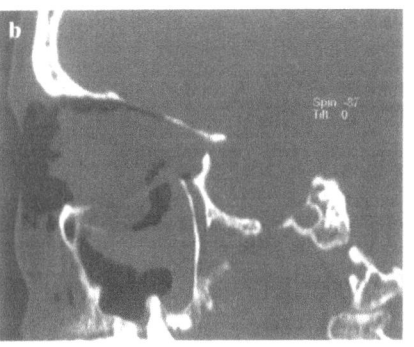 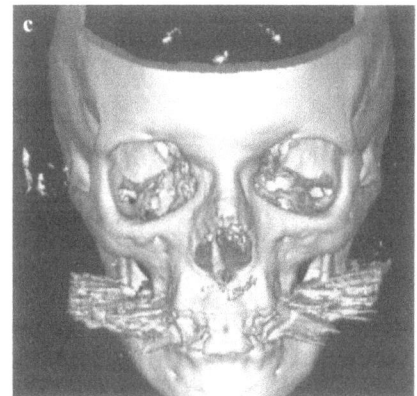

Fig. 4a-c. *Blow-out fracture of the right orbital floor.* **a** Coronal multidetector CT reformatted image, soft tissue window. **b** Sagittal multidetector CT reformatted image, bone window. **c** SSD display. The right orbital floor is fractured with displacement of small bone fragments and intraorbital fat into the maxillary sinus. The orbital rim is intact (c). The maxillary sinus is partially opacified (hematoma). There is orbital emphysema

blow to the midface, typically in proximity to the zygomaticomaxillary suture. The injury results in fractures of the zygomatic arch, the anterior wall of the maxilla, and the posterolateral wall of the maxilla. Isolated orbit fractures (Fig. 4), fractures of the orbital rims, nasal bones, zygomatic arch, maxillary and mandibular alveoli, and mandible may be seen. There is also wide acceptance of the value of 3D images in the review of these injuries. The ease with which these exams can be post-processed has led to an increased utilization in the acute trauma setting. We now routinely produce these images for our trauma service. They likely provide little new data, but the ability to see the entirety of the injury in few images is useful to surgeons, and of considerable importance when considering reconstruction.

Investigation of facial fractures should include careful review of the important skull base foramina, and of the soft tissue structures of the midface. A careful review of the soft tissue windows of the midfacial structures should always be performed. Evaluation of the orbital soft tissues is critical with injury in this region (Fig. 4). Particular attention should be paid to the carotid canal and optic canal. Involvement of either of these foramina may lead to surgical management or to additional investigations.

Temporal bone fractures are beyond the scope of this review, but can be divided into longitudinal or transverse fractures, depending upon the fracture orientation in relation to the axis of the temporal bone. Many of these fractures are complex, with orientation in both the longitudinal and transverse planes. Longitudinal fractures are more commonly associated with ossicular involvement and hearing loss, and transverse fractures are more commonly associated with facial nerve injury. There is considerable overlap, however. Previously, with single-slice CT units, questionable involvement of the skull base led to re-scanning this region with thin slices, and with a larger cumulative dose to the patient. In the era of MDCT, often the initial data set can be reformatted to permit a thorough evaluation of the temporal bone. Whenever the question is raised as to the possibility of temporal bone fracture, it is inherent in our responsibility to ensure that the examination is adequate to answer the question.

Severely injured patients with facial fractures may undergo MRI for other injuries, but review of the soft tissues of the face is rarely a concern that requires dedicated MRI. Injuries of the orbit, notably the question of involvement of the optic nerve, may on occasion necessitate MRI.

Intracranial Hypertension and Cerebral Herniation

Severe brain swelling or large intracranial mass lesions (e.g. hemorrhage) cause displacement of brain tissue. The cranial cavity is divided into anatomic compartments by combination of bony ridges and dural septa (falx cerebri and tentorium cerebelli). The three major compartments contain: (1) the right cerebral hemisphere, (2) the left cerebral hemisphere, and (3) the posterior fossa structures. The falx and the tentorium protect the brain against excessive motion but also limit the amount of compensatory shift and displacement that develops in response to increased intracranial pressure (ICP). When the pressure in one of the dural compartments increases beyond the physiological compensatory mechanisms, *increased ICP* or *intracranial hypertension* occurs and a pressure gradient ensues. This leads to a displacement of brain, cerebrospinal fluid (CSF) and blood vessels from one cranial compartment to another and a *cerebral herniation* follows.

Cerebral herniations are the most common secondary effects of an expanding intracranial mass. They can be due to an intra-axial process (e.g. intracerebral contusion or hematoma, edema, tumor) or an extra-axial mass (e.g. epidural or subdural hematoma). The subarachnoid spaces and basal cisterns become obliterated, hydrocephalus develops, vascular compression results in brain ischemia, and compression on vital brain tissue causes profound neurological deficits. Therefore, early detection of brain herniation can be of major clinical importance in patient management. Six types of brain herniation can be distinguished (Table 2).

Table 2. Cerebral herniation types

	Cerebral herniation					
	Subfalcial (cingulate)	Tonsillar	Descending transtentorial	Ascending transtentorial	Uncal	External
Definition	Medial displacement of cingulate gyrus under inferior free margin of the falx	Inferior displacement of cerebellar tonsil(s) through foramen magnum	Downward shift of diencephalon, mesencephalon and upper brain stem	Superior displacement of the vermis through the tentorial incisura	Herniation of medial temporal lobe through tentorial notch	Brain tissue extrudes externally through a skull defect
Cause	Supratentorial mass (e.g. EDH, SDH, hemispheric mass lesion)	Posterior fossa mass lesions or supratentorial mass effect	Increasing supratentorial mass effect	Posterior fossa mass lesion (tumor)	Temporal lobe mass lesion, e.g. focal focal hematoma	Increased ICP in association with a traumatic or surgical skull defect
Imaging	• Mass lesion • Bowing of falx • Compression of ipsilateral lateral ventricle • Contralateral ventricle enlarges due to obstruction of the foramen of Monro	• Downward displacement of cerebellar tonsils below level of foramen magnum • Obliteration of cisterna magna	• Obliteration of perimesencephalic cisterns with complete plugging of tentorial incisurea • Downward shift of pineal calcification • Brain stem is foreshortened (sagittal plane) and compressed (axial plane)	• Fourth ventricle becomes obliterated • Effacement of the superior cerebellar and quadrigeminal cisterns	• Obliteration of the suprasellar cistern • Shift of mesencephalon to opposite side • Widening of ipsilateral CPA cistern • Obstructive hydrocephalus (due to aqueductal obstruction)	• Extracranial displacement of brain tissue • Bone defect can be observed on CT
Compression of vascular structures	ACA infarction (pericallosal and callosomarginal arteries)	PICA infarction	PCA compression leads to occipital lobe ischemia or infarction	SCA compression may result in cerebellar infarction	Compression of the contralateral PCA against the tentorial edge	Venous obstruction may result in venous infarction (propensity to hemorrhage)
Other complications	Intracranial hypertension may cause descending transtentorial herniation	Hydrocephalus and syringomyelia	Duret's brain stem hemorrhage (disruption of perforating arteries to brain stem)	Hydrocephalus due to compression of the aqueduct	• Can progress to descending transtentorial herniation • Obstructive hydrocephalus	Pressure necrosis with swelling of the adjacent brain at the margins of the defect

EDH, epidural hematoma; *SDH*, subdural hematoma; *ICP*, intracranial pressure; *CPA*, cerebellopontine angle; *ACA*, anterior cerebral artery; *PICA*, posterior inferior cerebellar artery; *PCA*, posterior cerebral artery; *SCA*, superior cerebellar artery

Extra-axial Lesions

Four types of extra-axial hemorrhage can be considered: epidural, subdural, subarachnoid, and intraventricular hemorrhage.

Epidural hematoma (EDH) and subdural hematoma (SDH) are discussed in Table 3. Typical examples are illustrated in Figs. 5 and 6.

Traumatic Subarachnoid Hemorrhage

Traumatic traumatic subarachnoid hemorrhage (SAH) is common. Several etiologic mechanisms have been proposed: (1) superficial cerebral contusion with leakage of blood into the subarachnoid space; (2) direct injury to leptomeningeal vessels; and (3) intraventricular hemorrhage with reflux through the fourth ventricular foramina into the subarachnoid space. Traumatic SAH is an adverse independent prognostic factor in worsening outcomes. It appears that death among patients with traumatic SAH is related to the severity of the initial mechanical damage, rather than to the effects of delayed vasospasm and secondary ischemic brain damage.

Non-contrast CT is the preferred imaging technique for detection of acute traumatic SAH (accuracy, 90%-95%). Traumatic SAH is most often focal, overlying the site of cortical bruising, or subjacent to a subdural hematoma. Blood in the interpeduncular fossa is a reliable indicator of SAH. Diffuse spread of SAH throughout all the subarachnoid spaces is less common in head trauma. SAH is usually best seen on early CT scans and resolves over the following days.

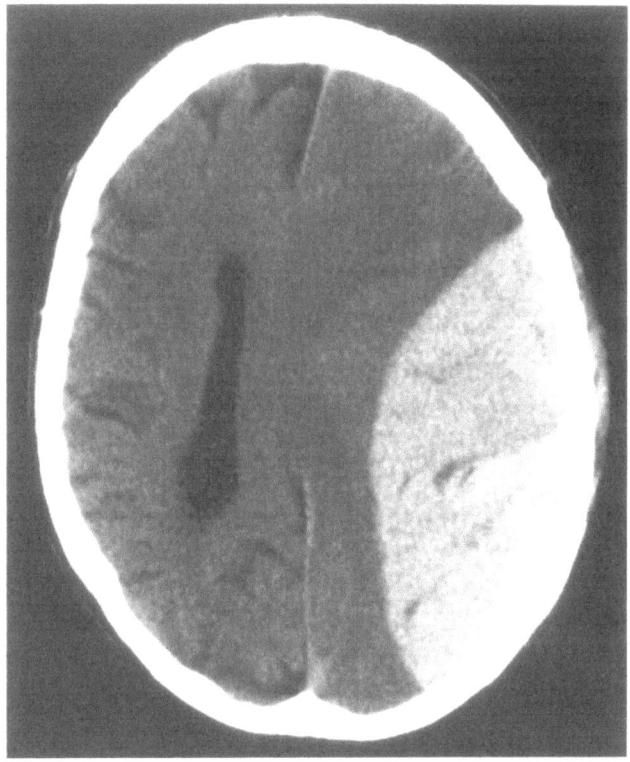

Fig. 5. Acute left epidural hematoma with subfalcial herniation. Non-contrast CT scan upon admission. The hematoma is biconvex, and is limited anteriorly by the coronal suture and posteriorly by the lambdoid suture (does not cross suture lines). The hematoma contains inhomogeneous hypodense areas, indicating blood that is not yet clotted. The mass effect causes a subfalcial herniation with compression of the left lateral ventricle and dilatation of the right lateral ventricle

Table 3. Epidural versus subdural hematoma

Epidural hematoma (EDH)	Subdural hematoma (SDH)
'Coup' side	'Contre-coup' side
Associated with skull fracture in approximately 90% of cases	No consistent relationship with skull fractures
Does not cross suture lines	Does cross suture lines
Not limited by falx or tentorium (may extend from supra- to infratentorial compartments or across midline)	Limited by falx and tentorium (confined to supra- or infratentorial compartment, does not cross midline)
Origin: • Arterial (majority, due to tearing of one or more branches of the meningeal arteries, most commonly the middle meningeal artery), • Venous (minority, due to laceration of a dural venous sinus, e.g. along the sphenoparietal sinus)	Origin: • Venous, due to laceration of superficial bridging cortical veins
Medical emergency	May be chronic
Magnitude of the mass effect caused by EDH is directly related to the size of the extracerebral collection	Magnitude of the mass effect caused by SDH is more often associated with underlying parenchymal injury
CT is preferred imaging technique because: • Rapid accessibility • Shows both the hemorrhage and the skull fracture	MRI is preferred imaging technique because: • MRI is more sensitive than CT, especially in the detection of so-called isodense SDHs which may be difficult to see on CT
MRI can be useful for: • Detection of parenchymal repercussions (edema, mass effect, herniations)	• Multiplanar imaging capability • Better definition of multicompartmental nature of SDH

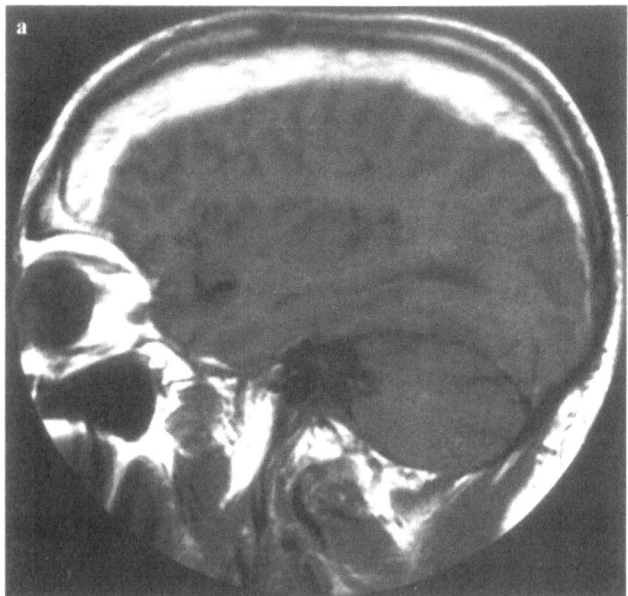

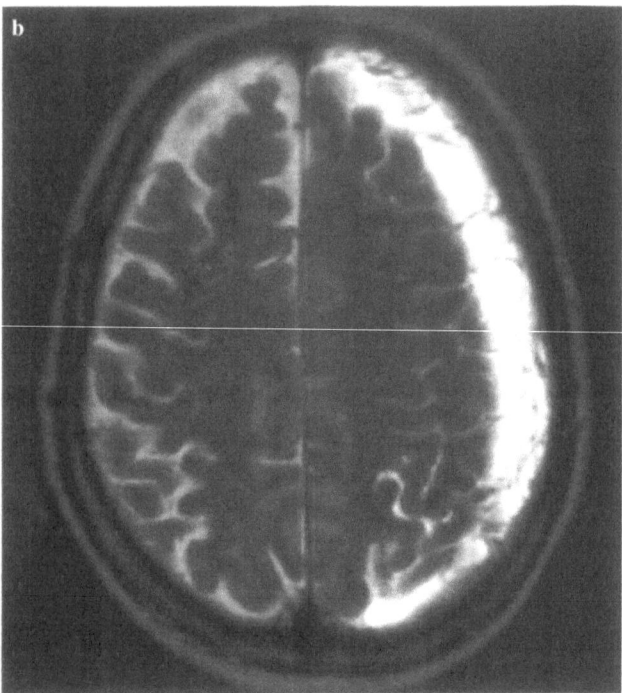

Fig. 6a, b. *Subacute subdural hematoma in a 75-year-old man.* **a** Sagittal SE T1-weighted image. **b** Axial TSE T2-weighted image. The MR images show the classic appearance of a crescent-shaped left subdural hematoma. There are multiple internal septations, representing strands of fibrovascular granulation tissue, derived from the inner (meningeal) layer of the dura. The hematoma extends over the surface of the left cerebral hemisphere from the frontal to the occipital region. The blood is hyperintense on the T1-weighted and T2-weighted images, indicating the presence of extracellular methemoglobin

MRI is less useful for the detection of acute traumatic SAH. The higher oxygen tension (pO_2) in the subarachnoid space slows the transformation of oxyhemoglobin (HbO_2) to paramagnetic breakdown products such as de-oxyhemoglobin (Hb) and methemoglobin (HbOH). Recent evidence suggests that FLAIR sequences are more useful than SE or turbo spin echo (TSE) sequences in the detection of SAH. Nevertheless, in most centers, CT remains the method of choice for the detection of SAH in the acute phase.

Intraventricular Hemorrhage

Traumatic intraventricular hemorrhage (IVH) can occur as a result of *tearing of subependymal veins* that line the ventricular cavities. Most commonly affected are the subependymal veins on the ventral surface of the corpus callosum and along the fornix and septum pellucidum. *Rupture of an intracerebral hemorrhage* into the adjacent ventricle can also cause IVH. The single cell layer, which forms the ependymal lining of the ventricles, does not constitute a significant barrier to the extension of an intraparenchymal bleed. Finally, IVH can be found due to reflux of SAH through the fourth ventricular foramina of Luschka and Magendie.

In trauma patients, one should look for a horizontally sedimented blood-CSF level, which is typically observed in the occipital horns. Even a small amount of IVH is well seen on CT. When the intraventricular thrombus matures, clot retraction occurs and a hyperdense intraventricular blood clot is observed adjacent to the intraventricular CSF. Signal intensities of IVH on MRI vary and depend on its age, presence or absence of clotting, and whether or not erythrocyte lysis has occurred.

Intra-axial Lesions

Post-traumatic Cerebral Edema

Post-traumatic cerebral edema with intracranial hypertension is a life-threatening secondary traumatic brain lesion. It starts immediately after injury, but massive edema usually takes 24-48 hours to develop. It can be associated with intra-axial or extra-axial lesions. Unilateral swelling of a cerebral hemisphere is most often secondary to an ipsilateral SDH or EDH.

Cerebral edema leads to compression of intracranial blood vessels, thereby causing underperfusion and ischemia of the edematous region or hemispheres. If the intracranial pressure is not relieved, the brain will gradually herniate through the tentorial incisure and the foramen magnum (Table 2). This results in compression of the brain stem with depression of breathing and cardiac function, and eventually leads to death. Cerebral edema is more common in children than in adults; in children, brain swelling may be the only identifiable feature of head injury.

CT is more sensitive than MRI for the detection of hyperacute cerebral edema. Early imaging findings in diffuse cerebral edema include: decreased cerebral attenuation values; diminished gray-white matter differentiation; increased density of the falx and tentorium (due to vascular stasis, associated SDH, SAH, or both); downward bowing of the tentorial leaflets, due to supratentorial mass effect; effacement of the cortical sulci of the cerebral surface; and obliteration of the subarachnoid cisterns near the skull base, particularly the suprasellar, quadrigeminal plate and ambient cisterns. The cerebellum may appear relatively hyperdense: this is called "white cerebellum" sign. Since the majority of relevant CT changes develop within 48 hours after injury, pathological categorization based on an early, control CT scan is useful for prognostic purposes.

Edema associated with intracerebral hemorrhagic contusions often increases dramatically during the days following the acute event. Therefore, it is not unusual for the initial CT scan to show no or only limited edema, and for the follow-up examination to reveal massive perilesional edema and associated mass effect.

Cerebral Contusion and Hematoma

The term *cerebral contusion* is used to indicate (punctate) hemorrhages within the brain parenchyma. Contusions are often multiple and located near the surface of the brain; associated SAH is a common finding. Traumatic cerebral contusions are most often encountered supratentorially. They are caused when the brain hits irregularities of the inner skull table or dural folds (falx, tentorium). Sites of predilection include anterior and inferior frontal lobes, anterior and inferior temporal lobes, and gyri around the sylvian fissure. Contusions are much less frequent in the cerebellar hemispheres, which are protected by the smooth inner surface of the thick occipital bone.

The term *cerebral hematoma* refers to a well-circumscribed parenchymal hemorrhage. Cerebral hematomas tend to be found in the deeper parts of the brain. Delayed development of a post-traumatic intracerebral hemorrhage is not uncommon, and should be suspected when the patient's neurologic condition worsens. As the hematoma matures, and clot retraction occurs, it becomes surrounded by a hypodense rim of edema; a hemorrhagic sedimentation level may develop. Cerebral hematomas can spontaneously decompress into the ventricles, thereby causing IVH. In trauma patients, a deep hematoma may be found along with one or more cortical contusions.

In acceleration and deceleration brain injuries, intraparenchymal bleeding sites can be categorized as "coup" or "contre-coup" injury. *Coup injury* occurs at the site of primary impact, which is identified by the associated scalp injuries or skull fractures. Epidural hematoma, contusion or laceration of the brain surface often occurs at the site of a fracture, especially if it is depressed. *Contre-coup injury* arises on the opposite side. Hemorrhagic cerebral contusions are more common at the contre-coup side, though both coup and contre-coup injuries can be hemorrhagic.

A severe impact on the stationary head (e.g. a blow with a blunt object) results in skull fractures, but generally does not cause contre-coup contusions. This is because in these cases, the head does not accelerate or decelerate, and there is no brain lag. This knowledge is useful in distinguishing head injuries due to falls from those due to blows.

On CT images, acute intraparenchymal hemorrhagic contusions are recognized as patchy, ill-defined frontal or temporal *low density* lesions, often containing small, hyperdense, punctate foci of *petechial hemorrhage*. Lesions may not be seen on an initial CT scan and *follow-up* scans are indispensable when the patient's clinical condition deteriorates. Over the next few days, as clot retraction occurs, the hemorrhagic area becomes surrounded by a rim of edematous brain. After surgical decompression of an EDH or SDH, hemorrhagic contusions may become more apparent. Over time, CT *density values decrease* as thrombolysis progresses; this may cause the affected area to become almost isodense with the surrounding normal brain tissue. The perilesional edema diminishes. A resolving hematoma may *enhance in a ring-like pattern* after intravenous contrast medium administration. In this stage of evolution, differentiation from an infarct or tumor may be extremely difficult.

On *MRI*, the appearance of intraparenchymal hemorrhage is extremely complex. Imaging findings are determined by many parameters, such as: age, location and size of the hematoma; pulse sequence; magnetic field strength; presence or absence of continued bleeding; local tissue pH; oxygen tension (pO_2). The MRI appearance of intracerebral hemorrhage follows the evolution as described in Table 4.

Diffuse Axonal Injury (Shearing Injury of the White Matter)

Even with closed head injury, the brain can suffer severe damage from shearing injuries caused by acceleration, deceleration or rotational forces. The lesions are determined by the magnitude of rotational acceleration and the difference in density and rigidity between two adjacent tissues, especially gray and white matter. Clinically, diffuse axonal injury (DAI) is characterized in the acute phase by impairment or complete loss of consciousness from the moment of impact. A typical example is the "uppercut" in boxing, which induces a sudden linear and rotational acceleration of the skull, causing a sudden loss of consciousness. Less severe hemispheric DAI can cause loss of telencephalic functions: decreased attention span, memory loss, concentration difficulties, lower intelligence quotient (IQ), headaches, seizures, less stress resistance, behavioral changes. DAI lesions can be found in the following sites of predilection (in decreasing order of frequency):

Table 4. Sequential signal intensity changes of intracranial hemorrhage on MRI (1.5 T)

	Intracranial hemorrhage				
	Hyperacute	Acute	Early subacute	Late subacute	Chronic
What happens	Blood leaves the vascular system (extravasation)	Deoxygenation with formation of DeoxyHb	Clot retraction and DeoxyHb is oxidized to MetHb	Cell lysis (membrane disruption)	Macrophages digest the clot
Time frame	< 12 hours	Hours to days (weeks in center of hematoma)	A few days	From 4-7 days to 1 month	Weeks to years
Red blood cells	Intact	Intact, but hypoxic	Still intact, severely hypoxic	Lysis (solution of lysed cells)	Gone; encephalomalacia with proteinaceous fluid
State of Hb	Intracelluar OxyHb (HbO$_2$)	Intracellular DeoxyHb (Hb)	Intracellular MetHb (HbOH) (first at periphery of clot)	Extracellular MetHb (HbOH)	Hemosiderin (insoluble) and ferritin (water soluble)
Oxidation state	Ferrous (Fe^{2+}) No unpaired e-	Ferrous (Fe^{2+}) 4 unpaired e-	Ferric (Fe^{3+}) 5 unpaired e-	Ferric (Fe^{3+}) 5 unpaired e-	Ferric (Fe^{3+}) 2000×5 unpaired e-
Magnetic properties	Diamagnetic ($\chi<0$)	Paramagnetic ($\chi>0$)	Paramagnetic ($\chi>0$)	Paramagnetic ($\chi>0$)	Superparamagnetic (FeOOH)
SI on T1-weighted images	$\approx$ or $\downarrow$	$\approx$ or $\downarrow$ No PEDD interaction	$\uparrow\uparrow$ PEDD interaction	$\uparrow\uparrow$ PEDD interaction	$\approx$ or $\downarrow$ No PEDD interaction
SI on T2-weighted images	$\uparrow$ (high water content)	$\downarrow$ T2 PRE (susceptibility effect)	$\downarrow\downarrow$ T2 PRE (susceptibility effect)	$\uparrow\uparrow$ No T2 PRE	$\downarrow\downarrow$ T2 PRE (susceptibility effect)

Hb, hemoglobin; *e-*, electrons; *FeOOH*, ferric oxyhydroxide; *SI*, signal intensity; *PEDD*, proton-electron dipole-dipole interaction; *PRE*, proton relaxation enhancement
$\approx$ same; $\uparrow$ increased, $\downarrow$ decreased SI relative to normal gray matter

1. The *hemispheric gray-white matter junction* is the most common location for DAI, because the peripheral location increases the vulnerability to trauma and because of the abrupt change in tissue density between the gray and white matter. The frontal and parietal lobes are most frequently involved.
2. The *corpus callosum* (CC) is the second most common location for DAI shearing lesions. The splenium is more commonly affected because of its closer proximity to the falx.
3. *Basal ganglia and internal capsule* shearing injuries.
4. *Brain stem and mesencephalon* shearing lesions are only observed with more severe injuries; they are always associated with multiple hemorrhages in the deep white matter and the corpus callosum. Most commonly involved is the dorsolateral quadrant of rostral brain stem adjacent to the superior cerebellar peduncle. Differential diagnosis includes: Duret's hemorrhage of the brain stem in transtentorial herniation.
5. *Cerebellar shearing injuries* are infrequent.

The *neuroradiological diagnosis* of DAI is difficult (Fig. 7). In the acute phase, a non-contrast CT scan may reveal small, punctate petechial hemorrhages (Fig. 7a), intraventricular blood (shearing of subependymal veins), and perimesencephalic subarachnoid hemorrhage. However, CT underestimates DAI lesions, because non-hemorrhagic lesions are difficult to identify. Therefore, when a patient's neurologic or psychiatric status is worse than predicted from the CT findings, MRI must be performed. MRI is far more sensitive for detecting DAI lesions. FLAIR sequences are useful for the detection of non-hemorrhagic lesions and areas of gliosis (Fig. 7b). Gradient echo sequences are used to detect the susceptibility effects of hemosiderin (Fig. 7d).

Recent evidence suggests that DAI lesions can be hyperintense on diffusion-weighted images, indicating restricted diffusion (Fig. 7e, f). Traumatic lesions can be classified into three categories depending on their signal characteristics on diffusion-weighted imaging (DWI) and apparent diffusion coefficient (ADC) maps: *type 1*, DWI- and ADC-hyperintense most likely representing lesions with vasogenic edema; *type 2*, DWI-hyperintense, ADC-hypointense indicating cytotoxic edema; *type 3*, central hemorrhagic lesion surrounded by an area of increased diffusion. It remains to be determined if this information is clinically useful in predicting final outcome and patient prognosis.

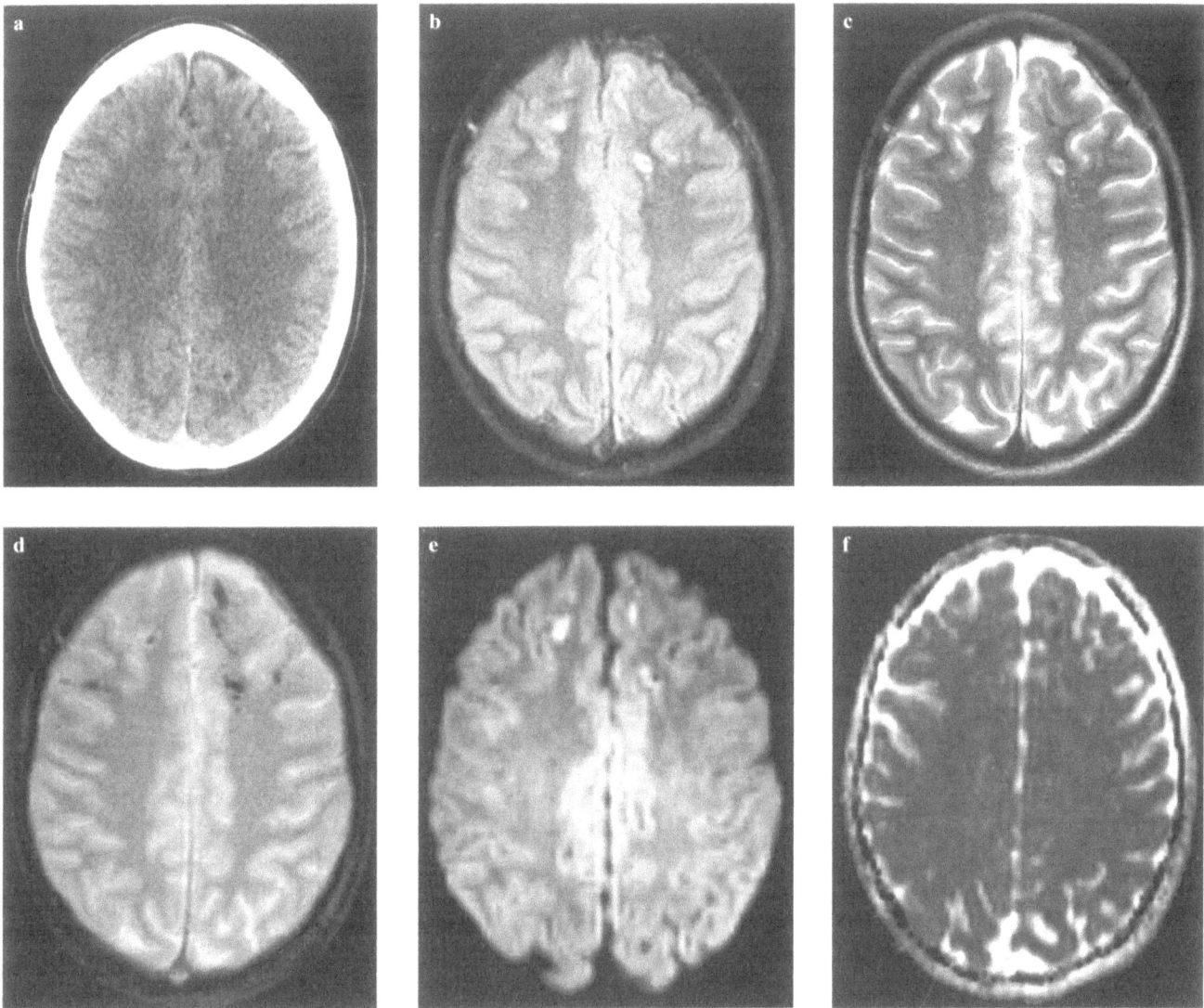

Fig. 7a-f. *Diffuse axonal injuries in a 14-year-old boy 4 days after a motor vehicle accident.* **a** Axial non-contrast CT scan. **b** Axial turbo FLAIR image. **c** Axial TSE T2-weighted image. **d** Axial spoiled gradient echo FLASH T2*-weighted image (TE=25 ms). **e** Axial diffusion-weighted trace image (b=1000). **f** Axial apparent diffusion coefficient map. The non-contrast CT scan shows several punctate petechial hemorrhages at the gray-white matter junction of the frontal lobes. On the turbo FLAIR and T2-weighted images, the lesions are hyperintense. On the gradient echo T2*-weighted image, multiple hypointense hemosiderin deposits are seen at the gray-white matter junction and in the corpus callosum. The appearance, multiplicity and topographical distribution are typical of hemorrhagic shearing injuries. On the diffusion-weighted scan, the lesions are hyperintense, and on the apparent diffusion coefficient map, the lesions are hypointense, indicating restricted diffusion, consistent with type 2 lesions

Ischemia and Infarction

Post-traumatic ischemia and infarction are common complications in patients with craniocerebral trauma. The causes of post-traumatic ischemia and infarction are:

- Vasospasm secondary to:
  - Subarachnoid hemorrhage
  - Direct vessel injury (laceration)
- Extrinsic compression of a blood vessel by:
  - Cerebral herniation (Table 2)
  - Extra-axial mass (e.g. EDH, SDH)
- Hypoxia and anoxia
- Thrombosis and distal embolization secondary to:

- Vascular dissection
- Fat embolization due to long bone fracture

Post-traumatic Sequelae

If trauma to the brain has been focal (e.g. cerebral contusions and hematomas), localized *encephalomalacia* (intraparenchymal tissue loss) may result. Areas of encephalomalacia are often surrounded by a rim of *gliosis* (Fig. 8). Findings on CT scans include one or more lucent areas of tissue loss; focal dilatation of the ventricle nearest to the traumatic lesion is common. On MRI, en-

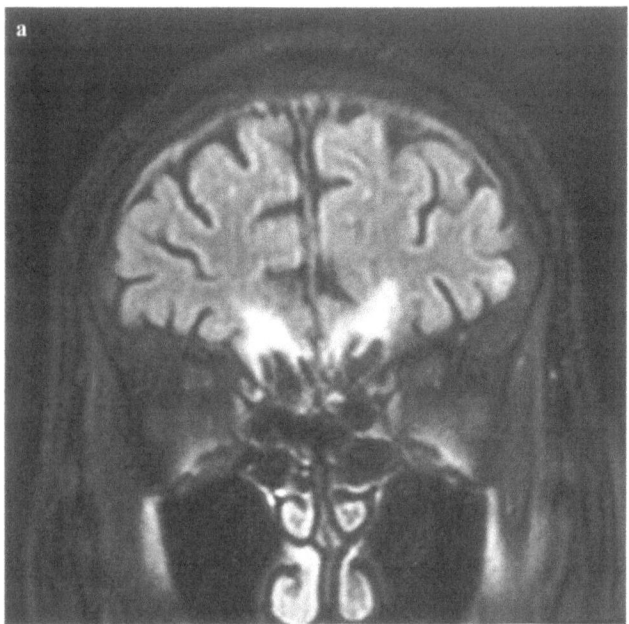

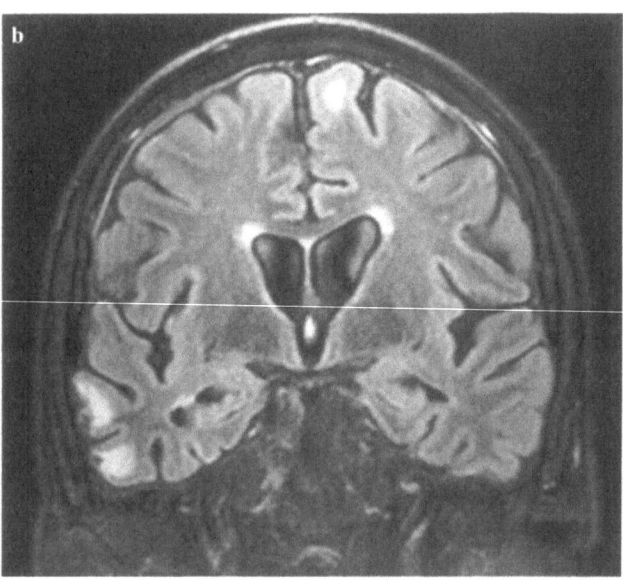

Fig. 8a, b. *Post-traumatic encephalomalacia and gliosis.* Coronal turbo FLAIR images through the frontal (**a**) and temporal (**b**) lobes. MRI performed 4 years after severe head injury. There are areas of post-traumatic tissue loss in the basal part of the frontal lobes bilaterally, and in the lateral portion of the right temporal lobe. The areas of tissue loss are surrounded by gliosis, which is hyperintense on the FLAIR images. In addition, there are old diffuse axonal injuries, seen as gliotic foci at the gray-white matter interface, e.g. in the upper part of the left frontal lobe

cephalomalacia and gliosis are of high signal intensity on T2-weighted images, and are often indistinguishable. FLAIR sequences are most helpful to differentiate tissue loss from gliosis. Moreover, a gradient echo sequence is of value to detect hemosiderin deposition.

More diffuse trauma can result in generalized atrophy of one or both hemispheres, with enlargement of sulci

and ventricles. Post-traumatic *atrophy* is observed as diffuse, non-focal enlargement of the intracranial CSF spaces. *Diffuse ventricular enlargement* can be due to communicating hydrocephalus (e.g. decreased CSF absorption due to adhesions in the subarachnoid space after SAH or meningitis). *Focal ventricular enlargement* is most often secondary to central tissue loss ("ex vacuo").

Vascular Injuries

Traumatic *carotid artery-cavernous sinus fistula* (CCF) is caused by a wall defect in the cavernous portion of the internal carotid artery (ICA), thus allowing a direct communication with the adjacent cavernous sinus. The increased arterial inflow into the cavernous sinus leads to dilatation of the superior ophthalmic vein, the facial veins, and the internal jugular vein. Clinical findings include pulsating exophthalmos, chemosis, conjunctival edema, restricted ocular mobility, and persistent bruit. The most common CT and MRI findings are widening of the affected cavernous sinus (convex lateral margin), and dilatation of the superior ophthalmic vein. MR angiography can be used to demonstrate the venous widening.

Post-traumatic aneurysms are infrequent complications of head trauma. The most common locations include the cervical, petrous, and cavernous ICA. The distal anterior and middle cerebral arteries are less commonly affected. Basal skull fractures, penetrating injuries, or shearing stress (e.g. against a dural margin) are the primary causes of post-traumatic cerebral aneurysms.

Traumatic *vascular dissections* are caused by the development of a hematoma within the intima; this results in splitting of the vessel wall and causes a false lumen within the media. Vascular dissection may lead to luminal occlusion or distal embolization. Dissections most commonly occur in the internal carotid (60%) or vertebral (20%) arteries; involvement of internal carotid and vertebral arteries is seen in up to 10% of cases. Traumatic dissection can be caused by blunt or, less frequently, penetrating trauma to the neck. In cases of "spontaneous" dissection, there is often a non-recalled or trivial trauma in the history, and if not, a primary arterial disease should be considered. The neuroradiological diagnosis can be established by different techniques:

- Catheter *angiography* shows a "flame-like" or "radish tail-like" tapering of the vessel lumen;
- *Duplex Doppler ultrasound* is being increasingly used for the diagnosis of intimal dissections;
- *Spiral CT* of the neck with surface rendering and maximum intensity projection (MIP) reconstructions can be used as an alternative to catheter angiography;
- MRI should include an axial T1-weighted sequence through the upper neck and skull. These images must be carefully studied to detect a crescentic area of high signal intensity, which represents the subintimal hematoma in the wall of the internal carotid artery. Findings can be confirmed by MR angiography.

CSF Leaks and Pneumocephalus

A post-traumatic CSF leak occurs as the combined result of a dural tear and a bone fracture. It can be the result of penetrating trauma (bullet wounds, stabbing) or blunt trauma (with skull base fractures). CSF leakage into the *paranasal sinuses or nasal cavity* is associated with fractures of the anterior cranial fossa: ethmoid, posterior wall of frontal sinus, planum sphenoidale or cribrifrom plate. CSF leakage into the *middle ear* is associated with fractures of the floor of the middle cranial fossa extending into the tegmen tympani. Otorrhea only occurs if the tympanic membrane is perforated or ruptured. If the tympanic membrane is intact, the CSF drains via the eustachian tube into the rhinopharynx, and rhinorrhea occurs. High-resolution CT images of the skull base and petrous bones with thin sections and bone algorithm images are useful for precise localization of the fractures. The presence of intracranial air bubbles (pneumocephalus) is an ominous finding.

Infections

In non-penetrating head trauma, meningitis can occur as the result of an open calvarial fracture, a skull base fracture, or a post-operative craniotomy defect. Meningitis may progress to cerebritis and brain abscess. If the abscess ruptures into the ventricular system, ventriculitis will develop. Ventriculitis and meningitis are frequently followed by obstructive hydrocephalus. In penetrating head trauma, infection is caused by debris (e.g. scalp, hair, foreign material) which is carried into the brain by a projectile.

Diabetes Insipidus

Pituitary dysfunction, especially diabetes insipidus, can occur as a result of trauma. *Transient diabetes insipidus* usually develops within the first week after trauma and is probably due to a contusion of the neurohypophysis. *Permanent diabetes insipidus* indicates structural damage to the pituitary gland, the pituitary stalk or the neurosecretory nuclei of the hypothalamus. One should look for fractures involving the floor of the sella, hemorrhage within the neurohypophysis, transection or laceration of the pituitary stalk, petechial hemorrhages in the hypothalamus and elevated intracranial pressure. *Delayed onset diabetes insipidus* arises months after trauma and should suggest the possibility of optochiasmatic arachnoiditis.

CT should be used to exclude hemorrhages in the suprasellar region or skull base fractures extending into the sellar floor. MRI shows absence of the normal hyperintense signal in the posterior pituitary lobe.

Leptomeningeal Cysts

Leptomeningeal cysts are rare complications of pediatric skull fractures. Herniation of the leptomeninges through the skull fracture and associated dural tear prevent normal healing of the fracture margins. The systolic-diastolic pulsation of the brain and CSF produces fracture diastasis. The result is a calvarial defect, which usually becomes visible 3-5 months after injury. Leptomeningeal cysts are also known as "growing fractures", because of their tendency to increase in size over time. On plain X-ray films, a skull defect with indistinct, scalloped margins is seen. On CT, a CSF density cyst adjacent to or in the skull is observed. The cyst is caused by subarachnoid fluid being trapped in the herniated tissue, probably secondary to arachnoidal adhesions. On MRI, the cyst is isointense with CSF and communicates with the subarachnoid space. Frequently, there is an underlying area of encephalomalacia, due to compression of the cerebral cortex by the cyst.

Spinal Injury

Spinal trauma is a potentially devastating form of trauma, which may be accompanied by significant neurologic injury, including paraplegia, quadriplegia, or death. Patients who present with complete spinal cord injuries, without discernable motor or sensory preservation on neurologic examination, have a diminishing hope for a positive outcome. On the other hand, patients who present with an incomplete injury may regain a large amount of useful function, or be spared the progression to complete injury with rapid diagnosis and treatment of fracture fragments, hematomas, or other lesions that compress the spinal cord. The role of the radiologist in this setting is clear: depict the spinal axis rapidly and accurately, and guide potential surgical decompression. Both CT and MRI have important roles to play.

The spine segment in which CT has played a critical role in the rapid assessment of the traumatized patient is the cervical spine. The difficulty in "clearing" the cervical spine in trauma patients is well known to most radiologists. Despite swimmers views, repeated attempts at open-mouth odontoid views, and other permutations of imaging, it is often difficult to depict the entirety of the cervical spine to a satisfactory extent, allowing the radiologist to exclude fractures which may prove significant. There was early adoption of the technique of thin-section CT with reformation into the sagittal or coronal plane to evaluate the spine, and the early literature was favorable. The widespread availability of first helical CT, and subsequently multidetector CT refined the technique, and allowed the rapid acquisition of data sets which provided confidence in diagnosis and increased utilization. It is the policy of many major trauma centers in this era to solely evaluate the cervical spine in the case of major trauma with an MDCT study (Fig. 9). We have utilized this technique in the setting of major trauma for several years now, without a significant misdiagnosis. The only limitation of this technique is the inability to provide screening for ligamentous injury. CT provides overall superior depiction of the bony anatomy of the spinal canal in the trauma patient. It also can depict significant soft tissue abnormalities, such as traumat-

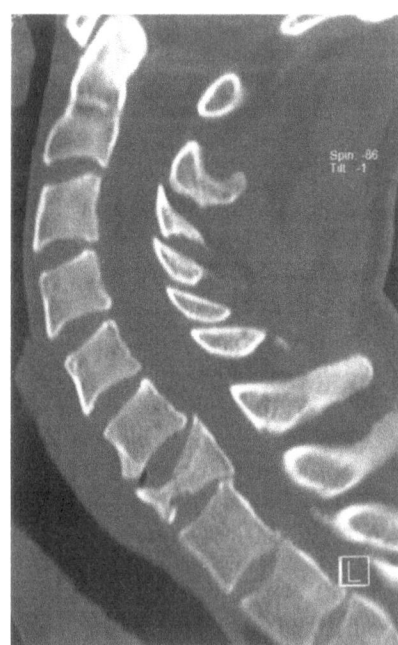

Fig. 9. Multidetector CT of the cervical spine (sagittal reformatted image) in a patient with a C7 fracture, not seen on plain radiographs. The height of the vertebral body is decreased, the posterior wall is displaced backwards, with narrowing of the anterior-posterior diameter of the spinal canal. It is now the policy of many major trauma centers to evaluate the cervical spine in the case of major trauma with a multidetector CT study

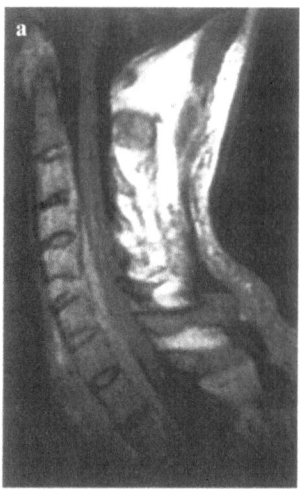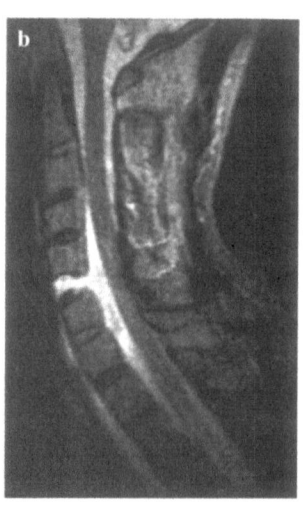

Fig. 10a, b. *Extension-distraction fracure at C5-C6 level with epidural hematoma.* The patient is a 54-year-old man, injured in a motor vehicle accident, with rapidly progressive neurologic deficit. MRI was performed on a 0.2 tesla open system. **a** Sagittal T1-weighted image. **b** Sagittal T2-weighted image. The anterior column of the spine is disrupted and the C5 and C6 vertebral bodies are distracted. Extension-distraction injury occurs when hyperextension forces are applied to the spine. This injury is unstable. An epidural hematoma is located in the anterior epidural space, displacing and compressing the spinal cord

ic disk herniations, significant epidural hemorrhage, and other injuries. It is clear that MRI is superior in this regard, but the review of spine CT in a trauma patient should include careful review of the soft tissue windows.

CT of the thoracic and lumbar spine is commonly performed to evaluate suspicious levels on plain film studies, or to evaluate the patient with a known level of injury. There is little literature on the utilization of CT to the exclusion of plain film studies in these areas, however, as has been the case in the cervical spine. We are often asked to reformat data sets on multitrauma patients who have undergone chest, abdomen and pelvic CT studies to evaluate the spine. The images that are obtained by reformatting this data are often adequate to exclude significant vertebral body fractures. As with the cervical spine, reformatted sagittal and coronal images are also helpful to demonstrate abnormalities in alignment, and to clarify the nature of fractures that are seen on the axial images.

MRI has also gained in importance with its increased availability for the emergency room physician. It is apparent that the depiction of the spinal cord is of primary importance, and with the adoption of MRI, the utility of myelography and post-myelography CT has diminished to the point of vanishing (in the absence of contraindications to MRI). MRI is capable of depicting the vertebra and supporting structures, intervetebral disks, the spinal cord and nerve roots, trauma-associated injuries such as hemorrhage (Fig. 10), traumatic disk herniations, and primary cord injury such as hematomas, edema, and even cord transection. Any patient with presumed spinal cord injury should undergo emergent MRI study. MRI is superior at depicting the previously mentioned lesions and guides surgical management in these patients. Careful clinical examination with a determined level of injury is an excellent means of directing the level to be studied. Many trauma protocols may also mandate evaluation of the other spinal segments to exclude additional injury which may be masked by a higher level spinal cord injury. The sensitivity of MRI for not only the soft tissue injuries associated with trauma is well known, but MRI may also demonstrate changes within the bone marrow of traumatized vertebrae which are inapparent on plain film studies, such as bone contusions. MRI is also sensitive and specific for ligamentous injury in the trauma setting. We have used MRI to provide a "ligament screen" exam for major trauma patients for several years now, with consistent results. The typical exam protocol for this purpose includes sagittal T1-weighted, sagittal gradient recalled T2*-weighted, and sagittal short inversion-time inversion recovery (STIR) images, as well as axial images. Edema in the interspinous or supraspinous ligaments is particularly conspicuous on STIR images. Some observers may prefer fat-suppressed T2-weighted images, which provide similar conspicuity of the changes of ligamentous injury. Typical fast spin echo T2-weighted images are not adequate for the purpose of ligament evaluation, as the high signal of fat in the posterior paraspinous region obscures the edema.

Suggested Reading

Gean AD (1994) Imaging of head trauma. Raven, New York

Gentry LR (2002) Head trauma. In: Atlas SW (ed) Magnetic resonance imaging of the brain and spine, 3rd edn. Lippincott-Raven, Philadelphia New York, pp 1059-1098 (Chapter 20)

Nontraumatic Neuroemergencies

J.R. Hesselink[1], S. Atlas[2]

[1] Neuroradiology Section, UCSD Medical Center, San Diego, CA, USA

[2] Department of Radiology, Stanford University Medical Center, Stanford, CA, USA

Introduction

Several clinical presentations require emergent neuroimaging to determine the cause of the neurological deficit and to institute appropriate therapy. Time is critical because neurons that are lost cannot be replaced. Generally, the clinical symptoms are due to ischemia, compression, or destruction of neural elements. The two primary imaging modalities for the central nervous system (CNS) are computed tomography (CT) and magnetic resonance imaging (MRI). CT is fast and can readily visualize fractures, hemorrhage, and foreign bodies. Otherwise, in patients who can cooperate for the longer imaging study, MRI provides better contrast resolution and has higher specificity for most CNS diseases. This paper discusses the five major categories of nontraumatic neuroemergencies.

Seizure or Acute Focal Neurological Deficit

Arterial Thrombosis and Occlusion

Thrombotic strokes may occur abruptly but the clinical picture often shows gradual worsening over the first few hours. Primary causes of arterial thrombosis include atherosclerosis, hypercoagulable states, arteritis, and dissection. Secondary compromise of vascular structures can result from traumatic injury, intracranial mass effect, neoplastic encasement, meningeal processes, and vasospasm.

Arterial Embolus

Embolic strokes characteristically have an abrupt onset. After a number of hours, there may be sudden improvement in symptoms as the embolus lyses and travels more distally. The source of the embolus is usually either the heart (in patients with atrial fibrillation or previous myocardial infarction) or ulcerated plaques at the carotid bifurcation in the neck.

Arterial Dissection

Relatively minor trauma is sufficient to cause an arterial dissection, or the dissection can occur spontaneously. Spin echo images, especially T1-weighted images with fat suppression, should also be obtained because they are sensitive for detecting intramural hemorrhage. The typical appearance of an oval-shaped hyperintense area with an eccentrically placed flow void may provide convincing evidence for a dissection. Magnetic resonance angiography (MRA) may demonstrate complete occlusion or only narrowing of the arterial lumen. MRA is useful for following a dissection to look for recanalization of a complete occlusion or resolution of the vascular compromise caused by the intramural thrombus [1].

Hypotension and Hypoxia

Hypotension can be cardiac in origin or result from blood volume loss or septic shock. Anoxic or hypoxic events are usually related to respiratory compromise from severe lung disease, perinatal problems, near drowning, high altitude exposure, carbon monoxide inhalation, or CNS-mediated effects.

Venous or Sinus Occlusion

Thrombosis of the cerebral venous sinuses has multiple etiologies, including hypercoagulable states, pregnancy, sepsis, dehydration, paranasal sinus infection, and neoplastic invasion. Occlusion of the venous sinuses results in cerebral venous engorgement, brain swelling, and increased intracranial pressure. If the thrombosis extends retrogradely and involves the cortical veins, secondary cerebral infarction can occur.

Acute thrombus is hyperdense on CT and may be detected within one of the major sinuses or cortical veins. The other classic sign is the "empty delta" sign due to nonfilling of the superior sagittal sinus on a contrast scan. Nonetheless, MRI is far superior for diagnosing abnormalities of the cerebral veins and sinuses. Normally, the dural sinuses have sufficient flow to exhibit a flow void.

If that flow void is missing or if the sinuses are hyperintense, thrombosis should be suspected. One must be careful to exclude the possibility of any in-flow enhancement effect. The diagnosis must be confirmed with gradient echo techniques or MRA. Phase-contrast MRA is the preferred technique because it is not adversely affected by intraluminal clot.

Associated parenchymal infarcts are found in the areas of venous abnormalities, and the infarcts are often hemorrhagic because arterial perfusion to the damaged tissue is maintained. In cases of superior sagittal sinus thrombosis, the infarcts are typically bilateral and in a parasagittal location.

Cortical Mass Lesion

Any lesion that irritates the cortical neurons can be a source of seizures. Neoplasms, encephalitis, meningitis, abscess, and hemorrhage are the more common causes of new-onset seizures.

Worst Headache of Life

Subarachnoid Hemorrhage

The incidence of congenital aneurysms in the general population is about 1%-2%. Clinically, a ruptured aneurysm presents as sudden onset of severe headache. In cases of subarachnoid hemorrhage, the most common aneurysms (38% of all cases) are posterior-communicating, while anterior-communicating anerysms represent 36% and middle cerebral aneurysms represent 21%. These three locations account for 95% of all ruptured aneurysms. The basilar artery accounts for only 2.8% and posterior fossa aneurysms are even less common.

The CT scan is important, first of all, to document the subarachnoid hemorrhage and to assess the amount of blood in the cisterns. Detection of subarachnoid blood is dependent on how early the scan is obtained. Data in the literature vary from 60% to 90%. If the scan is obtained within 4-5 days, the detection rate is high. Second, CT helps localize the site of the aneurysm. This can be done by the distribution of blood within the cisterns and also with dynamic scanning following an intravenous bolus of contrast medium. Third, CT is important to evaluate complicating factors such as cerebral hematoma, ventricular rupture, hydrocephalus, cerebral infarction, impending uncal herniation and re-bleed.

Conventional MRI sequences are insensitive for detecting subarachnoid hemorrhage. Clots within cisterns can be detected, but in general, MRI is not the procedure of choice in the workup of patients with subarachnoid hemorrhage. Due to the flow void phenomenon, aneurysms about the circle of Willis can be identified on spin echo MR images [2]. With fluid-attenuated inversion recovery (FLAIR) sequences, the cerebrospinal fluid (CSF) is dark, so that subarachnoid hemorrhage can be seen more easily. These sequences may be helpful for detecting subarachnoid blood in the posterior fossa where CT has difficulty [3].

Acute Meningitis

Bacterial meningitis is an infection of the pia and arachnoid and adjacent cerebrospinal fluid. The most common organisms involved are *Haemophilus influenzae*, *Neisseria meningitidis* (meningococcus) and *Streptococcus pneumoniae*. Patients present with fever, headache, seizures, altered consciousness and neck stiffness. The overall mortality rate ranges from 5% to 15% for *H. influenzae* and meningococcal meningitis to as high as 30% with streptococcal meningitis. In addition, persistent neurologic deficits are found in 10% of children after *H. influenzae* meningitis and in 30% of patients with streptococcal meningitis.

The ability of nonenhanced MRI to image meningitis is extremely limited, and the majority of cases appear normal or have mild hydrocephalus. In severe cases, the basal cisterns may be completely obliterated, with high signal intensity replacing the normal CSF signal on proton density images. Intermediate signal intensity may be seen in the basal cisterns on T1-weighted images in these cases. Meningeal enhancement often is not present, unless a chronic infection develops [4].

Fungal organisms can start as meningitis or cerebral abscess, or can invade directly from an extracranial compartment. Coccidioidomycosis is endemic to the Central Valley region of California and desert areas of the southwestern United States. Infection occurs by inhalation of dust from soil usually heavily infected with arthrospores. Primary coccidioidomycosis, a pulmonary infection, is followed by dissemination in only about 0.2% of immunocompetent patients. Central nervous system involvement most often represents meningitis, but cerebral abscess and granuloma formation can also occur [5]. Other fungal infections are primarily found in immunocompromised hosts.

Migraine

Migraine headaches can be severe and unrelenting. At presentation, the severity of the headache may raise the clinical question of possible subarachnoid hemorrhage or acute meningitis. Patients with known migraine may also develop atypical headaches.

Acute or Increasing Confusion and Obtundation

Obstructive Hydrocephalus

Acute obstructive hydrocephalus is caused by compression of the ventricular system to the point of obstructing the outflow of CSF. The common locations of blockage are at the foramina of Monro, the cerebral aqueduct, and the outlets of the fourth ventricle. Possible causes include tumor, abscess, ventriculitis, and hemorrhage. Brain injury or cerebral infarction with massive vasogenic edema can also cause obstructive hydrocephalus.

Brain Stem or Basal Ganglia Hemorrhage

Most large deep hemorrhages in the brain are associated with hypertension. The criteria for diagnosing hypertensive hemorrhage include a hypertensive patient, 60 years of age or older, and a basal ganglia or thalamic location of the hemorrhage. CT or MRI is the procedure of choice for evaluating these patients. Arteriography is necessary only if one of these criteria is missing. Hypertensive hemorrhages are often large and devastating. Since they are deep hemorrhages and near ventricular surfaces, ventricular rupture is common. One-half of hypertensive hemorrhages occur in the putamen, 25% in the thalamus, 10% in the pons and brainstem, 10% in the cerebellum, and 5% in the cerebral hemispheres.

Brain Herniation

As with hydrocephalus, any large mass lesion or process with prominent vasogenic edema can produce brain herniation. With large frontal or parietal lesions, subfalcine herniation is common. Also, any large hemispheric lesion can result in medial migration of the temporal lobe and subsequent inferior herniation through the tentorial incisura. Subfalcine herniation can compress the ipsilateral anterior cerebral artery, leading to brain infarction, whereas temporal lobe herniation commonly compresses the contralateral posterior cerebral artery, causing an occipital infarct. Diffuse brain swelling or posterior fossa masses can result in herniation of the cerebellar tonsils and brain stem inferiorly through the foramen magnum.

Encephalitis

Encephalitis refers to a diffuse parenchymal inflammation of the brain. Acute encephalitis of the non-herpetic type presents with signs and symptoms similar to meningitis but with the added features of any combination of convulsions, delirium, altered consciousness, aphasia, hemiparesis, ataxia, ocular palsies and facial weakness. The major causative agents are arthropod-borne arboviruses (Eastern and Western equine encephalitis, St. Louis encephalitis, California virus encephalitis). Eastern equine encephalitis is the most serious but fortunately also the least frequent of the arbovirus infections. The Enteroviruses, such as coxsackievirus and echoviruses, can produce a meningoencephalitis, but more benign aseptic meningitis is more common with these organisms. MRI reveals hyperintensity on T2-weighted scans within the cortical areas of involvement, associated with subcortical edema and mass effect.

Herpes simplex is the commonest and gravest form of acute encephalitis with a 30%-70% fatality rate and an equally high morbidity rate. It is almost always caused by type 1 virus except in neonates where type 2 predominates. Symptoms, including hallucinations, seizures, personality changes and aphasia, may reflect the propensity to involve the inferomedial frontal and temporal lobes. MRI has demonstrated positive findings in viral encephalitis as soon as 2 days after symptoms onset, more quickly and definitively than CT. Early involvement of the limbic system and temporal lobes is characteristic of herpes simplex encephalitis. The cortical abnormalities are first noted as ill-defined areas of high signal on T2-weighted scans, usually beginning unilaterally but progressing to become bilateral. Edema, mass effect and gyral enhancement may also be present. Since MRI is more sensitive than CT for detecting these early changes of encephalitis, we hope that it will improve the prognosis of this devastating disease [6].

Meningitis

As described previously, in addition to severe headache, patients with acute meningitis commonly present with fever, seizures, altered consciousness and neck stiffness. Most of these cases are bacterial in origin, but tuberculosis and fungal infections can also present acutely.

Metabolic and Toxic Disorders

Whenever a patient presents to the emergency department, the possibility of ingestion of drugs or other toxic substances must be considered. Narcotics and sedatives generally produce respiratory depression, which can lead to global cerebral hypoxia. Some toxic agents specifically target the basal ganglia or the white matter. In diabetic patients, the possibility of an insulin overdose and hypoglycemia must be considered.

Acute or Progressive Visual Deficit

Monocular Deficit

Monocular visual loss can be caused by anything anterior to the optic chiasm that blocks light from the retina or compresses the optic nerve. Ocular diseases, such as retinal detachment and ocular hemorrhage, are generally first evaluated by direct visualization with fundoscopy or by ultrasound. A mass compressing the optic nerve or causing severe proptosis can cause a visual deficit. Severe proptosis and stretching of the optic nerve can compromise the arterial supply to the nerve. Finally, intrinsic optic nerve lesions, such as tumors, ischemia and inflammation, are other causes of visual loss. Intraorbital diseases are evaluated equally well by CT and MRI. For intracranial disease, MRI is the imaging procedure of choice.

Bitemporal Hemianopsia

This visual deficit is caused by chiasmatic compression, usually by a mass in the suprasellar cisterns. Differential diagnosis includes all tumors and inflammatory conditions that can occur in the suprasellar region.

Homonymous Hemianopsia

The most common cause of homonymous hemianopsia is ischemia in the distribution of the posterior cerebral artery that supplies the calcarine cortex of the occipital lobe. Mass lesions can also compress the geniculate ganglion or the optic radiations in the temporo-occipital region.

Acute and Progressive Myelopathies

Epidural Hemorrhage

Most epidural hemorrhages are post-traumatic or postoperative events. Patients who are receiving anticoagulatants are at increased risk for epidural hemorrhage. The introduction or presence of an epidural catheter also increases the risk of both hemorrhage and infection.

Epidural Abscess

Most epidural abscesses are associated with diskitis or osteomyelitis, however, isolated infections of the epidural space can occur. The diagnosis of epidural abscess can be a challenge for both the clinician and radiologist. Patients may present with back pain or radicular pain. Fever and leukocytosis may be mild. Early diagnosis and prompt therapy are critical for favorable patient outcome.

The imaging findings can be quite subtle on plain T1- and T2-weighted images. During the cellulitis stage, the first sign of infection is thickening of the epidural tissues, which are initially isointense on T1-weighted images and moderately hyperintense on T2-weighted images. When liquefaction occurs, the abscess cavity becomes hypointense and more hyperintense on T1- and T2-weighted images, respectively. Detection of the infectious process is easier on gadolinium-enhanced scans. The inflamed tissues are vascular and enhance with gadolinium. On both T2-weighted images and enhanced T1-weighted images, fat suppression increases the contrast between the infectious process and normal tissues. The abscess cavity does not enhance, and appears as thin linear region of hypointensity surrounded by the enhancing cellulitis on sagittal images. The abscess cavity has an oval configuration on axial images.

Tumor

Epidural tumor usually extends from the spine, and the vast majority of spine tumors are metastases. The common primary tumor sites are lung, breast, and prostate. Occasionally, the epidural space may be directly seeded by lymphoma or leukemia. Spinal cord tumors and other intradural tumors (schwannoma and meningioma) may present with progressive myelopathy.

Inflammatory Diseases

Several demyelinating diseases are associated with transverse myelitis and acute myelopathy. In addition to classic multiple sclerosis, post-viral syndromes and Guillain-Barré syndrome are in the differential diagnosis. In patients infected with human immunodeficiency virus (HIV), the two primary diseases to consider are epidural abscess and cytomegalovirus (CMV) polyradiculopathy.

Ischemia

Spinal cord ischemia is rare. It is usually associated with spinal and paraspinal tumors or surgical procedures on the spine and aorta that may compromise the blood supply to the cord.

Cervical or Thoracic Disk Extrusion

Disk extrusions in the cervical and thoracic spine, if sufficiently large, can compress the spinal cord and produce a myelopathy. Accompanying cord edema can exacerbate the problem. Emergent laminectomy and diskectomy may be necessary to relieve the cord compression.

References

1. Levy C, Laissy JP, Raveau V et al (1994) Carotid and vertebral artery dissections: three-dimensional time-of-flight MR angiography and MR imaging versus conventional angiography. Radiology 190:97
2. Bondi A, Scialfi G, Scotti G (1988) Intracranial aneurysms: MR imaging. Neuroradiology 30:214
3. Noguchi K, Ogawa T, Inugami A, Totoshima H et al (1995) Acute subarachnoid hemorrhage: MR imaging with fluid-attenuated inversion recovery pulse sequences. Radiology 196:773-777
4. Chang KH, Han MH, Roh JK et al (1990) Gd-DTPA enhanced MR imaging of the brain in patients with meningitis: comparison with CT. AJNR Am J Neuroradiol 11:69
5. Wrobel CJ, Meyer S, Johnson RH et al (1992) MR findings in acute and chronic coccidioidomycosis meningitis. AJNR Am J Neuroradiol 13:1241
6. Tien RD, Felsberg GJ, Osumi AK (1993) Herpesvirus infections of the CNS: MR findings. AJR Am J Roentgenol 161:167

Imaging the Patient with Seizures

P. Ruggieri[1], A. Nusbaum[2]

[1] Section of MRI, Cleveland Clinic Foundation, Cleveland, OH, USA

[2] Department of Radiology, New York University Medical School, New York, NY, USA

Introduction

Seizures occur as a result of excessive, prolonged and synchronous electrical discharges of neurons within the brain parenchyma that alter neurologic function. Seizures may be acute or provoked such as in the case of a patient with a recent closed head injury, acute intracranial inflammatory process, or an acute cerebral infarct. The term "epilepsy" is applied to chronic, recurrent seizures. These seizures may be partial or focal in onset from a certain region of the brain such as the parenchyma adjacent to a neoplasm. Alternatively, the seizures may be generalized with simultaneous onset of the abnormal electrical activity from both cerebral hemispheres. If the data are insufficient to make these distinctions, the seizures are listed as unclassified. There is a higher incidence of partial seizures among all patients with epilepsy, but this varies with age. Generalized seizures are more common in early childhood while partial seizures increase in incidence with age such that partial seizures account for 75% of seizures in the elderly [1].

Imaging studies are requested in patients with seizures in order to reveal a causative underlying disease process. Identifying an underlying structural lesion (e.g., neoplasm) on imaging studies in patients with intractable partial epilepsy dramatically increases the likelihood of a seizure-free surgical outcome if the lesion correlates in location to the epileptogenic zone suspected on the basis of the clinical history, seizure semiology, and electroencephalographic findings. In patients with generalized seizures, imaging may identify developmental abnormalities, intracranial manifestations of a neurocutaneous syndrome, the sequelae of a remote insult (e.g. closed head injury, perinatal hypoxic or ischemic event), or an acute process that may ultimately have an impact on overall prognosis or may lead to the use of alternative medications for seizure control and treatment of the acute inciting process.

Neuroimaging of patients with seizures largely relies on magnetic resonance imaging (MRI) for routine clinical studies but may also include computed tomography (CT), positron emission tomography (PET), single photon emission computed tomography (SPECT), magnetic resonance spectroscopy (MRS), and magnetoencephalography (MEG). While noncontrast head CT is frequently requested for patients who present to the emergency room with new-onset seizures, studies have shown that the efficacy is quite limited for both adult and pediatric populations in this setting [2, 3]. CT is falsely negative in up to 40% of epilepsy patients with seizures and small underlying neoplasms or developmental abnormalities that account for the seizures [4]. These studies suggest that CT should be reserved for patients with new-onset seizures who also present with new neurologic deficits, a persistent change in neurologic status, fever, known malignancies, anticoagulation therapy, recent trauma, persistent headaches, or a suspicion of acquired immunodeficiency syndrome.

As outlined previously, MRI has assumed a dominant imaging role in the clinical evaluation of patients with partial (focal onset) epilepsy or poorly controlled generalized epilepsy. Modalities such as PET, SPECT, and MRS are largely reserved for problem solving when the MRI studies are negative or the clinical and imaging findings are somewhat discordant. PET and SPECT have recently gained popularity with the new availability of PET CT machines. PET is most frequently performed with [^{18}F]2-deoxyglucose (FDG) in epilepsy patients to measure cellular glucose metabolism and glucose uptake [5]. Studies in epilepsy patients demonstrate regional hypermetabolism during the ictal period (radiopharmaceutical injected during the seizure or within 2 minutes of the end of the seizure) and hypometabolism if the study is performed during the interictal period. PET is clearly more sensitive for localization when the epileptogenic foci are temporal rather than extratemporal in location but, in either case, PET demonstrates regional variations in cerebral metabolism so the localization of seizure onset is generally overestimated by PET. SPECT studies utilize Tc^{99m}-hexamethyl amine oxime (Tc^{99m}-HMPAO) or Tc^{99m}-ethyl cysteinate dimer (Tc^{99m} ECD) to evaluate the relative changes in local blood flow during the ictal and interictal periods to localize epileptogenic foci. SPECT studies also demonstrate regional variations in seizure patients, are more helpful in temporal lobe epilepsy, and demand precise data about the timing of the seizure onset and the radiopharmaceutical injection for accurate interpretation. MRS also measures cerebral metabolism but can only investigate a specific area of the brain. Therefore, a priori knowledge about the location of the epileptogenic site is necessary to perform the study. MEG is still primarily implemented as a research tool in a few larger institutions.

The strong soft tissue contrast and multiplanar capabilities of MRI are particularly advantageous for the identification and characterization of structural abnormalities in patients with epilepsy. Information on the lesion's signal intensity characteristics on T1- and T2-weighted and FLAIR (fluid attenuated inversion recovery) images, pattern of enhancement with intravenous gadolinium (when appropriate) and morphology, together with the age and clinical presentation of the patient, may be sufficient for clinical management. Not infrequently, the cortical or subcortical epileptogenic lesions responsible for the seizures are rather subtle or small and are thus difficult to characterize with conventional spin echo studies. It has therefore become standard practice to incorporate high resolution imaging (e.g. MPRAGE, fast or turbo spin echo T2) along with the more conventional pulse sequences to enhance the sensitivity of MRI and to permit additional image elaboration.

Adult Epilepsy

The electroencephalograms of patients with partial seizures demonstrate a focal onset of abnormal electrical activity, so the primary clinical question is whether there is a focal structural abnormality that is inciting the seizure activity in the adjacent brain parenchyma. Because epilepsy is a chronic process by definition, the parenchymal lesions causing the epilepsy are generally slowly progressive or static in nature, and supratentorial and cortical or subcortical in location. Such lesions in the adult population commonly include mesial temporal sclerosis, low-grade neoplasms, vascular malformations, encephalomalacia related to prior insults (e.g. infarcts) and, in young adults, developmental abnormalities.

Mesial temporal sclerosis, commonly seen in patients with temporal lobe epilepsy, consists of neuronal cell loss and reactive gliosis in the hippocampal formation, amygdala, entorhinal cortex, and parahippocampal gyrus. There is a strong association with the history of a prolonged febrile convulsion during early childhood but it remains controversial whether this is a cause or an effect of the seizures. The imaging hallmarks (Fig. 1) include asymmetric atrophy and loss of the normal internal architecture of the head and body of the hippocampal formation and prolonged T2-relaxation times in this same distribution [6]. There may also be asymmetric volume loss in the ipsilateral amygdala, mammillary body, column of the fornix and the parahippocampal gyrus, and hypointensity

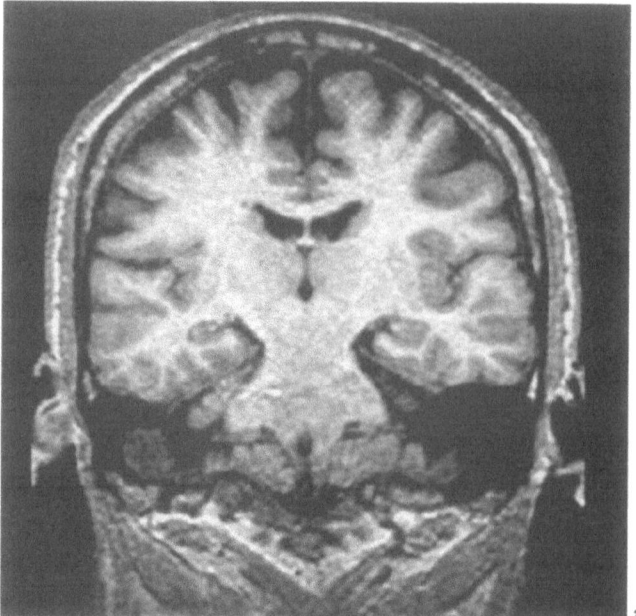

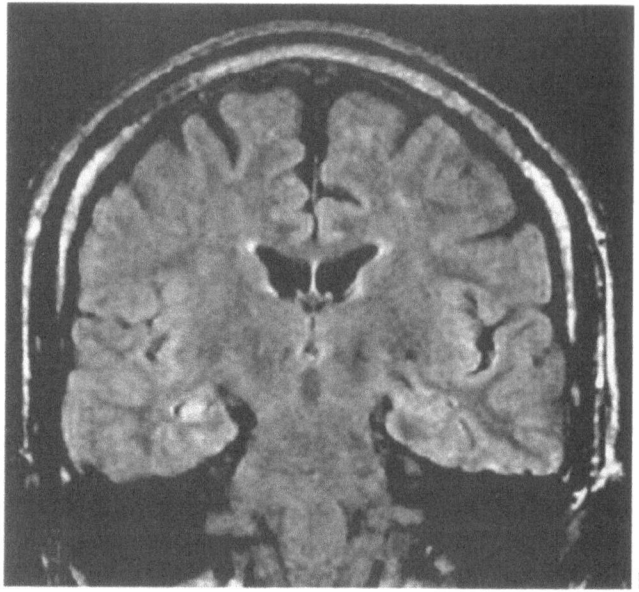

Fig. 1a, b. *Mesial temporal sclerosis.* **a** Severe volume loss of the body of the right hippocampal formation compared to normal left side. **b** Prolonged T2 relaxation time seen as moderate hyperintensity in the same distribution on coronal TSE FLAIR

in the previously mentioned gray matter structures on the T1-weighted gradient echo volume sequence. In view of the size of these structures, the abnormal morphology is best appreciated on high-resolution, three-dimensional (3D) coronal, T1-weighted gradient echo images perpendicular to the long axis of the hippocampal formations. The T2 findings are best appreciated on coronal FLAIR or T2-weighted turbo spin echo images.

Neoplastic processes are typically low-grade masses that are more apt to cause seizures than symptoms related to local mass effect, hydrocephalus, increased intracranial pressure, or focal neurologic deficits. Neoplasms account for seizures in 10%-30% of patients with chronic epilepsy [7]. Most commonly, such masses include astrocytomas, gangliogliomas, oligoden-drogliomas (Fig. 2), and dysembryoplastic neuroepithe-lial tumors (DNETs). It may be difficult to distinguish between some of these neoplasms on preoperative MRI but it is more important to determine that the structural lesion is neoplastic and to define the extent of the mass and the relationship to eloquent cortex for surgical plan-

ning purposes. In general, these masses are relatively small and infiltrative, account for only mild localized mass effect, have little or more commonly no surround-ing vasogenic edema, are variably hyperintense on FLAIR and T2-weighted images, and enhance mildly or not at all with gadolinium. Notable exceptions to these generalizations include pilocytic astrocytomas and pleo-morphic xanthoastrocytomas, both of which prominently enhance with gadolinium, tend to be better defined, and are surrounded by mild edema (Fig. 3). The DNETs are

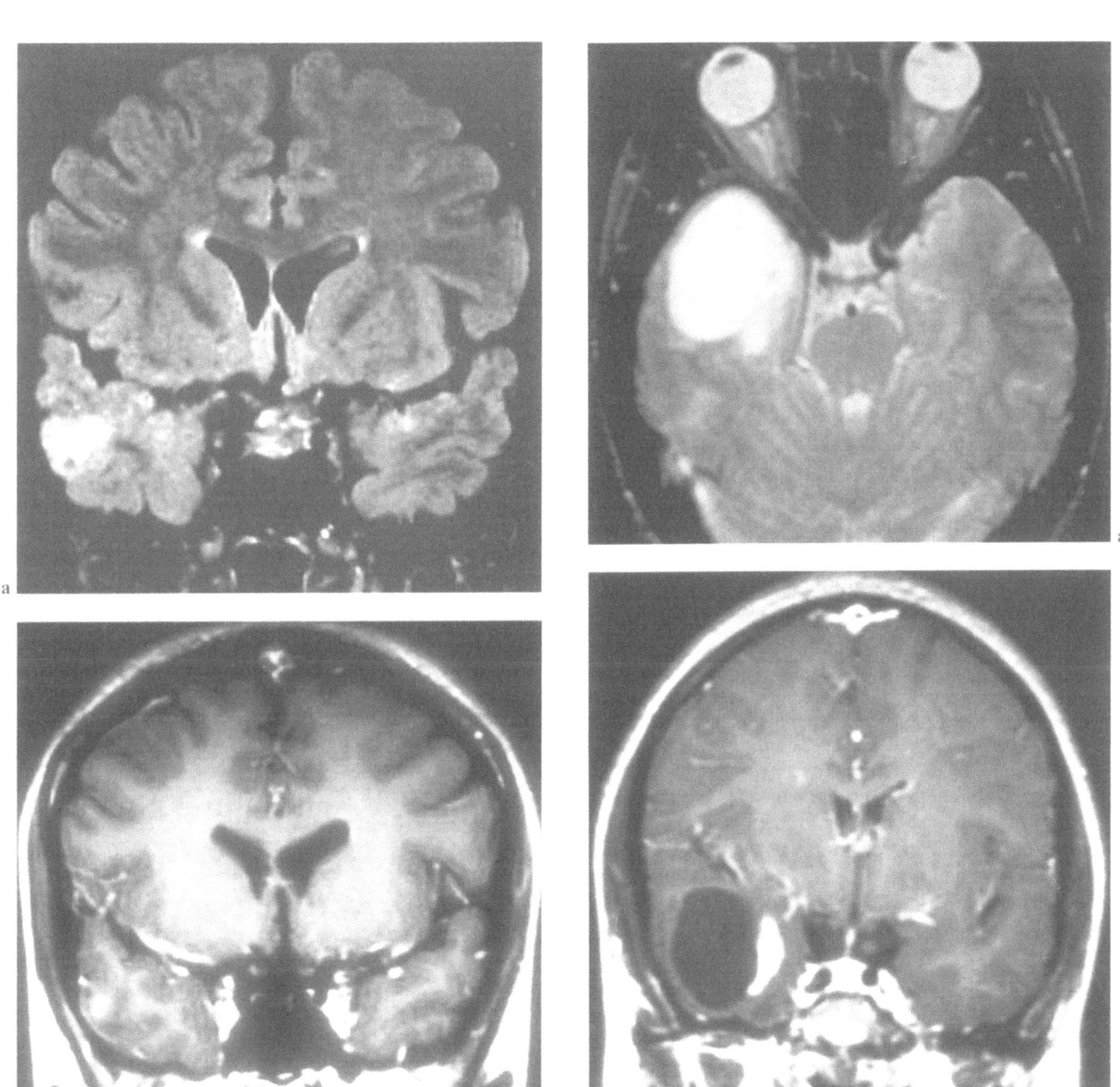

Fig. 2a, b. *Oligodendroglioma.* **a** Relatively well defined, irregu-lar focus of hyperintensity in the gray and white matter of the tem-poral pole on coronal FLAIR. **b** Mild irregular enhancement pe-ripherally with gadolinium administration

Fig. 3a, b. *Pilocytic astrocytoma.* **a** Large well-defined right tem-poral lobe mass with mild surrounding edema relative to size. **b** Large cystic component with crescentic medial rim of soft tissue that enhanced very prominently with gadolinium

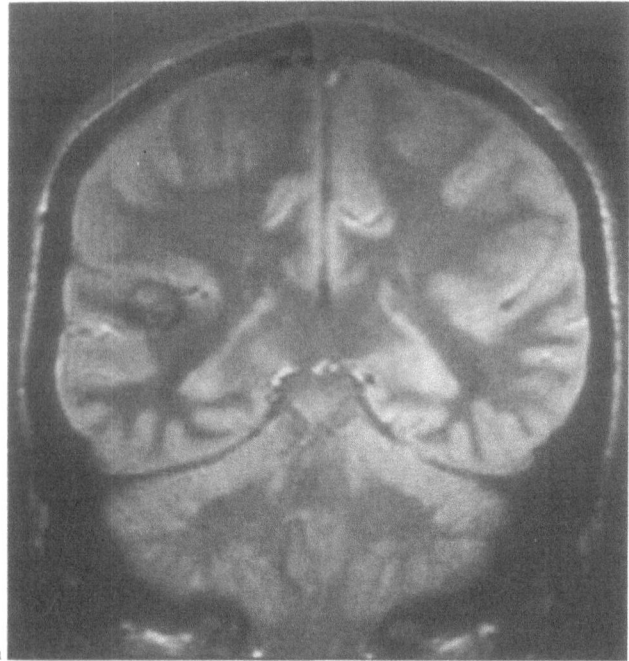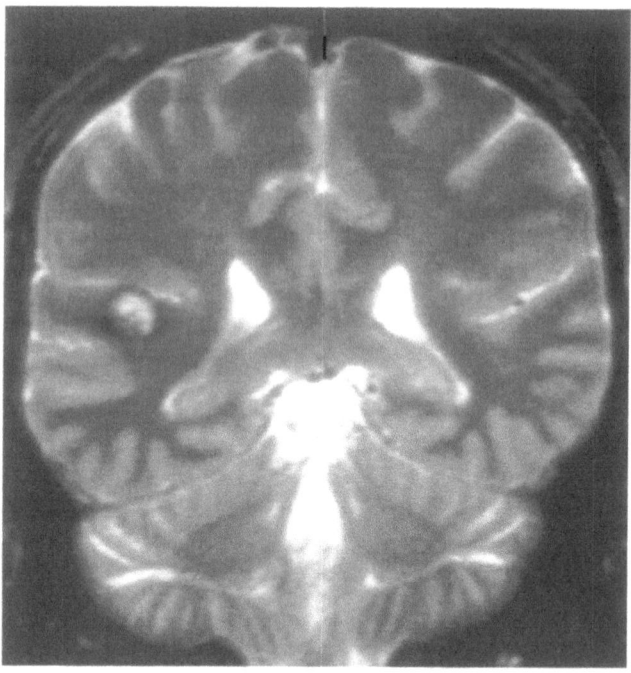

a   b

Fig. 4a, b. *Cavernous angioma.* **a** Nodular heterogeneously hyperintense mass in the left superior temporal gyrus without significant mass effect. **b** Peripheral rim of hypointensity more obvious on T2 weighted image related to prior hemorrhage

also somewhat atypical as they may demonstrate stigmata of malformations of cortical development (characteristic ion histological analysis), in addition to the characteristics of a primary mass.

Vascular malformations that cause seizures may be true arteriovenous malformations (AVMs) or, more commonly, occult vascular malformations. True AVMs are a direct communication between the arterial and venous circulations whose nidus is recognized as a cluster of serpiginous flow voids that are commonly supratentorial and superficial and may cause localized volume loss in the parenchyma due to a steal phenomenon or prior hemorrhage. Preoperatively, these AVMs are classified by the size of the nidus, location relative to eloquent cortex, and the presence of deep venous drainage [8]. Cavernous angiomas are occult vascular malformations that commonly present with seizures or headaches, are generally identified in young adults, and are typically supratentorial and subcortical in location. They typically appear as a nodular focus of heterogeneous hyperintensity on T1- and T2-weighted images with a peripheral rim of hypointensity on the T2-weighted images due to ferritin and hemosiderin deposition from prior repeated parenchymal hemorrhage (Fig. 4). A gradient echo study will make the hemorrhagic byproducts more obvious and help to identify additional similar foci elsewhere that are easily masked on the turbo spin echo images.

Encephalomalacia is potentially epileptogenic if it is supratentorial and cortical or subcortical. Such lesions can be recognized by localized or more generalized volume loss on a variety of sequences and by the hyperin-

tense signal on FLAIR and T2-weighted images. The etiology can be quite variable and may occur as the chronic sequelae of prior intracranial infections, ischemia, trauma or metabolic disorders (Fig. 5). On occasion, the

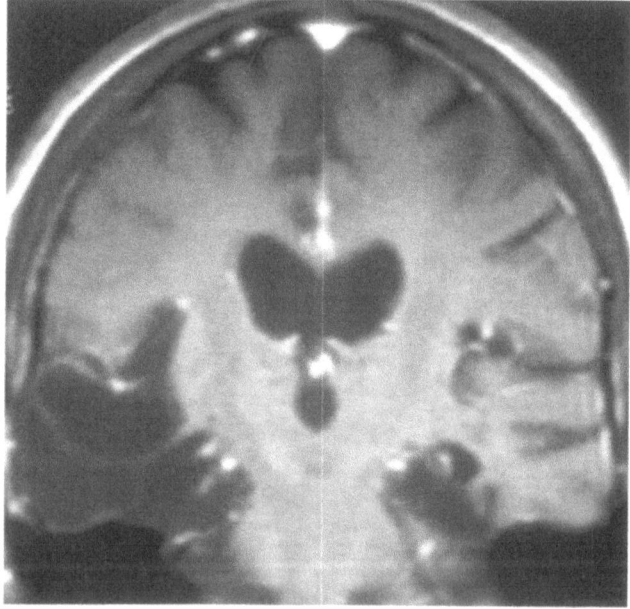

Fig. 5. Encephalomalacia from remote HSV infection. Extensive volume loss in the right temporal lobe suggestive of prior contusion but extensive involvement of the mesial temporal structures in each temporal lobe, characteristic of herpes simplex virus (HSV) infections

imaging findings can be more specific such as cortical volume loss and evidence of old hemorrhage in the subfrontal regions or temporal poles, which implies the residua of prior contusions from a closed head injury. More commonly, the imaging findings are non-specific and it is necessary to rely on the clinical history to define the etiology. The history and clinical characteristics of the epilepsy also provide a sense of the likely extent of involvement that may not be obvious on imaging and therefore demands closer inspection of the volume acquisition. The most important issues are to recognize the lesions as encephalomalacia and to define the extent and severity of the parenchymal involvement for prognostic and surgical planning purposes. The parenchymal damage from insults such as prior meningitis or closed head injuries may be more extensive than would be suggested upon cursory review of the spin echo images. If supported by clinical parameters, such data frequently indicate that the patient is unlikely to be a good surgical candidate.

Pediatric Epilepsy

All of the structural lesions discussed previously can certainly account for seizures in the pediatric population as well. In contrast, the encephalomalacia causing seizures in infants and young children may stem from insults during the intrauterine or perinatal period and are frequently considerably more extensive than the typical cortical infarct that may cause seizures in the adult population (Fig. 6). Moreover, insults that occur before the beginning of the third trimester will not result in reactive astrocytosis that is typical of insults in older children and adults. Hence, the hyperintense T2-signal abnormalities cannot necessarily serve as imaging cues for encephalomalacia in these children. If present, the T2 signal abnormalities can be more difficult to recognize in infants due to the reversal of normal contrast in the brain on conventional MR pulse sequences in infants with immature myelin. The prior insult may also result in a delay in normal myelination, further complicating the diagnosis and potentially causing more diffuse imaging abnormalities. Alternatively, the insult to the developing brain may cause a malformation of cortical development so there may be more than one type of pathology accounting for the child's seizures (dual pathology).

Malformations of cortical development can be focal, lobar, multilobar, hemispheric or more generalized. The dysplasia can arise from an insult to the developing brain but may be genetically predetermined. A malformation of cortical development can arise due to an alteration of the normal pattern of programmed cell death, disruption of the normal neuronal migration, or defective cortical maturation or organization [9-12]. If secondary, the ultimate type and extent of dysplasia likely depends on the nature of the insult during development, the timing of the event relative to the normal developmental processes that are taking place, and whether there is a local or global effect

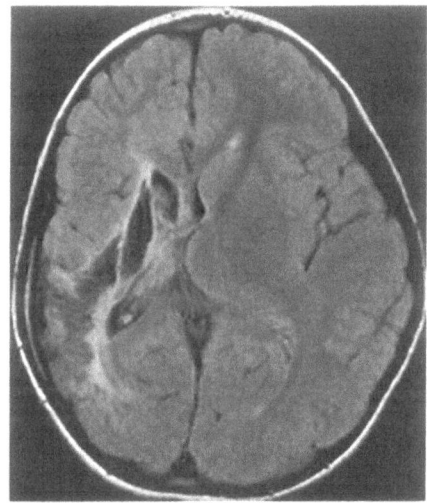

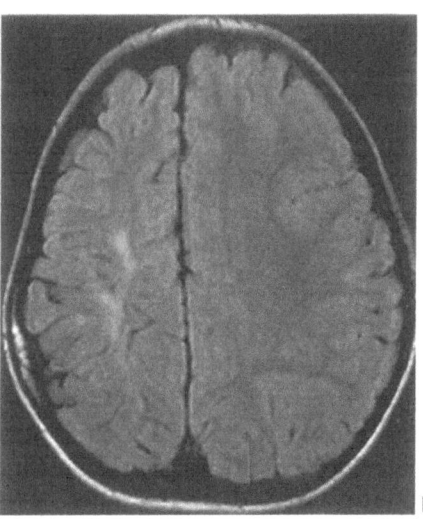

Fig. 6a, b. *Perinatal infarct.* **a** Full-term infant with uncomplicated pregnancy and caesarian section delivery due to position of fetus but apneic episode shortly after delivery. Right middle cerebral artery (MCA) infarct compromising corpus striatum, insular cortex and occipital lobe. **b** Small right cerebral hemisphere with diffuse subtle FLAIR hyperintensity and hemispheric hypometabolism on PET

on the developing brain. These considerations would naturally suggest a wide variety of developmental dysplasias that may be encountered in children and young adults with chronic epilepsy. The various classifications of cortical malformations will not be discussed in this chapter. Instead, this discussion will provide generalizations about their imaging characteristics.

A malformation of cortical development may be suspected by recognizing a significant variation in the normal sulcation pattern in one or multiple regions of the brain. This demands not only familiarity with the normal surface anatomy of the brain but also with the extent of normal variations as many asymmetries likely simply represent sulcation "anomalies" rather than "abnormalities." This detail is generally only apparent on the thin contiguous slices of a high-resolution, gradient echo volume acquisition.

The level of confidence can be improved on imaging findings alone if closer inspection of the cortical architecture demonstrates other asymmetries beyond the sulcation pattern. For example, thickened cortex may be apparent on the conventional spin echo sequences but correlation with the high-resolution 3D acquisition may reveal numerous small gyri or broad flat gyri (suggesting polymicrogyria or pachygyria) that may not be distinguished on the thicker spin echo slices. Even the sagittal T1-weighted images may be especially helpful over the lateral convexities (Fig. 7). Alternatively, the cortex may be more subtly dysmorphic, such as unusually deep or complex cortical infolding compared to the corresponding region in the opposite hemisphere, possibly with localized enlargement of the overlying cerebrospinal fluid (CSF) space or the underlying ventricle.

When cortical developmental abnormalities are isointense to normal tissues, the only visual clue to their presence is a morphologic abnormality. In other cases, the morphologic abnormalities are subtly evident if at all and the dysplasia is recognized by slight differences in signal intensity characteristics in the subcortical white matter with or without similar findings in the overlying cortex. Importantly, there should be no localized mass effect as this might imply neoplasm. The signal abnormalities are generally most evident on FLAIR images in mature brains but can also be seen on T2-weighted spin echo and gradient echo volume studies. The latter two sequences are frequently more helpful during the first year of life when the signal abnormalities may be reversed on these sequences. More commonly, the mild hyperintensity in the cortex and subcortical white matter on FLAIR or T2-weighted images and hypointensity on the gradient echo volume images in older patients may cause blurring of the gray-white matter junction (Fig. 8). The FLAIR and T2-weighted images may also show curvilinear bands of hyperintensity in the region

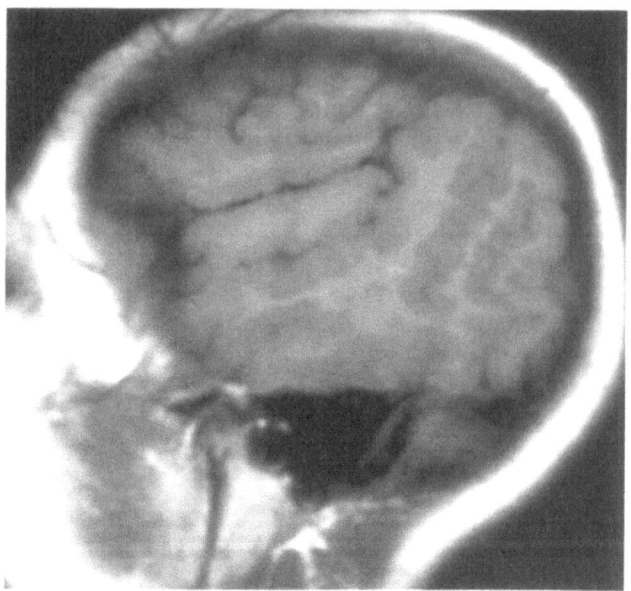

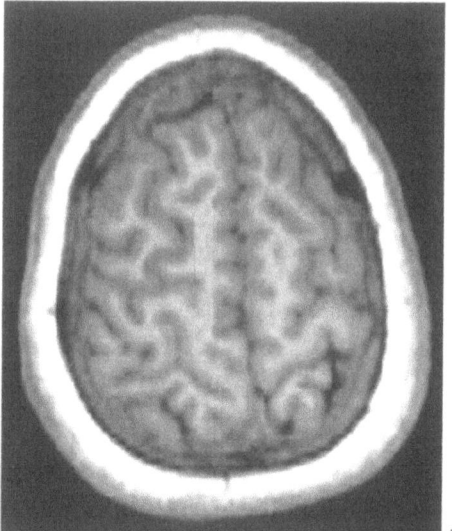

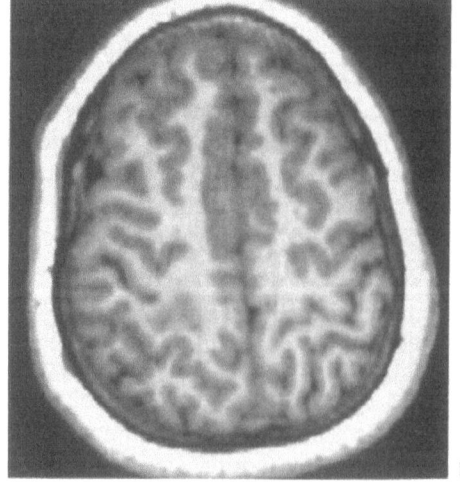

Fig. 7a, b. *Polymicrogyria.* **a** Axial T2-weighted image with asymmetric gyri in the right sylvian region with slight loss in gray-white distinction. **b** Parasagittal T1-weighted image clearly reveals multiple small gyri with thickened cortical mantle reflecting polymicrogyria

Fig. 8a, b. *Focal malformation of cortical development.* **a** Anomalous anterior extension of the superior aspect of the right central sulcus may just be normal variant. **b** Further axial reconstructions of coronal volume sequence show blurring of gray-white junction, distinctly different from adjacent cortex and suggesting focal dysplasia of the subcortical association fibers. When these signal abnormalities extend centrally to the ependymal surface of the underlying ventricle in a conical configuration (apex centrally), the dysplasias are termed transmantle malformations of cortical development (Fig. 9). When the malformations of cortical development are more extensive such as in lesions involving the whole cerebral hemisphere, there may be a combination of different imaging findings in the same patient in view of the variable underlying histology.

Another group of extensive parenchymal disorders in children with epilepsy includes the various neurocutaneous syndromes such as Sturge-Weber syndrome and tuberous sclerosis. Sturge-Weber syndrome or encephalotrigeminal angiomatosis is thought to arise from the persistence of the primordial vasculature present early in the first trimester when the ectoderm responsible for the skin of the face and the neural tube is contiguous. Sturge-Weber syndrome is characterized by a facial port-wine nevus, angioma of the choroid, and angioma of the leptomeninges. The MRI findings are most commonly evident in the parietal occipital region of one cerebral hemisphere but can be frontal, holohemispheric or rarely bilateral and generally correlate with the distribution of the port-wine nevus. Leptomeningeal enhancement on gadolinium-enhanced T1-weighted or FLAIR images indicates the extent of the pial vascular malformation [13, 14]. Generally, there is also evidence of less extensive preferential cortical volume loss, hypointensity in the subcortical white matter on T2-weighted images, enlarged medullary veins, absence of the overlying cortical veins, thickening of the overlying calvarium, and enlarge-

ment of the ipsilateral choroid plexus in the atrium of the lateral ventricle (Fig. 10).

Tuberous sclerosis (Bourneville's disease) is a disorder with autosomal dominant transmission characterized by mental retardation, epilepsy and adenoma sebaceum, but the primary diagnostic criteria include facial angiofibro-

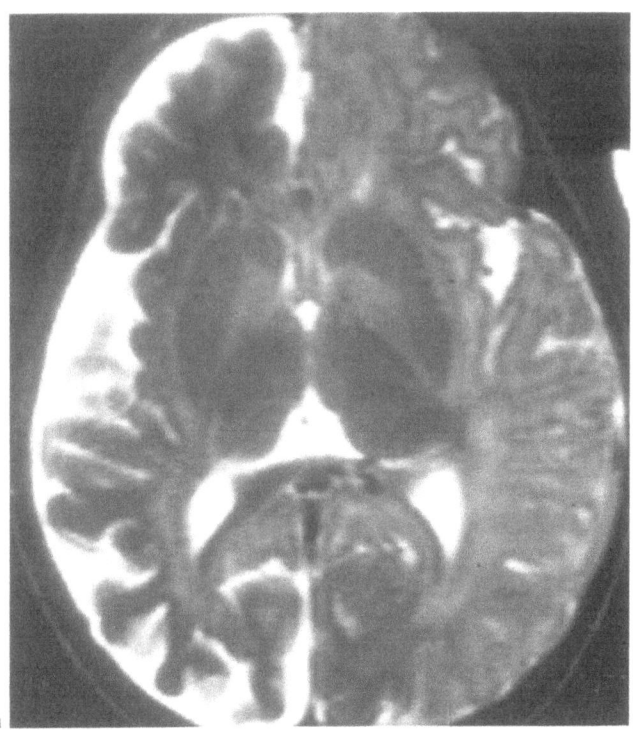

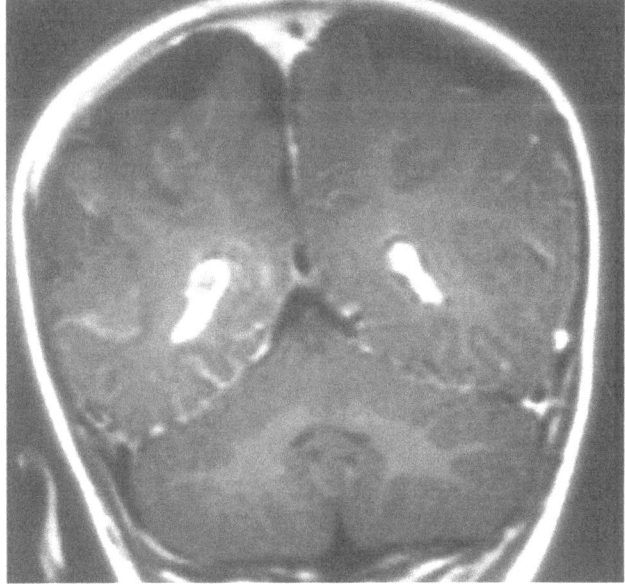

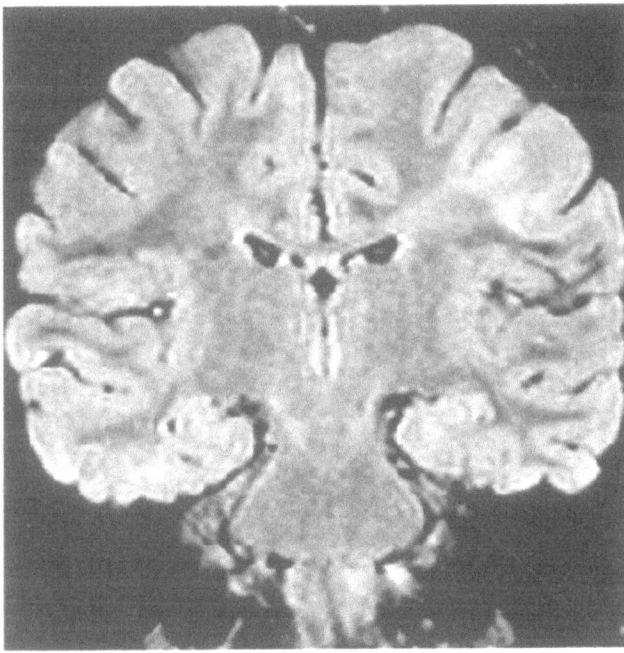

Fig. 9. Transmantle malformation of cortical development. FLAIR image demonstrates band of hyperintensity radiating from the ependymal surface to the cortex and more extensive subcortical hyperintensity along the central sulcus without local mass effect

Fig. 10a, b. *Sturge-Weber syndrome.* **a** Asymmetric volume loss throughout the right hemisphere with preferential cortical involvement and hypointensity in the subcortical white matter on T2-weighted image. **b** Diffuse mild leptomeningeal enhancement of angioma, asymmetrically large choroid plexus in the atrium, and prominent medullary veins

mas, ungual fibromas, retinal astrocytomas, cortical tubers, and subependymal nodules or giant cell astrocytomas. MRI findings include subependymal hamartomas, giant cell tumors, cortical tubers, and radiating white matter lesions [15, 16]. Subependymal hamartomas are recognized as small nodules protruding into the ventricles, most commonly along the course of the caudate nucleus. In the unmyelinated infant brain, these hamartomas are hyperintense on T1-weighted images and hypointense on T2-weighted images. In the older child and adult, these nodules are isointense to white matter on T1-weighted images, iso- or hypointense on T2-weighted images, and demonstrate mild if any enhancement with gadolinium. Giant cell astrocytomas are similar in appearance but occur in the region of the foramina of Monro, enhance prominently with gadolinium or iodinated contrast medium, and increase in size over time. These masses can rarely degenerate into more aggressive neoplasms while the location and propensity for growth may cause obstructive hydrocephalus. Cortical tubers are centered in the subcortical white matter; in unmyelinated brain they are hyperintense on T1-weighted images and hypointense on T2-weighted images, while in mature brain they are iso- or hypointense on T1-weighted images and hyperintense on T2-weighted images. There is generally negligible mass effect and no enhancement with gadolinium. The white matter lesions are hyperintense on T2-weighted images in mature brain and hyperintense on T1-weighted images in immature brain; they may appear nodular or as radiating bands extending from the periventricular region to the overlying cortex (Fig. 11)

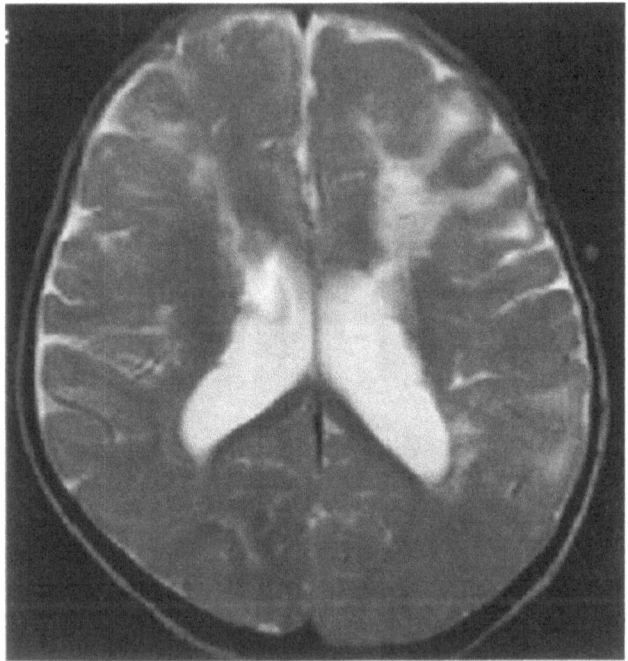

Fig. 11. Tuberous sclerosis. Axial T2-weighted image demonstrates small hypointense subependymal nodular hamartomas, hyperintense subcortical tubers, and hyperintense radiating foci in the intervening deep white matter throughout both cerebral hemispheres

References

1. So EL (1995) Classifications and epidemiologic considerations of epileptic seizures and epilepsy. Neuroimaging Clin N Am 5(4):513-526
2. Greenberg MK, Barsan WG, Starkman S (1996) Neuroimaging in the emergency room patient presenting with seizure. Neurology 47:26-32
3. Maytal J, Krauss JM, Novak G, Nagelberg J, Patel M (2000) The role of brain computed tomography in evaluating children with new onset of seizures in the emergency department. Epilepsia 41(8):950-964
4. Shields WD (1993) Neuroimaging in the diagnosis and management of pediatric epilepsy. In: Dodson WE, Pellock JM (eds) Pediatric epilepsy: diagnosis and therapy. Demos, New York, pp 99-106
5. Spencer SS (1994) The relative contributions of MRI, SPECT, and PET imaging in epilepsy. Epilepsia 35[Suppl 6]:S72-S89
6. Jack CR Jr (1993) Epilepsy: surgery and imaging. Radiology 189:635-646
7. Britton JW, Cascino GD, Sharbrough FW et al (1994) Low-grade glial neoplasms and intractable partial epilepsy: efficacy of surgical treatment. Epilepsia 35:1130-1135
8. Spetzler RF, Martin DDA (1986) A proposed scheme for grading intracranial arteriovenous malformations. J Neurosurg 65:476-483
9. Raymond AA, Fish DR, Sisodiya SM et al (1995) Abnormalities of gyration, heterotopias, tuberous sclerosis, focal cortical dysplasia, microdysgenesis, dysembryoplastic neuroepithelial tumour and dysgenesis of the archicortex in epilepsy: clinical, EEG and neuroimaging features in 100 adult patients. Brain 118:101-131
10. Dobyns WB, Truwitt CL (1995) Lissencephaly and other malformations of cortical development: 1995 update. Neuropediatrics 26:132-147
11. Barkovich AJ, Kuzniecky RI, Dobyns WB et al (1996) A classification scheme for malformations of cortical development. Neuropediatrics 27:59-63
12. Barkovich AJ, Kuzniecky RI, Jackson GD et al (2001) Classification system for malformations of cortical development: update 2001. Neurology 57(12): 2168-2178
13. Benedikt RA, Brown DC, Walker R et al (1993) Sturge-Weber syndrome: cranial MR imaging with Gd-DTPA. AJNR Am J Neuroradiol 14:409-415
14. Griffiths PD, Coley SC, Romanaowski CA et al (2003) Contrast-enhanced fluid-attenuated inversion recovery imaging for leptomeningeal disease in children. Am J Neuroradiol 24:719-723
15. Braffman BH, Bilaniuk LT, Naidich TP et al (1992) MR imaging of tuberous sclerosis: pathogenesis of this phakomatosis, use of gadopentetate dimeglumine, and literature review. Radiology 183:227-238
16. Baron Y, Barkovich AJ (1999) MR imaging of tuberous sclerosis in neonates and young infants. AJNR Am J Neuroradiol 20:907-916

Infectious Diseases of the Central Nervous System

V. Dousset

Neuroradiology Service, CHU Pellegrin, Bordeaux, France

Introduction

Infectious diseases affecting humans have greatly decreased in the past decades because of the use of antibiotics and the increased level of hygiene. However, the central nervous system (CNS) must be seen has a potential target for many organisms that are able to cause severe diseases with striking symptoms.

Imaging technology including computed tomography (CT) and especially magnetic resonance imaging (MRI) have enhanced our ability to characterize infectious processes. MRI techniques such as T2-weighted fast imaging and fluid-attenuated inversion-recovery (FLAIR) make it possible to depict lesions in the brain, spinal cord and meninges. More recently, techniques such as diffusion-weighted imaging and magnetic resonance spectroscopy (MRS) have been applied to inflammatory and infectious lesions, bringing new capabilities for in vivo characterization [1-4]. They have an impact on making the diagnosis and understanding the disease process.

The appearance of inflammatory lesions is a reflection of multiple factors, including the type of organism, mode of spread, host response, and histopathologic findings. Infections spread to the CNS by three potential ways:

1. Hematogenously, either through the choroid plexus or through the blood-brain barrier (BBB). It is now the most frequent origin of infection in the CNS.
2. Direct spread from adjacent structures, such as the sinuses, nasopharynx, or mastoid air cells.
3. Retrograde axoplasmic flow along cranial or peripheral nerves by some viral agents such as herpes.

The imaging features of CNS infections can be classified by the type of organism, location of the lesion, and host response. Organisms infecting the CNS include viruses, mycotic agents, parasites and bacteria. The lesions may be located in one or several of the following sites: cerebrospinal fluid (CSF), meninges, parenchyma, arteries, veins and cranial cavities (e.g. sinuses, mastoid). It is important in an imaging study to look for several locations.

Finally, the host response depends on the host's characteristics:

(a) *Immunocompetent patients (children and adults).* The response is immunologic and most often symptoms and imaging findings are related to the response rather than to the infectious agent. This means that similar imaging features are observed for several organisms, making a specific diagnosis somewhat difficult. There is now evidence for a strong role of the individual's genetic background in the development of an infection in the CNS. Just as prions are infectious only in susceptible individuals, many organisms are probably infective for some individuals and not for others. A transient decrease in the level of immunity may also be responsible for disease development.

(b) *Immunocompromised patients.* This group includes patients with particular conditions or pathologies that lead to an immunodeficient state; these conditions include anticancer chemotherapy, long-term steroid therapy, infection with human immunodeficiency virus (HIV) and diabetes mellitus. These patients are susceptible to infections with opportunistic agents, i.e. pathogens that do not cause disease in immunocompetent persons [5]. HIV has infected more than 60 million people in the world, including 26 million persons in Africa. In the CNS of HIV positive patients, numerous and some very specific agents may develop: HIV virus, *Toxoplasma gondii*, JC virus, tubercolosis, cytomegalovirus (CMV), cryptococcus for the most frequent. CNS type B lymphoma can also develop. In immunocompromised non-HIV patient as in HIV patients, agents such as *Candida albicans*, mucormycosis or nocardia may become pathogenic for the CNS.

(c) *Newborns.* During birth and the first few weeks afterwards, newborn infants can be infected by agents present in the mother's birth channel, for example herpesvirus type 2, Listeria monocytogenes, and urinary germs such as E. coli, *Proteus* and *Candida albicans*.

(d) *Embryo and fetus.* Several infections may develop in utero, sometimes leading to death of the embryo or to

CNS malformations in the fetus. The most frequent agents are *Toxoplasma gondii*, CMV, rubella virus, herpesviruses and HIV [6].

(e) Finally, the immune system may be the origin of CNS manifestations of systemic infections when the immune response to the infectious agent cross-reacts with constitutive proteins of the CNS. The infectious organism is usually absent from the CNS. The most sensitive targets are myelin proteins, leading to acute disseminated encephalomyelitis (ADEM). ADEM is caused by cross-reaction to viruses or bacteria following systemic infection or vaccination. Vasculitis may also be of immunologic origin; in this case a response to a systemic infection leads to cerebral infarct. Some granulomatous diseases (e.g. inflammatory pseudotumor, sarcoidosis) lead to the abnormal collection of normal immune cells in the CNS, mostly in the meninges, facial cavities and cavernous sinus.

I now describe the infections by type of organism affecting the CNS: viruses, prions, bacteria, parasites, fungi, granulomatous infections and immunologic diseases. The immunologic state of the host and the location of the infection are discussed in each section.

Viral Infections

The two main types of viral infections of the CNS are meningitis and encephalitis. Neurological symptoms depend on the location of the infection:

1. *Meningitis due to viruses*, the most frequent infectious disease of immunocompetent hosts, has few imaging manifestations. Waiting for imaging manifestations may unnecessarily delay the time for lumbar puncture and treatment. Enhancement of meninges is rare.

2. *Viral encephalitis* is usually associated with seizure, a decrease of consciousness or focal symptoms such as sensorimotor deficits. Mild mass effect may be seen during the acute phase of encephalitis. Enhancement is often absent early in the course of acute encephalitis unless there is associated meningitis.

Viruses in Immunocompetent Patients

Some viruses may affect both immunocompetent and immunocompromised patients, children, adults and neonates. These virus belong to the groups of herpesviruses, enteroviruses and arboviruses.

Herpesviruses are DNA viruses, and many can cause CNS infections in humans, including herpes simplex viruses 1 and 2, varicella-zoster virus, Epstein-Barr virus, and cytomegalovirus [7, 8].

– *Herpes simplex virus* (HSV1) is the most common cause of sporadic viral meningo-encephalitis. Clinical manifestations include fever, headache, neck stiffness, seizures, focal deficits, and depressed mental state. Because acyclovir therapy is safe, it is recommended that the drug be given on the basis of clinical findings. Encephalitis results from reactivation of latent viral infection of the gasserian (fifth cranial nerve) ganglion. From here, the infection spreads to the parenchyma. The virus has a predilection for the medial area of the temporal, frontal and insular lobes. On CT, low densities are seen on affected areas. There is no enhancement, and only the adjacent meninges may show some congestive changes with little contrast agent uptake. On MRI, hyperintensities are encountered in the temporal, frontal and insular areas, and the bilateral nature of the process is frequently apparent. Initially, the infection may appear unilateral on imaging studies, but over time, involvement of the contralateral temporal and frontal lobes becomes apparent.

– *Herpes simplex virus 2* is the most common cause of neonatal encephalitis. Infection occurs when the fetus passes through the birth canal of a mother with genital herpes. Imaging findings reflect rapid brain destruction. In adults, infections with extension to the spinal cord have been observed.

– *Varicella-zoster virus* produces two distinct clinical syndromes, chicken pox and herpes zoster. Diffuse encephalitis is a rare complication of chicken pox; it is more common in adults and is usually mild. Herpes zoster may lead to an involvement of peripheral and cranial nerves. The affected cranial nerve appears edematous and swollen, and it will enhance at MRI with gadolinium.

– *CMV* infection in adults, seen almost exclusively in immunocompromised patients, leads to ventriculitis and leptomeningitis. Ventriculitis is diagnosed on MRI by the presence of enhancement of ventricle surfaces. The differential diagnosis is subependymal lymphoma. CMV is also the most common cause of congenital encephalitis. It produces massive brain destruction. Infections acquired in the second trimester produce cortical dysplasias.

– *Epstein-Barr virus* has been linked to diverse entities, such as Guillain-Barré syndrome and lymphoma in patients with acquired immune deficiency syndrome (AIDS). About 5% of the patients with infectious mononucleosis develop acute, usually self-limiting encephalomyelitis. This disorder may be responsible for hyperintensities on T2-weighted images of the deep supratentorial gray matter and central gray matter of the spinal cord. Rapid resolution of the lesions has been reported in this disease.

– *Human herpesvirus 6* has been identified as a cause of encephalitis and febrile seizure [8].

Enterovirus may be responsible for meningitis and rarely for encephalitis [1]. In the latter, the spinal cord, medulla, pons, mesencephalon, dentate nucleus of the cerebellum, and occasionally the thalamus may be affected. These structures appear hyperintense on T2-weighted images.

Location of infection in the rhombencephalon and mesencephalon is the predilection of one species of bacteria, *Listeria monocytogenes*.

West Nile virus has emerged in the United States as a new pathogen causing encephalitis [8].

Viruses in Immunocompromised Patients

The CNS of immunocompromised patients may be infected by the same viruses affecting immunocompetent patients. Additionally, other viruses only develop in immunocompromised patients [5, 9]. The human immunodeficiency virus that causes the depletion in immunity may be responsible for encephalitis. Another virus, JC virus, can also cause multifocal encephalitis with destruction of oligodendrocytes.

HIV Encephalitis

HIV-1 is the human RNA retrovirus that causes AIDS. The brain is one of the most commonly affected organs. Almost all patients have the virus in the CNS, and 10%-15% may develop a decrease in mental status or dementia.

The primary infection with HIV may lead to focal abnormal deep white matter spots recognized as hyperintensities on T2-weighted images [10]. These nonspecific signs should be interpreted cautiously since they are frequent in many other conditions such as aging, hypertension, tabacco use and diabetes.

The brain parenchyma is one of the sites of residency of HIV for several years. During the latency phase, before a patient is diagnosed with AIDS, some degree of atrophy may occur.

When immunodepression is strong, HIV itself causes subacute progressive encephalitis. The organism replicates within multinuclear giant cells and macrophages in the white matter [9], causing atrophy, water accumulation in the interstitium but no demyelination, inflammatory changes or focal destruction.

The most common finding on CT or MRI is generalized atrophy without focal abnormalities. Some degree of nonatrophic brain shrinkage is caused by systemic effects of the disease. In severe cases, diffuse symmetric hyperintensity is seen in the supratentorial white matter, predominantly in the periventricular region. Mass effect and enhancement are absent. On T1-weighted images, the white matter appears almost normal or slightly hypointense.

Progressive Multifocal Leukoencephalopathy

Progressive multifocal leukoencephalopathy (PML) is caused by a papovavirus, the JC virus. This virus is ubiquitous in the adult population. It is present in lymph nodes and may reside in the kidneys. When a deep immunodepression is present, usually with CD4 cells below $100/mm^3$, the virus infects the myelin-producing oligodendrocytes, which results in severe demyelination with little inflammatory reaction. Patients complain of focal and progressive neurological impairment with motor or visual function loss or cerebellar syndrome. Demyelination starts at the subcortical white matter, in the U fibers. Areas of demyelination are seen as hypointense signal on T1-weighted images, with high signal intensity on T2-weighted and FLAIR images, without mass effect or enhancement [5]. There is always a strong correlation between the symptoms and the location of the abnormalities on MRI.

In the past, PML was inevitably fatal, with death occurring within 6-12 months of disease onset. The administration of drugs developed to treat HIV, such as protease inhibitors, can stabilize the lesions produced by PML, probably by improving the function of the immune system. Additionally, the incidence of PML, around 5% before the development of antiretroviral drugs, has dropped significantly [11].

Prion Diseases

A group of CNS diseases called transmissible spongiform encephalopathies (TSE) is characterized by spongiform degeneration of neurons in the cortex and subcortical nuclei. TSE have been known to be transmissible since the 1920s, when it was observed that humans in Borneo eating the brain of defeated warriors were affected by a fatal dementia called kuru. Several human and animal diseases produce this distinctive pattern, including kuru, bovine spongiform encephalopathy ("mad cow disease"), scrapie (sheep). There are 4 forms of TSE according to the way of contamination:

1. Creutzfeldt-Jakob disease (CJD), the most frequent (80%) form of TSE, has a spontaneous and sporadic origin. Although spontaneous, tissues from patients affected by CJD may transmit the disease to other humans when injected or grafted. Patients with CJD usually present late in life (>50 years of age) with rapid onset of dementia and myoclonic jerks [12]. Most patients die within a year of the onset of symptoms.
2. Heritable TSE affect families and are known as Gertsmann-Strausler disease and fatal familial insomnia.
3. Iatrogenic TSE are of medical transmission, when patients receive blood transfusions or are grafted with contaminated tissues (hypophysial extracts, dura mater, cornea) from infected donors
4. CDJ variant (vCDJ) is believed to affect patients who have eaten meat from affected cows. The epidemic has affected mostly the United Kingdom with more than 1000 cases and France with 4 cases since 1996. The epidemic is now stopped.

This classification shows the role of an infectious agent which become pathogenic in particular genetic settings. Stanley Prusiner and others have partially elucidated the origin of TSE [13]. Although still controversial, the transmissible agents are likely to be proteins called prions. The normal protein (PrP^c) becomes pathogenic when misfolded, thus becoming insoluble and resistant to heat (PrPres). PrPres are capable of inserting themselves into the cell membrane of neurons and inducing their own reproduction. They produce the spongiform degeneration of the brain.

MRI is becoming the technique of choice for diagnostic orientation. The earliest MRI signs are symmetric basal ganglia and cortical hyperintensities on FLAIR and diffusion-weighted images [14]. In the clinical setting, these signs are quite specific, although not constant. Most cases of Creutzfeldt-Jakob disease are bilateral and symmetric, but the disease may be unilateral. Infarct and Creutzfeldt-Jakob disease can be differentiated on a clinical basis in most cases. Bilateral hyperintensities of the basal ganglia may be seen in deep venous thrombosis, in acute exposure to toxic agents, and in some metabolic disorders. Usually the clinical setting is far different from CJD, making these diagnoses unlikely.

vCJD shows a peculiar MRI sign with a high signal intensity in the pulvinar of the thalami [15]. This sign is however sometimes seen in cases of non-variant CDJ. Lately, atrophy and high signal intensities in white matter are present on MRI studies. Electroencephalography may reveal the presence of triphasic waves that strongly suggest the disease. This sign is however of low sensitivity. CSF may be normal or have increased protein concentration. The 14-3-3 protein may be suggestively, although not specifically, high. The identification of PrPres protein in different organs (e.g. lymphoid organs, amygdala) is necessary to confirm the diagnosis.

Bacterial Infections

Many bacteria enter the CNS via a hematogenous route, by contiguity from the paranasal sinuses, inner ear or middle ear, or through a traumatic or surgical opening in the dura [1]. The infection may affect one or several compartments of the brain at the same time: subdural (empyema) or CSF spaces (meningitis) and the brain parenchyma (encephalitis followed by a circumscribed abscess). Arteries, veins and perivascular Virchow-Robin spaces contribute to the spread of the bacteria from one compartment to another. Furthermore, acute or rapidly progressive thromboses of these vessels lead to additional abnormalities. The infection may also gain the surface of the endothelial wall, making the so-called distal mycotic aneurysms that have a high risk of rupture.

Staphylococcus and *Streptococcus pneumoniae* spread to the CNS either by a hematogenous route or via adjacent cranial structures. Meningococci follow a hematogenous way and produce acute meningitis with high risk of death. Koch's bacilli causing tuberculosis (TB) usually are of hematogenous origin, leading to acute or subacute meningitis or brain abscess. TB affects many people in underdeveloped countries and patients with AIDS worldwide. *Nocardia* affects immunocompromised patients (with AIDS or other conditions)

and causes in many cases brain abscesses, usually contemporarily with chest infection. *Listeria monocytogenes* may affect newborns or patients eating a large amount of bacteria in contaminated foods. The distribution of *L. monocytogenes* is usually the meninges and the rhombencephalum (brain stem and cerebellum) [16]. In neonates, brain abscesses may also be due to urinary germs such as *E. coli* and *Proteus*. *Tropheryma whippelii* causing Whipple's disease is a rare infection, usually but not constantly encountered in patients with digestive malabsorption. Syphilis is becoming a rare cause of CNS infection. It produces mostly chronic meningitis and, in a few cases, granulomas have been described along the cranial nerves. Lyme disease is caused by *Borrelia burgdorferi* and usually produces an infectious and granulomatous involvement of the white matter resembling multiple sclerosis (MS).

Clinical and Imaging Features

Systemic signs of infection (e.g. fever and leukocytosis) may be present. Signs of CNS contamination include the following: neck stiffness and photophobia when meninges are affected, and seizures and focal deficit or cerebellar signs when the parenchyma is involved.

Imaging features are a reflection of the host and are vary according to the type and location of the infection. Techniques such as FLAIR and diffusion-weighted imaging, including the calculation of apparent diffusion coefficient (ADC) maps, are now used routinely in the imaging of inflammatory CNS diseases. On diffusion-weighted images, purulent material is usually hyperintense and the decreased ADC shows the restriction of water motion [2, 17]. Conversely, necrotic tumor debris has variable and heterogeneous intensity and usually an increased ADC. There is of course some overlap, especially in parasitic toxoplasmic abscesses or in punctured bacterial abscesses, which may show increased ADC. Although less routinely used, MRS reveals the presence of amino acids from extracellular proteolysis and bacterial metabolism (e.g. fermentation products), including succinate, acetate, leucine, valine, and alanine that are not seen in necrotic neoplasms [2-4].

Bacterial Meningitis

The diagnosis of bacterial meningitis is confirmed with lumbar puncture, and imaging does not play a primary role in the detection or treatment of this disorder. It is recommended to treat the patients as early as possible without waiting for imaging results. CT may be used to exclude increased intracranial pressure prior to lumbar puncture only when there are clinical doubts. T2-weighted images are usually normal. FLAIR imaging may be helpful in the diagnosis of meningitis, if the clinical presentation is not straightforward. FLAIR shows diffuse subarachnoid hyperintensity while the CSF in the ventricles is dark. Enhancement in the CSF space evokes granulomatous diseases, described later. Tuberculous meningitis may be seen as an enhancement in the cisterna and along the sylvian fissures.

Subdural Empyema

Subdural empyemas produce an acute progressive syndrome characterized by fever, leukocytosis and the rapid development of neurologic abnormalities (e.g. seizure and hemiparesis) [18]. Subdural empyemas may result from direct spread of infection from the paranasal sinuses or the middle ear; they may also be of hematogenous origin or subsequent to meningitis or cerebritis, through the venous structures. Retrograde venous thrombosis leads to cortical venous stasis with marked cortical swelling.

A complete imaging study of the brain and cranial structures is necessary in case of subdural empyema. Subdural empyemas can be difficult to detect, particularly on nonenhanced CT images. The collection is typically narrow. There is disproportionate mass effect, with diffuse swelling of the hemisphere adjacent to the collection [1]. The cortex may appear thickened because of venous stasis. There may be evidence of sinusitis or mastoiditis.

On MR images, the subdural collection is more conspicuous, in particular on FLAIR images where it appears hyperintense to adjacent brain. On diffusion-weighted images, the content may appear bright and ADC values are low. MRS reveals the presence of amino acids. Contrast-enhanced CT and MRI reveal thin enhancement of the deep and superficial membranes of the subdural empyema.

Brain Abscesses

An abscess is the result of the host defense against bacteria that initially produce diffuse cerebritis or encephalitis. Macrophages produce a true collagenous capsule that marks the passage from cerebritis to the abscess phase. On CT, the capsule may appear with a slight increased density. Contrast enhancement with iodine contrast agents shows a regular ring appearance. The capsule made of fibrin and collagen has a typical appearance on MRI: low signal intensity on T2-weighted images and FLAIR, and ring enhancement with gadolinium. Additionally, on FLAIR and T2-weighted images, vasogenic edema (hyperintensity in the subcortical white matter) is present [19].

The central necrotic region is hyperintense on FLAIR images, and isointense to CSF on T2-weighted images. On diffusion imaging the center appears bright, which may be due to "T2 shine-through" effects. On ADC maps, the central necrotic material is hypointense, which confirms the restriction of water motion. In at least two circumstances, the ADC may be increased: in toxoplasmic abscesses and in bacterial abscesses that have been punctured. Nevertheless, the decreased ADC values help to differentiate abscess from necrotic brain tumors or metastases that have increased ADC values. In brain abscesses, MRS with long repetition time (TR) sequences reveals the presence of amino acids that are the proteolytic breakdown and fermentation products unique to bacterial infection. Enhancement persists for up to 8 months.

A peculiar feature of brain abscesses observed on CT and MRI is a miliary pattern, which corresponds to innumerable, small abscesses in the parenchyma. This radiographic pattern develops following the hematogenous spread of Koch's bacillus i.e. *Mycobacterium tubercolosis* producing TB or nocardia.

Mycotic Aneurysms

Intracranial infectious aneurysms are important conditions that are not rare. They usually occur in patients with staphylococcal endocarditis and are called "mycotic" aneurysms [20]. They also develop in intravenous drug abusers [21]. Their imaging presentation is usually a small mass in the subarachnoid space near the cortex with strong enhancement. They may rupture, leading to subarachnoid hemorrhage with high risk of death. They also can be revealed by focal infarcts or seizures. Stroke may occur without infective aneurysms in patients with valve endocarditis [22]. Nonruptured aneurysms may disappear with antibiotic therapy. Ruptured and sometimes nonruptured aneurysms need endovascular treatment or surgical clipping.

Parasitic Infections

The most common parasites that infect the CNS are [23]:
1. *Taenia solium* from undercooked pork, responsible for neurocysticercosis
2. *Taenia echinococcus granulosus* from the dog, responsible for hydatid cysts
3. *Taenia echinococcus multilocularis* from the fox
4. *Toxoplasma gondii* that develops in the CNS of HIV-infected patients
5. *Toxocara canis* and *Toxocara cati* that produce CNS manifestations in children
6. *Paragonimus*, from infected crabs or crayfish

Other parasitic infections, including sparganosis, trichinosis and amebiasis, may also develop or manifest in the CNS.

The three taenia usually produce cystic lesions; symptoms often arise only after the death of the parasite, when the host response occurs. Thus, the cystic wall is completely different from the capsule of a brain abscess. The cystic wall has a parasitic origin (not from the host) and it is not detectable by the host immunologic system until the larva dies. However, the location of the cyst may be responsible for symptoms such as seizures, mass effect or CSF occlusion, before the death of the parasite.

Cysticercosis

The larvae of *Taenia solium* enter the intestinal wall and develop in the brain, subarachnoid space or ventricles

[24]. Once the scolex is established, it makes itself immunologically invisible to the host and therefore incites no inflammatory reaction. Live cysts are isointense to CSF on all pulse sequences. No enhancement is seen within the cyst wall while the organism is alive. The scolex may be seen as a 2- to 4-mm mural nodule in the cyst wall. There is no associated edema [1].

When the organism dies, an inflammatory granulomatous response occurs. The clinical manifestations are seizures or focal deficits. The wall enhances, and there is associated vasogenic edema. The dead cyst commonly calcifies. Patients treated with praziquantel may develop acute symptoms because of the simultaneous death of all live cysts. Subarachnoid cysts may often produce secondary obstructive hydrocephalus.

Hydatid Cysts

Human echinococcis occurs by accidental ingestion of contaminated dog feces. The disease is endemic. The most common sites of development in humans are the liver, lung and bone. Brain is affected in less than 5% of patients. It is usually a single, unilocular and quite large cyst. When the cyst ruptures it produces an inflammatory reaction.

Echinococcus multilocularis causes a rare parasitic infection that usually has a fatal outcome. The cysts are recognized because they resemble a bunch of grapes.

Toxoplasmosis

Toxoplasma gondii is distributed worldwide and infects more than 500 million humans [25]. It does not cause intracranial infections in immunocompetent hosts and therefore was rarely seen prior to the onset of the AIDS epidemic. However, toxoplasmosis may infect the embryo, producing cerebral malformations and intracranial calcifications.

Toxoplasmosis is the most common cerebral mass lesion encountered in the HIV-positive patient [25]. This is the first diagnosis to consider when CNS manifestations occur with rapid progression in HIV-infected patients. The imaging appearance may be ubiquitous but antibiotic treatment is efficient. Thus, AIDS patients with rapid CNS manifestations should be treated for toxoplasmosis regardless of the imaging features. The diagnosis may be reconsidered if treatment is inefficient. With HAART treatment, the incidence of toxoplasmosis has dropped [11]. Now, toxoplasmosis is encountered in patients who ignore their viral status for HIV. It is not rare that patients presenting inaugural seizures and several brain lesions are positive for HIV. This diagnosis must be considered by the radiologist.

Although grossly identical to an abscess, the lesion is not encapsulated, which accounts for the histologic classification of encephalitis rather than abscess [1]. In the majority of cases, multiple mass lesions are present, and they may be located anywhere within the brain.

The imaging findings at the beginning include a mass effect without or with slight, not well demarcated, contrast enhancement. Lately, the enhancement is quite similar to an abscess, like a ring. The central necrosis is typically hyperintense on FLAIR and T2-weighted images. Diffusion-weighted imaging reveals heterogeneous intensity and the ADC is usually increased. Hemorrhage is not present at the time of initial diagnosis. Signs of hemorrhage appear when the patient is treated with antibiotics. High signal intensity from methemoglobin is seen on nonenhanced T1-weighted images, leading to confirmation of the diagnosis in patients under treatment.

In patients who are not improving with antibiotics, the diagnosis of toxoplasmosis must be reconsidered with the primary goal of differentiating toxoplasmosis from lymphoma. Although it is rare, lymphoma is the second most common cause of mass lesions in patients with AIDS [25]. Lymphoma lesions are usually single and located in the deep gray and white matters (basal ganglia and corpus callosum). Lymphoma is often hypointense on T2-weighted images. There is mild adjacent edema with a mass effect lower than expected. Enhancement is usually diffuse but may be of a ring appearance, especially when the lesion is superior to 3.5 cm. Single photon emission CT (SPECT) with radioactive thallium can be used to confirm the diagnosis of lymphoma prior to therapy. Inflammatory lesions, including toxoplasmosis, are negative on SPECT, while lymphoma is positive. When the diagnosis cannot be established noninvasively, biopsy is necessary. Non-Hodgkin's lymphoma type B is the most common. Its outcome is unfortunately fatal.

Infections with *Toxocara canis* and *Toxocara cati*

These parasites are dog and cat nematodes. Human infection occurs by accidental ingestion of their eggs passed from pet animals. The liver, lung and peritoneum are most frequently involved. They produce focal lesions in the white matter that spontaneously resolve. Vasculitis or ganulomas around the larvae may form in the parenchyma.

Fungal Infections

Fungal CNS infections are possible in susceptible populations, such as immunocompromised patients with AIDS, patients with leukemia, diabetes mellitus or renal diseases, those under aggressive chemotherapy, and intravenous drug abusers using unsterilized materials [26]. The most frequent fungal infections are cryptococcosis due to *Cryptococcus neoformans*, aspergillosis, mucormycosis, candidiasis and histoplasmosis.

The patient with *cryptoccocosis* usually presents with meningoencephalitis [26]. The infection is fatal without appropriate treatment using amphotericin B. Lumbar puncture is the single most useful test. After infecting the CSF, the organisms may extend along the perforating arteries in the perivascular Virchow-Robin spaces. The signal intensity is similar to that of the cerebrospinal fluid. Cerebral edema rarely occurs.

Aspergillosis is relatively rare in the AIDS population, but is more common in patients under corticosteroid therapy. The organisms invade the lung parenchyma and spread hematogenously. Aspergillus may also gain the CNS via direct spread from the paranasal sinuses or orbits. Aspergillous abscesses have a non-specific appearance.

Most patients with *mucormycosis* are diabetic. The pathology of infection is similar to that of aspergillosis. Rhinocerebral mucormycosis is a common feature.

Granulomatous Infections and Immunoreactive Diseases

Granulomatous Infections

Granulomas correspond to cellular mass with T cells, macrophages and histiocytes without liquefied necrotic debris. Caseous ("cheesy") necrosis is typical of tuberculous granulomas.

Granulomatous infections can result from diverse pathogens, including bacteria (*Mycobacterium*, *Nocardia*, *Actinomyces*, spirochetes), fungi (*Aspergillus* or *Mucorales*), and parasites. Sarcoidosis is an idiopathic granulomatous disease that most commonly affects young, otherwise healthy adult patients [27]. Most granulomatous infections affect the meninges. The brain parenchyma may be involved, usually by the spread of the granuloma along the perivascular Virchow-Robin spaces. Inflammatory pseudotumor may also affect the cavernous sinuses, the orbits and rarely the hypophysial sellae.

CT and MRI features of granulomatous meningitis are cisternal enhancement, usually following the vessel routes. Thus, contrast-enhanced images are critical in establishing the diagnosis of granulomatous meningitis. Basal meningitis often leads to hydrocephalus. There is often compromise of the vascular system with secondary infarction or hemorrhage. The combination of hydrocephalus and deep infarction in a young adult should therefore always raise the suspicion of granulomatous meningitis [1].

The differential diagnosis of granulomatous infectious meningitis is neoplastic carcinomatous meningitis [28]. It has a predilection for the retrocerebellar cisterns. Sarcoidosis has a predilection for the suprasellar cistern, often producing thickening of the pituitary stalk [27]. Enhancement along the course of the cranial nerves is characteristic of sarcoidosis but can also be seen in lymphoma.

Vasculitis

Vasculitis may be the result of direct spread from the leptomeninges along the perivascular spaces or from direct invasion and growth within the vessel lumen. It also can be the result of an immune reaction at the endothelial level without infectious agents. Infarcts occur in the deep gray matter or in the cortex.

Acute Disseminated Encephalomyelitis

Acute disseminated encephalomyelitis (ADEM) is an autoimmune disorder that is similar to multiple sclerosis except that it is monophasic [29]. ADEM occurs with a latency of one to several weeks after viral exposure or vaccination. In most of the cases, multiple lesions are present at the same time in the white matter, affecting the gray matter in at least one-third of cases. The disease may produce multifocal demyelination similar to viral encephalitis or multiple sclerosis. Enhancement is inconstant, although frequent. In most cases the evolution is good with steroid therapy. Death is possible in the most severe cases.

References

1. Zimmerman RD (2000) Infection. In: RSNA categorial course in diagnostic radiology: neuroradiology. Radiological Society of North America, Chicago, pp 45-63
2. Lai PH, Ho JT, Chen WL et al (2002) Brain abscess and necrotic brain tumor: discrimination with proton MR spectroscopy and diffusion-weighted imaging. AJNR Am J Neuroradiol 23:1369-1377
3. Cecil KM, Lenkinski RE (1998) Proton MR spectroscopy in inflammatory and infectious brain disorders. Neuroimaging Clin N Am 8:863-880
4. Burtscher IM, Holtas M (1999) In vivo proton MR spectroscopy of untreated and treated brain abscesses. AJNR Am J Neuroradiol 20:1049-1053
5. Post MJD, Sheldon JJ, Hensley GT et al (1986) Central nervous system disease in acquired immunodeficiency syndrome: prospective correlation using CT, MR imaging, and pathologic studies. Radiology 158:141-148
6. Osborn RE, Byrd SE (1991) Congenital infections of the brain. Neuroimaging Clin N Am 1:105-118
7. Tien RD, Felsberg GJ, Osumi AK (1993) Herpesvirus infections of the CNS: MR findings. AJR Am J Roentgenol 161:167-176
8. Bonthius DJ, Karacay B (2002) Meningitis and encephalitis in children. An update. Neurol Clin 20:1013-1038
9. Dal Canto MC (1997) Mechanisms of HIV infection of the central nervous system and pathogenesis of AIDS-dementia complex. Neuroimaging Clin N Am 7:231-242
10. Trotot PM, Gray F (1997) Diagnostic imaging contribution in the early stages of HIV infection of the brain. Neuroimaging Clin N Am 7:243-260
11. Gray F, Chretien F, Vallat-Decouvelaere AV, Scaravilli F (2003) The changing pattern of HIV neuropathology in the HAART. J Neuropathol Exp Neurol 62:429-440
12. Martindale JL, Geschwind MD, Miller BL (2003) Psychiatric and neuroimaging findings in Creutzfeldt-Jakob disease. Curr Psychiatry Rep 5:43-46
13. Prusiner SB (1987) Prions and neurodegenerative disease. N Engl J Med 317:1571-1581
14. Collie DA, Sellar RJ, Zeidler M, Colchester AC, Knight R, Will RG (2001) MRI of Creutzfeldt-Jakob disease: imaging features and recommended MRI protocol. Clin Radiol 56:726-739

15. Collie DA, Summers DM, Sellar RJ et al (2003) Diagnosing variant Creutzfeldt-Jakob disease with the pulvinar sign: MR imaging findings in 86 neuropathologically confirmed cases. AJNR Am J Neuroradiol 24:1560-1569

16. Maezawa Y, Hirasawa A, Abe T et al (2002) Successful treatment of listerial brain abscess: a case report and literature review. Intern Med 41:1073-1078

17. Desprechins B, Stadnik T, Koerts G, Shabana W, Breucq C, Osteaux M (1999) Use of diffusion-weighted MR imaging in differential diagnosis between intracerebral necrotic tumors and cerebral abscesses. AJNR Am J Neuroradiol 20:1252-1257

18. Rich PM, Deasy NP, Jarosz JM (2000) Intracranial dural empyema. Br J Radiol 73:1329-1336

19. Zimmerman RD, Weingarten KW (1991) Neuroimaging of cerebral abscess. Neuroimaging Clin N Am 1:1-16

20. Phuong LK, Link M, Widjdicks E (2002) Management of intracranial infectious aneurysms: a series of 16 cases. Neurosurgery 51:1145-1151

21. Tunkel AR, Pradhan SK (2002) Central nervous system infections in injection drug users. Infect Dis Clin North Am 16:589-605

22. Anderson DJ, Goldstein LB, Wilkinson WE et al (2003) Stroke location, characterization, severity, and outcome in mitral vs aortic valve endocarditis. Neurology 61:1341-1346

23. Chang KH, Cho YS, Hesselink JR, Han MH, Han MC (1991) Parasitic diseases of the central nervous system. Neuroimaging Clin N Am 1:159-178

24. Del Brutto OH, Rajshekhar V, White AC Jr et al (2001) Proposed diagnostic criteria for neurocysticercosis. Neurology 57:177-183

25. Ramsey RG, Dean AD (1997) Central nervous system toxoplasmosis. Neuroimaging Clin N Am 7:171-186

26. Harris DE, Enterline DS (1997) Fungal infections of the central nervous system. Neuroimaging Clin N Am 7:187-198

27. Ulmer JL, Elster AD (1991) Sarcoidosis of the central nervous system. Neuroimaging Clin N Am 1:141-150

28. Aparicio A, Chamberlain MC (2002) Neoplastic meningitis. Curr Neurol Neurosci Rep 2:225-235

29. Talbot PJ, Arnold D, Antel JP (2001) Virus-induced autoimmune reactions in the CNS. Curr Top Microbiol Immunol 253:247-271

Cerebral Infections

D. Mikulis

University of Toronto, Toronto, Canada

Introduction

The broad categories of diseases that afflict human beings continue to evolve as do the methods used to detect and evaluate them. Although most of the infectious diseases that affect the brain remain the same, there are a number of unusual infections that have appeared. Infectious agents are opportunists and will take advantage of weaknesses in the immune system that appear under a variety of conditions. Medical advances have lead to treatments and therapies that compromise the immune system. How, and under what setting, these defects in the immune system appear influences the type of organism that invades and how the host responds to it. Manipulation of the immune response in the setting of transplantation and the appearance of acquired immune deficiency syndrome (AIDS) are examples in which unusual infections occur.

Conventional magnetic resonance imaging (MRI) methods have become the mainstay for evaluation of cerebral infections. Functional MRI methods, such as diffusion imaging and proton spectroscopy, that look at specific characteristics of the tissues have further improved this capability. In view of these considerations, the information provided here focuses on the broad categories of infectious diseases that affect the brain, including those infections that appear in the immunocompromised host. The contribution that diffusion imaging and magnetic resonance spectroscopy (MRS) offer are also discussed.

Cerebral Abscess

In the pre-antibiotic era, brain abscesses were most commonly caused by direct extension from infected paranasal sinuses. Now, the most common source is blood-borne bacterial seeding originating from infections elsewhere in the body. The abscess initially begins as a region of cerebral inflammation or cerebritis that progresses to form a pus-filled cavity with a fibro-glial capsule. The typical abscess has a relatively thin, smooth wall showing intense contrast enhancement on computed tomography (CT) or MRI. Edema in the adjacent white matter is common. The abscess wall can appear bright on T1-weighted images. This is thought to be the result of a T1-shortening effect related to constituents in white cells [1]. The critical imaging issue, however, revolves around the similarity that a brain abscess can have with neoplastic diseases, especially metastases. Both commonly show ring enhancement following contrast medium administration. How then, can they be distinguished? In general, the enhancing ring of an abscess is thin and quite smooth as opposed to a neoplasm where some irregularity or nodularity is present. The deepest portion of the abscess wall that "points" to the ventricular system may be thinner than other portions of the rim. However, these features are not reliable as metastases can have "perfect" enhancing rims, and abscesses can often have irregular margins.

Increases in diagnostic specificity can be gained through application of diffusion methods and MRS. Abscess cavities on MR diffusion imaging typically show restricted water movement similar to that seen with acute ischemic stroke. Although the reason for this restriction has not been established, it is tempting to assume that it is related to dead or dying white cells "absorbing" any available extracellular water, analogous to the proposed mechanism for ischemic neurons and glia in ischemic stroke. One caveat is that metastases composed of cells with high nuclear to cytoplasmic ratios or cells that produce large amounts of proteinaceous material (mucin) can also have ring enhancement and restricted water movement.

Perhaps the most important contribution that MRS has made in the diagnosis of cerebral diseases is the ability to detect bacteria by their metabolic signatures. Certain byproducts of bacterial metabolism are not seen in mammals in spectroscopically significant concentrations. Proton MRS is capable of detecting some of these substances such as succinate and acetate as unique peaks in the spectra. However, treatment with antibiotics prior to MRS may reduce these metabolites to undetectable levels. Amino acids, produced by proteases released by white cells as part of the inflammatory response, can also be detected using proton MRS (Table 1). This is rele-

Table 1. Amino acid peaks on proton magnetic resonance spectroscopy (MRS) and their resonant frequencies in parts per million (ppm)

Metabolite	Resonant frequency (ppm)
Broad amino acid peak (valine, leucine, and isoleucine)[a]	0.9
Alanine[b]	1.4 and 1.6, doublet
Succinate	2.4
Acetate	1.9
Pyruvate	2.4

[a] Shows phase reversal at echo time (TE) = 135 ms
[b] Shows phase reversal at TE = 135 ms; peak at 1.4 ppm overlaps with peak of lactate doublet; can be seen in meningiomas and in cases of demyelination

vant since large amounts of amino acids are not seen in normal brain or in other disease processes. They are present even if antibiotics have been administered.

The expected utility of MRS should therefore be quite high in screening patients suspected of having brain abscesses. However, in modern practice, most patients have already been started on antibiotic treatment by the time MRI is performed. In my experience, the presence of bacterial metabolites in patients previously treated with antibiotics is null. My colleagues and I have also failed to consistently detect amino acids. From the practical point of view, these deficiencies coupled with the difficulty in acquiring adequate spectra in sick patients who are unable to cooperate for long spectroscopic acquisitions have diminished the value of MRS. The promise of faster acquisitions through new multicoil parallel imaging techniques should improve the applicability of MRS in these patients.

In spite of these issues, the value of MRS may ultimately be in the ability to monitor therapeutic efficacy. Declines in acetate and pyruvate have been reported one week after aspiration and medical treatment in 5 patients with bacterial abscesses. Furthermore, these declines correlated with positive responses to treatment [2]. Experience with MRS for the assessment of brain abscesses is at an early stage and additional prospective investigation with larger studies is needed. Information concerning the incidence and the effect of antibiotics on specific spectral peaks would be useful in determining the sensitivity and specificity of MRS in general.

Tuberculoma and Tuberculous Abscess

Tuberculoma by definition is a parenchymal infection in which granulomas are found, whereas a tuberculous abscess contains pus devoid of granulomas and caseation. Both may show ring enhancement. Tuberculomas usually have decreased T2 signal surrounded by T2-bright edema in the adjacent brain, whereas the tuberculous abscess is bright on T2-weighted images with a hypointense wall.

There is some evidence that diffusion-weighted images and apparent diffusion coefficients (ADC) are normal in tuberculomas whereas restriction of water movement is seen in tuberculous abscesses [3]. MRS has shown that there are differences between bacterial and mycobacterial brain abscesses. Although both can have elevations in lipid and lactate, there is a conspicuous absence of the peaks indicated in Table 1 in mycobacterial infections [4]. Tuberculomas may also show an elevated lipid peak related to caseation.

Meningitis

The diagnosis of bacterial meningitis is almost always based on clinical presentation that consists of high fever, signs of meningismus, and a rapidly decreasing level of consciousness. Imaging is usually performed to assess the status of the ventricles prior to lumbar puncture since hydrocephalus is a relative contraindication to this procedure. CT can show evidence of increased attenuation in the basal cisterns and sulci due to high concentrations of inflammatory cells. This must not be confused with subarachnoid hemorrhage since both can show increased attenuation in the basal cisterns [5]. Vessels in the subarachnoid space can become directly involved in the inflammatory process with necrotizing panarteritis and septic thrombophlebitis causing ischemic injury to the brain. In addition, the inflammatory process can extend directly into the brain resulting in meningoencephalitis. Hydrocephalus occurs in most patients, resulting in increased intracranial pressure that further compromises blood flow. These secondary manifestations of the meningeal infection can be detected with diffusion imaging which shows the extent of acute cortical ischemic injury. However, direct infection causing cerebritis can have a similar appearance with evidence of restricted water movement [6]. We have rarely performed MRI in the assessment of acute meningitis since all patients initially receive broad-spectrum antibiotics and imaging would not alter subsequent management.

Imaging does play a role in the detection and management of less fulminant forms of meningitis. Tuberculous meningitis, for example, can initially be quite indolent with patients presenting with headache and cranial neuropathies. Untreated, the disease can progress rather suddenly with high mortality. Lumbar puncture may show no growth of the bacillus, but there is usually an elevation in the white cell count and protein level. Precontrast MRI can be normal although FLAIR images may show increased signal in the sulci when cerebrospinal fluid (CSF) protein is sufficiently elevated [7]. Gadolinium-enhanced acquisitions can show striking enhancement of the leptomeninges. Tuberculous pachymenigeal involvement can also occur [8].

Patients with immune deficiencies are also susceptible to tuberculous meningitis, but in addition, fungal, viral and treponemal forms of the disease must be considered, including cryptococcal, varicella-zoster, cytomegalovirus, and neurosyphilis. Although these other agents can be associated with leptomeningeal enhancement [9, 10], tuberculous meningitis typically produces an intense diffuse or nodular pattern of enhancement in the basal cisterns. Meningeal enhancement is uncommon in viral meningitis with MRI giving normal results unless an encephalitic component develops with signal changes in the parenchyma.

Encephalitis

Encephalitis can be divided into two groups (Table 2). In the first group, the virus is transmitted to humans via an insect vector (e.g. ticks and mosquitoes). Viruses in the second group infect the brain primarily. Brain inflammation can also occur as a complication of viral infections such as measles, mumps and chicken pox, or in autoimmune disorders such as multiple sclerosis or Rasmussen's encephalitis, but these diseases are not considered here. Although Creutzfeldt-Jacob disease (CJD) may not be infectious disease in the true sense, the behavior of this agent mimics an infection and is discussed.

In view of the number of viruses that can infect the central nervous system (CNS), time and space limitations impose limits on the subsequent discussion. Emphasis is therefore placed on adult herpes encephalitis. However, in order to stay current, I draw from my own experience to discuss the recent outbreak of West Nile virus in North America. Viral infections that occur in immunodeficient individuals are discussed in a separate section.

Table 2. Some agents causing encephalitis, by infectious route. Group 1 agents require an insect vector, while group 2 agents infect the brain directly

Group 1.	Arbovirus encephalitic agents:
	St. Louis encephalitis virus
	Japanese B virus
	Equine encephalomyelitis virus
	Russian spring-summer encephalitis virus
	Louping ill virus
	Powassan virus
	Colorado tick fever virus
	California encephalitis virus
	West Nile virus
Group 2.	Primary infective agents:
	Herpes simplex
	Cytomegalovirus
	Epstein-Barr virus
	JC virus (progressive multifocal leukoencephalopathy, PML)
	Rabies
	Human immunodeficiency virus (HIV), LAV/HTLV-III or AIDS virus
	Subacute sclerosing panencephalitis (from reactivation of latent measles virus)

Herpes Simplex Virus

Herpes simplex encephalitis is the most common sporadic viral infection in the Western world [11]. The virus resides in the trigeminal ganglion and is usually benign except when it produces lesions in the oral mucosa. Rarely does the virus re-activate to produce encephalitis. In general terms, the disease should be considered in any patient presenting with acute mental status changes and parenchymal signal abnormalities in the temporal lobe. Clinical outcome depends on early recognition and institution of antiviral treatment (e.g. acyclovir). Unilateral presentation is common. I have even observed redevelopment of the infection in the contralateral temporal lobe several months after successful treatment of the initial infection.

CT in the early stages of the infection gives normal images. MRI is capable of showing decreased T1 and increased T2 involving the mesial temporal lobes and insular cortex. As the disease progresses, signal enhancement with gadolinium can develop and the lesions can become hemorrhagic. Diffusion imaging can show evidence of both increased and decreased water mobilities. The areas of the parenchyma with restricted water movement, presumably representing cytotoxic edema, were often associated with lesions that had minimal T2 signal changes, while those areas that showed increased water movement, indicating vasogenic edema, had prominent increases in T2 signal [12].

Although not proven, there is some evidence that cytotoxic edema is seen early in viral encephalitis, perhaps as a result of premorbid changes in the cell (swelling) as the virus takes over cellular machinery [13]. Vasogenic edema appears later as the cells rupture. Alternatively, infectious load may be the controlling factor. This concept is supported by findings observed in vitro when cells are infected with West Nile virus [14]. If the cells are exposed to a high infectious load, they become swollen and rupture due to high viral budding and to loss of membrane integrity. High mobility group 1 (HMGB1) protein, a proinflammatory cytokine, is then released into the extracellular space. This protein is a proinflammatory cytokine that in vivo leads to inflammation and vasogenic edema. If the infectious load is low, delayed cell death occurs due to apoptosis. This model therefore supports a similar temporal pattern of cytotoxic edema followed by vasogenic edema.

West Nile Virus

Prior to 1999, West Nile virus (WNV) was confined to Africa, the Middle East, and Asia. The first North American cases occurred in New York in 1999. The first Canadian case was reported in Ontario in 2001 [15]. As of 2002, WNV had spread to 44 states across the US and to 5 Canadian provinces. In 2002, there were 4156 cases of West Nile virus reported to the Centers for Disease Control in Atlanta, with 284 fatalities. In 2003, there were 8912 cases with 211 deaths [16]. Spread to Europe is now becoming a significant concern [17].

Fortunately, most WNV infections are mild with no clinical symptoms. Approximately 20% of cases have mild illness lasting 3-6 days and consisting of malaise, headache, anorexia, myalgia, nausea, vomiting, or rash. One in 150 cases develop severe neurological disease consisting of meningitis or encephalitis.

Imaging reports of these severe cases are now becoming available. The type of CNS involvement is different from that seen with herpes. WNV tends to involve the brain stem, cerebellum, and thalami. CT images are frequently normal, however MRI shows increased T2 signal with evidence of swelling within these structures. As opposed to herpes infection, the neocortex is not usually involved by WNV infection. Gadolinium enhancement is not usually present except in the setting of meningitis where leptomeningeal enhancement occurs. The spinal cord and cauda equina can also be affected. Some patients present with myeloradiculopathy similar to that seen with Guillain-Barré syndrome. Enhancement of the pia along the spinal cord and cauda equina has been observed. Parenchymal signal changes can also occur within the spinal cord. Pathologic changes in the spinal cord resemble poliomyelitis [18]. My colleagues and I reported a case in which diffusion imaging during the early phase of the disease showed marked restriction of water movement in the pons at a time when conventional sequences were normal. Later in the disease water diffusion became markedly increased in pons [13]. As suggested previously, this changing pattern of water diffusion may be a signature of viral brain infections, but much work needs to be done to confirm this.

Little information is available concerning MRS and encephalitis. Acquiring diagnostic spectra from the temporal lobe, brain stem, cerebellum, and thalamus is challenging due to shimming problems that arise from tissues near the skull base. This is made even more difficult in uncooperative patients. Spectral similarities with brain tumors, showing elevations in choline and reductions in N-acetylaspartic acid (NAA), have been reported [19]. However, there are no specific spectroscopic features diagnostic of encephalitis. Clearly, much more work needs to be done in this area.

Prion Diseases

Scrapie, bovine spongiform encephalopathy, kuru, and CJD are examples of prion (from "proteinaceous" and "infectious") diseases causing spongiform encephalopathy. Scrapie occurs in sheep and goats. Kuru is found in New Guinea tribes that practice cannibalism. Bovine spongiform encephalopathy has been linked with variant Creutzfeldt-Jakob disease that occurs in humans. In addition to the variant form, which is probably of greatest concern since it may be propagated through food (eating contaminated beef), sporadic and familial forms also exist.

These diseases have a common theme in that the responsible agent is thought to be a misfolded prion protein that induces further misfolding of normal prion proteins into protease-resistant aggregates. These accumulate and cause progressive cerebral degeneration over a period of 3-6 months leading to death. A viral etiology or carrier, however, has not been completely ruled out as the cause of this disease [20].

The most important neuropathological feature from the neuroimaging standpoint is cytoplasmic vacuolization which is most likely responsible for the decreases in water diffusion observed on MR diffusion imaging [21]. Ultrastucturally, the cytoplasmic vacuoles contain a proliferation of membranes in a "labyrinth-like manner" explaining the restriction in water movement [22]. There is also extensive gliosis in areas of neuronal loss, explaining the elevations in T2 relaxation [23]. However, these theories may not be correct as there is evidence that T2 and ADC signal abnormalities correlate with sites of abnormal prion protein deposition and not the presence of vacuoles or gliosis [24]. T2 and ADC abnormalities do evolve as the disease progresses. It has been suggested that in the initial phase of the disease, signal behavior is influenced by vacuoles in intact neurons, with diffusion imaging more sensitive than T2-weighted or FLAIR imaging. Later in the disease, as neurons disappear and are replaced by gliotic tissue, ADC may normalize and T2 abnormalities gain prominence [25].

Many unanswered questions remain. For example, it is not known if imaging can be used to distinguish the different types of prion diseases. In my experience, there are two different imaging patterns. The first is the more classic pattern in which there is involvement of the striatum and thalamus (especially the pulvinar and dorsomedial nuclei). The second is a somewhat random involvement of the cortex. As we gain more experience with the disease, we may find that the first pattern evolves into the second as the disease progresses. Table 3 summarizes the

Table 3. Imaging findings observed in prion disease

Imaging technique	Observations
T2-weighted and FLAIR MR imaging	Pattern 1: Increased SI in striatum and thalamus Pattern 2: Increased SI in cortex (patchy)[a]
Diffusion-weighted imaging	Increased SI (may change with disease progression)
Apparent diffusion coefficient	Decreased (may change with disease progression)
Post-gadolinium T1-weighted MR imaging	No enhancement
Magnetic resonance spectroscopy	Decreased NAA
Brain morphology	Atrophy develops as disease progresses

[a] Pattern 1 may evolve into or be coexistent with pattern 2
SI, signal intensity; NAA, N-acetylaspartate

imaging findings observed in prion disease. There are few MRS studies in patients with prion disease. It appears that MRS can detect neuronal loss, showing areas of reduced NAA, but there are no specific metabolites unique to prion disease [26].

Parasites

Parasites infecting the brain typically affect individuals living in the undeveloped world. Parasitic CNS diseases include cysticercosis, malaria, neuroschistosomiasis, paragonimiasis, angiostrongyliasis, hydatid disease, sparganosis, trypanosomiasis, and gnathostomiasis. Toxoplasma is also considered to be a parasite, but since it is infective in immunocompromised hosts it is therefore discussed in the subsequent section. Since most parasitic infections of the CNS are rarely seen clinically, they are not discussed. Cysticercosis, however, is seen frequently enough to merit attention.

The larval stage of the pork tapeworm (*Taenia solium*) infects the human nervous system, causing neurocysticercosis. The larvae have a variable appearance on imaging depending on whether they are: (1) viable and not under attack by the host's immune defenses, (2) under immune attack, or (3) dead. It must be kept in mind that the larvae can infect the parenchyma directly or can seed the CSF spaces including the ventricles, sulci and cisterns. The larvae typically form cysts with a central scolex. The cysts are very thin-walled with a small central solid component representing the scolex. I have even observed the scolex enhance following gadolinium administration, a finding that is difficult to explain since it infers that some connection with the host blood supply exists for the contrast agent to find its way to the parasite in the cyst. The cysts can be multiloculated especially in the subarachnoid space, resulting in a "raccmose" appearance. If present in strategic locations of the ventricular system, obstructive hydrocephalus may ensue. Some ventricular cysts can even move into dependent locations based on head position. When the cysts are viable, the intracystic fluid matches CSF on CT and all MRI pulse sequences although some cysts can have slightly different signal on MRI, especially on FLAIR sequences. No adjacent edema is seen.

The average size of the cysts is 0.5–1.0 cm in diameter but they can be much larger. When a host immune reaction is present (typically associated with seizures), the cyst wall thickens and enhances. There is edema in the adjacent parenchyma. When the immune response is successful, the cysts begin to disappear and nodular areas of enhancement remain. These areas eventually become densely calcified.

The cysticerci in this intermediate phase can be difficult to distinguish from other nodular enhancing lesions. They may also be hypointense on T2-weighted images. A soft tissue radiographic survey of the patient's muscles may reveal calcified cysticercal lesions, indicating the correct diagnosis. Occasionally, even calcified lesions may show some adjacent edema and contrast enhancement, probably reflecting continued host reaction to residual larval antigens. Diffusion imaging does not play a significant role in establishing the presence of cysticerci since the diagnosis is predominantly based on morphological characteristics alone. MRS may play a significant role especially in the nodular form of the disease when the etiology is uncertain, since elevations in alanine, succinate, acetate, and amino acids point to an infectious etiology [27, 28]. Since nodular cysticercous lesions can be hypointense on T2-weighted images and may appear virtually identical to tuberculomas. MRS should be helpful in distinguishing between these similar lesions.

Infections in Immunocompromised Patients

Not only are immunocompromised patients prone to infections that are seen in normal hosts, but they also become infected quite commonly by agents that are easily controlled by the normal immune system. This section focuses on two of the most common agents that infect the immunocompromised patient: toxoplasma and JC virus. Finally, cryptococcal infection, encephalitis, and neurosyphillis are addressed.

Toxoplasma Infection

These infections tend to present as enlarging irregular mass lesions with perilesional edema, variable signal characteristics, and variable contrast enhancement. They can be difficult to distinguish from lymphoma, a significant diagnostic consideration in immunocompromised individuals, although some evidence exists that ADC values are higher than those seen with lymphomas but also tend to be lower than in normal brain [29]. Toxoplasma has a predilection for the basal ganglia; any mass seen to involve this structure in an immunocompromised individual should be considered to represent toxoplasmosis until proven otherwise, since it is easily treatable and responds to appropriate treatment. Multiple lesions are usually present and involvement of the frontal and parietal lobes is common. As opposed to other infectious agents, no specific or unique metabolite peaks are present in toxoplasma lesions. In fact, MRS is unable to distinguish between lymphoma and toxoplasmosis.

Progressive Multifocal Leukoencephalopathy

PML is caused by JC virus infection of oligodendrocytes in the immunocompromised host and typically involves only white matter structures. It has the appearance of a demyelinating lesion and is associated with little or no contrast enhancement except along the margins of the lesion. It can involve white matter in the posterior fossa and, like multiple sclerosis (MS), has a predilection for the middle cerebellar peduncle. Both increased and decreased water diffusion values have been seen in these lesions. It has recently been suggested that ADC is reduced in early infections (indicating swelling of infected cells) and later reverses to increased values as cells are lost and gliosis develops [30]. Decreased ADC is also observed in the advancing edge of older lesions. Tissue injury tends to be more severe in patients with AIDS compared to other immunocompromised patients, most likely because of co-existent injury from HIV. MRS shows a decrease in NAA that is usually greater than that seen with HIV encephalopathy alone. Choline is frequently elevated [31]. No spectral peaks unique to this infection have been identified with proton spectrosocopy.

Cryptococcal Infection

Cryptococcal infections occur in the form of meningitis or mass lesions (cryptococcomas) in the CSF spaces or brain parenchyma. The typical infection is that of meningitis with spread into the Virchow-Robin (VR) spaces at the base of the brain into the basal ganglia. The enlarged VR spaces show increased T1 and T2 relaxations without contrast enhancement. However, enhancement in the meninges and in cryptococcomas can occur. Secretion of an external polysaccharide capsule by these yeast-like organisms gives rise to large gelatinous pseudocysts that form in the ventricular system or subarachnoid space. Surprisingly, there is a paucity of information concerning diffusion imaging and MRS in patients with these lesions.

HIV Encephalitis

HIV enters the CNS via infected macrophages that cross the blood-brain barrier (BBB). Direct neuronal infection, as seen in other viral encephalitides, is thought not to occur, although this has not been entirely ruled out. Since there is initial preservation of neurons, CNS symptoms consisting of dementia are delayed.

It has been proposed that the pathogenesis of dementia proceeds along noninflammatory and inflammatory pathways. In the noninflammatory pathway, infection of the microglia inhibits the supportive function of these cells. Inhibition of growth factor and impaired clearance of excitotoxic neurotransmitters lead to neuronal loss. In the inflammatory pathway, production of proinflammatory cytokines and the ensuing inflammatory process injure neurons directly, leading to gliosis and brain atrophy [32].

MRI findings include white matter lesions and generalized cerebral atrophy. MRS shows elevations in choline and myoinositol markers of glial proliferation. There is also a reduction in NAA, indicating neuronal loss. Diffusion imaging is generally non-contributory, although diffusion tensor analysis may provide information at a time when diffusion-weighted imaging (DWI) is normal.

CMV Encephalitis

Ependymitis with periventricular enhancement suggests infection with cytomegalovirus (CMV) but parenchymal lesions can also be seen.

Neurosyphillis

Neurosyphilis is typically a meningovascular disease producing meningeal inflammation as well as ischemic brain injury from vasculitis and vascular occlusion. The meninges may show enhancement following contrast medium administration. Occasionally meningeal granulomas or "gummas" can form. These gummas can rarely be seen in the parenchyma as enhancing nodules with increased T2 signal intensity surrounded by edema. Ischemic brain infarction can occur due to vascular compromise by the inflammatory process. In fact, significant vascular narrowing can be seen at angiography.

A form of encephalitic involvement that is becoming increasingly recognized mimics the appearance of herpes encephalitis, in which there is increased T2 signal and mild swelling of the mesial temporal lobes [33]. This emphasizes the need to maintain an open mind concerning the differential diagnosis of temporal lobe infections. The classic progression of neurosyphilis from meningeal to cerebrovascular and to encephalitic phases over decades can be considerably foreshortened in immunocompromised patients. Diffusion imaging can help to establish evidence of acute ischemic injury to the brain parenchyma as a result of vascular compromise. The role of MRS is unclear as there are no published cases in this disease.

References

1. Haimes AB, Zimmerman RD, Morgello S, Weingarten K, Becker RD, Jennis R, Deck MD (1989) MR imaging of brain abscesses. Am J Roentgenol 152(5):1073-1085
2. Dev R, Gupta RK, Poptani H, Roy R, Sharma S, Husain M (1998) Role of in vivo proton magnetic resonance spectroscopy in the diagnosis and management of brain abscesses. Neurosurgery 42(1):37-43
3. Basoglu OK, Savas R, Kitis O (2002) Conventional and diffusion-weighted MR imaging of intracranial tuberculomas. A case report. Acta Radiol 43(6):560-562
4. Gupta RK, Vatsal DK, Husain N, Chawla S, Prasad KN, Roy R, Kumar R, Jha D, Husain M (2001) Differentiation of tuberculous from pyogenic brain abscesses with in vivo proton MR spectroscopy and magnetization transfer MR imaging. Am J Neuroradiol 22(8):1503-1509
5. Chatterjee T, Gowardman JR, Goh TD (2003) Pneumococcal meningitis masquerading as subarachnoid haemorrhage. Med J Aust 178(10):505-507
6. Tung GA, Rogg JM (2003) Diffusion-weighted imaging of cerebritis. Am J Neuroradiol 24(6):1110-1113
7. Kuwahara S, Kawada M, Uga S (2001) Cryptococcal meningoencephalitis presenting with an unusual magnetic resonance imaging appearance – case report. Neurol Med Chir (Tokyo) 41(10):517-521
8. Goyal M, Sharma A, Mishra NK, Gaikwad SB, Sharma MC (1997) Imaging appearance of pachymeningeal tuberculosis. Am J Roentgenol 169(5):1421-1424

9. Erly WK, Bellon RJ, Seeger JF, Carmody RF (1999) MR imaging of acute coccidioidal meningitis. Am J Neuroradiol 20(3):509-514

10. Berkefeld J, Enzensberger W, Lanfermann H (1999) Cryptococcus meningoencephalitis in AIDS: parenchymal and meningeal forms. Neuroradiology 41(2):129-133

11. Lipkin WI (1997) European consensus on viral encephalitis. Lancet 349:299-300

12. Heiner L, Demaerel P (2003) Diffusion-weighted MR imaging findings in a patient with herpes simplex encephalitis. Eur J Radiol 45:195-198

13. Agid R, Ducreux D, Halliday WC, Kucharczyk W, terBrugge KG, Mikulis DJ (2003) MR diffusion-weighted imaging in a case of West Nile virus encephalitis. Neurology 61(12):1821-1823

14. Chu JJ, Ng ML (2003) The mechanism of cell death during West Nile virus infection is dependent on initial infectious dose. J Gen Viro 84(Pt 12):3305-3314

15. Environmental Risk Analysis Program, Cornell University. http://environmentalrisk.cornell.edu/WNV/ (accessed 20 January 2004)

16. http://www.cdc.gov/ncidod/dvbid/westnile/index.htm (accessed 20 January 2004)

17. Gould EA (2003) Implications for Northern Europe of the emergence of West Nile virus in the USA. Epidemiol Infect 131(1):583-589

18. Jeha LE, Sila CA, Lederman RJ, Prayson RA, Isada CM, Gordon SM (2003) West Nile virus infection: a new acute paralytic illness. Neurology 61(1):55-59

19. Calli C, Ozel AA, Savas R, Kitis O, Yunten N, Sener RN (2002) Proton MR spectroscopy in the diagnosis and differentiation of encephalitis from other mimicking lesions. J Neuroradiol 29(1):23-28

20. Manuelidis L (2003) Transmissible encephalopathies: speculations and realities. Viral Immunol 16(2):123-139

21. Bahn MM, Parchi P (1999) Abnormal diffusion-weighted magnetic resonance images in Creutzfeldt-Jakob disease. Arch Neurol 56:577-583

22. Liberski PP, Gajdusek DC, Brown P (2002) How do neurons degenerate in prion diseases or transmissible spongiform encephalopathies (TSEs): neuronal autophagy revisited. Acta Neurobiol Exp (Wars) 62(3):141-147

23. Urbach H, Klisch J, Wolf HK et al (1998) MRI in sporadic Creutzfeldt-Jakob disease: correlation with clinical and neuropathological data. Neuroradiology 40:65-70

24. Haik S, Dormont D, Faucheux BA, Marsault C, Hauw JJ (2002) Prion protein deposits match magnetic resonance imaging signal abnormalities in Creutzfeldt-Jakob disease. Ann Neurol 51(6):797-799

25. Tschampa HJ, Murtz P, Flacke S, Paus S, Schild HH, Urbach H (2003) Thalamic involvement in sporadic Creutzfeldt-Jakob disease: a diffusion-weighted MR imaging study. Am J Neuroradiol 24(5):908-915

26. Pandya HG, Coley SC, Wilkinson ID, Griffiths P (2003) Magnetic resonance spectroscopic abnormalities in sporadic and variant Creutzfeldt-Jakob disease. Clin Radiol 58(2):148-153

27. Pandit S, Lin A, Gahbauer H, Libertin CR, Erdogan B (2001) MR spectroscopy in neurocysticercosis. J Comput Assist Tomogr 25(6):950-952

28. Chang KH, Song IC, Kim SH, Han MH, Kim HD, Seong SO, Jung HW, Han MC (1998) In vivo single-voxel proton MR spectroscopy in intracranial cystic masses. AJNR Am J Neuroradiol 19(3):401-405

29. Camacho DL, Smith JK, Castillo M (2003) Differentiation of toxoplasmosis and lymphoma in AIDS patients by using apparent diffusion coefficients. Am J Neuroradiol 24(4):633-637

30. Bergui M, Bradac GB, Oguz KK, Boghi A, Geda C, Gatti G, Schiffer D (2003) Progressive multifocal leukoencephalopathy: diffusion-weighted imaging and pathological correlations. Neuroradiology

31. Hurley RA, Ernst T, Khalili K, Del Valle L, Simone IL, Taber K (2003) Identification of HIV-associated progressive multifocal leukoencephalopathy: magnetic resonance imaging and spectroscopy. J Neuropsychiatry Clin Neurosci 15(1):1-6

32. Avison MJ, Nath A, Berger JR (2002) Understanding pathogenesis and treatment of HIV dementia: a role for magnetic resonance? Trends Neurosci 25(9):468-473

33. Bash S, Hathout GM, Cohen S (2001) Mesiotemporal T2-weighted hyperintensity: neurosyphilis mimicking herpes encephalitis. Am J Neuroradiol 22(2):314-316

Diseases of the Sella

J.F. Bonneville[1], W. Kucharczyk[2]

[1] Hôpital J. Minjoz, CHU Besançon, France
[2] Medical Imaging, University of Toronto, Toronto, Canada

Introduction

Pituitary adenomas are by far the most common pathology in the region of the sella turcica. Accordingly, a large part of this synopsis is devoted to them, while the remainder discusses other common lesions in this area. The emphasis is on imaging diagnosis and differential diagnosis.

Pituitary Adenomas

Magnetic resonance imaging (MRI) is usually the only imaging method needed for the morphological investigation of pituitary adenomas. Computed tomography (CT) is occasionally helpful to complement the MRI examination for better delineation of the bony skull base, anatomic variants, calcification and osseous malformations. Classically, pituitary adenomas are divided into two categories: microadenomas are less than 10 mm in diameter, and macroadenomas are over 10 mm in diameter. Occasionally the term "picoadenoma" is used to describe lesions smaller than 3 mm; these pose diagnostic problems due to their small size.

Clinically, microadenomas usually present with endocrine dysfunction. Rarely they may be a serendipitous discovery. On T1-weighted images, pituitary microadenomas are usually hypointense compared to the unaffected anterior pituitary gland, and round or oval in shape. In approximately 25% of cases, however, the adenoma is isointense on T1-weighted images. Pituitary microadenomas can also cause high signal intensity on T1-weighted images, probably due to internal hemorrhagic transformation of all or parts of the adenoma, a rather frequent phenomenon in prolactinomas. On T2-weighted images, the signal intensity of microadenomas typically resembles that of the temporal lobe cortex, slightly hyperintense to that of the normal adenohypophysis, which is close to that of white matter. The signal intensity on T2-weighted images varies, in particular, with the type of endocrine activity. The diagnosis of microadenomas is simple when they demonstrate high intensity on T2-weight-

ed images, although this signal may only represent a part of the adenoma. Increased intensity on T2-weighted images is found in over 80% of microprolactinomas. Conversely, iso- or hypointensity on T2-weighted images occurs in two-thirds of all growth hormone-secreting microadenomas. T2-weighted images are particularly helpful when looking for picoadenomas for which T1-weighted images, and even gadolinium-enhanced sequences, are negative. When both the T1- and T2-weighted images corroborate the diagnosis, which is the usual case with prolactinomas, gadolinium enhancement is unnecessary. On the contrary, when the diagnosis has not been established, enhanced imaging is mandatory. A half-dose of gadolinium-chelate (0.05 mmol/kg) is usually adequate. Contrast-enhanced images typically show a hypointense lesion surrounded by the intense enhancement of the normal pituitary gland, but even the contrast-enhanced images may be negative if the tumor is extremely small, the dose of gadolinium is too high, or the visualization window is too large. Delayed images taken 30-40 minutes after injection of contrast medium may show late enhancement of the adenoma. Dynamic images are useful in the diagnosis of adenomas secreting adrenocorticotrophic hormone (ACTH), or are used as a complementary investigation when clinical signs are strongly evocative of a pituitary adenoma, but conventional MR images are not convincing.

Pituitary macroadenomas are intrasellar masses with extrasellar extension, which is usually upwards into the suprasellar cistern or laterally into the cavernous sinus. It is important to delineate this extension in relation to the various surrounding anatomical structures, and whether the tumor is likely to be firm, cystic, necrotic or hemorrhagic, based on its signal intensity and enhancement. Macroadenomas with suprasellar extension are often polycyclic in shape with one or two extensions into the suprasellar cistern. Macroadenoma signal intensity is often inhomogeneous, particularly on T2-weighted images, with disseminated areas of hyperintensity reflecting cystic or necrotic portions of the adenoma. The adenomatous tissue usually enhances slightly after contrast medium injection, but the object of enhanced imaging is to visualize normal pituitary tissue. It usually forms a strongly enhancing pseudocapsule around the adenoma: above it, behind it, rarely below or in front of it, and usually unilaterally. The coronal section of the enhanced T1-weighted image generally reveals a unilateral layer of normal pituitary tissue located between the adenoma and the elements of the cavernous sinus, of crucial importance to neurosurgeons. The hyperintense posterior lobe is modified: it appears either flattened or displaced and is well seen on the axial sections, or an ectopic hyperintensity is located within the pituitary stalk, which is compressed by the superior pole of the macroadenoma. The pituitary stalk is tipped laterally. When the suprasellar extension is large, the chiasm itself may be difficult to identify. In such cases, T2-weighted coronal sections help because the optic chiasm is clearly hypointense. After gadolinium injection, discrete meningeal enhancement is usually noticeable near the area where the meninges are in contact with the adenoma, and particularly so in the anterior part of the posterior cranial fossa, along with a possible dural tail, which has previously been described with meningiomas. In our experience, the enhanced dura has no specificity whatsoever.

Involvement of the cavernous sinus can modify the prognosis, but compression and invasion remain difficult to differentiate. The best sign of invasion is complete encircling of the intracavernous carotid by the tumor. The diagnosis can practically be eliminated if it can be demonstrated that a strip of normal pituitary tissue lies between the tumor and the cavernous sinus. Large pituitary adenomas can apply pressure onto the cavernous sinus and cause convex deformation of its external wall without necessarily involving it.

Other Considerations: Gender, Age, Hormone Secretion, Pregnancy

Prolactin-secreting microadenomas are common in young women. Some may spontaneously remain dormant over long periods. They do not develop after menopause. When prolactin-secreting adenomas are discovered in male patients, they have usually reached the stage of macroadenomas. This is probably due in part to the fact that clinical signs are less obvious in men than in women, and in part to the fact that their development is probably different. Cavernous sinus involvement is far from exceptional. Pediatric pituitary adenomas are not only exceptional but also potentially active. Prolactin-secreting adenomas can be responsible for late puberty.

Prolactinomas are usually discovered at the stage of microadenomas owing to distinctive clinical signs found in young women, including amenorrhea, galactorrhea, and hyperprolactinemia (over 30 or 40 µg/l). Most of the time, the prolactinoma is hypointense on T1-weighted images, while it is hyperintense on T2-weighted images in 4 cases out of 5. This hypersignal may only be exhibited by a portion of the adenoma. Correlation between prolactin levels and adenoma size is usually good. However, given two prolactinomas of equal size, the hypointense tumor on T2-weighted images secretes more than its counterpart. Medical treatment based on bromocriptine decreases adenoma volume drastically. As a result, diagnosis becomes difficult. We strongly recommend MRI documentation before instituting the medical treatment. In some cases when prolactinomas are imaged long after medical treatment with bromocriptine is started, peculiar scarred tissue can be seen, which is evocative of a former pituitary adenoma: it is due to the local remodeling of the pituitary gland, forming a "V" on its superior aspect.

While prolactinomas and growth hormone (GH)-secreting adenomas are usually located laterally in the sella turcica, ACTH-secreting adenomas in Cushing's disease, usually smaller in size, are more often located in the midline. Because of the severe prognosis of this disease and the surgical possibilities, ACTH-secreting lesions require the most detailed and exhaustive imaging. GH-secreting adenomas have the unique characteristic of exhibiting hypointensity on T2-weighted images in two-thirds of cases. Spontaneous infarction or necrosis of GH-secreting adenomas is far from exceptional. Some cases of acromegaly that were detected late in the course of the disease exhibited an enlarged, partially empty sella turcica, lined with adenomatous tissue that proved difficult to analyze. Medical treatment based on octreotride analogs (somatostatin) decreases the size of the adenoma by an average of 35% and brings the level of somatomedin C back to normal in 50% of cases. It is useful before surgery.

Macroadenomas can be nonfunctioning, but they can also be prolactin-secreting adenomas, gonadotrope adenomas, and growth hormone-secreting adenomas. The greater their size, the more heterogeneous they are, as areas of cystic necrosis are caused by poor tumoral blood supply. Gonadotrope adenomas are often massive and have a strong tendency to recur.

Hemorrhage occurs in all or parts of 20% of all pituitary adenomas, but it is usually occult. Pituitary apoplexy, with the usual headache, pseudomeningeal syndrome, cranial nerve paralysis and severe hypopituitarism, is generally caused by massive hemorrhage within a pituitary macroadenoma. Smaller scale hemorrhage occurs much more often, and can be seen within pituitary adenomas. Bromocriptine is held responsible, to a certain degree, for intratumoral hemorrhages in prolactinomas, although the phenomenon is sometimes revealed on MR images before the treatment has been instituted. Recurrent hemorrhage is possible, and can cause repeated headaches. Intratumoral hemorrhages are revealed by hyperintensity on the T1-weighted image, sometimes with a blood-fluid level in the mass.

Normal pituitary tissue has a longer T1 in women during pregnancy. Normal pituitary tissue increases in height during pregnancy (0.08 mm per week, i.e. almost 3 mm during the whole pregnancy). Pituitary adenomas also increase in volume, especially prolactinomas. The increased volume of the prolactinoma is especially visible when medical treatment has been interrupted. Vision and tumor size should be closely monitored during this period.

Postoperative Sella Turcica and Pituitary Gland

The surgical cavity is often filled with packing material after transphenoidal resection of a pituitary adenoma. Surgicel is frequently used, and is impregnated with blood and secretions. The presence of packing material, secretions and periadenomatous adhesions usually keeps the cavity from collapsing in the days and weeks that follow surgery. Blood, secretions and packing material slowly involute over the following 2-3 months. Even after a few months, fragments of blood-impregnated Surgicel can still be found in the surgical cavity. If the diaphragm of the sella turcica is torn in the course of surgery, fat or muscle implants are inserted by the surgeon to prevent the occurrence of a cerebrospinal fluid fistula. Their resorption takes much longer. Implanted fat involutes slowly and may exhibit hyperintensity on the T1-weighted image up to 2-3 years after surgery. Postoperative MRI 2-3 months after surgery is useful to monitor further development of a resected adenoma. An earlier MRI examination performed 48 hours after surgery checks for potential complications and may visualize residual tumor, i.e. a mass of intensity identical to that of the adenoma before surgery that commonly occupies a peripheral portion of the adenoma. This early investigation is extremely helpful to interpret the follow-up MR images. At this stage, the remaining normal pituitary tissue can be characterized: it is usually asymmetrical, and a hyperintense area is frequently observed at the base of the deviated hypophyseal stalk, due to an ectopic collection of neurohypophyseal secretory vesicles. The 2-month follow-up MRI examination is essential to check for residual tumor. Late follow-up MRI, after 1-2 years or more, usually demonstrates adenoma recurrence as a rounded or convex mass that is isointense with the initial tumor.

Craniopharyngioma

Craniopharyngiomas are epithelial-derived neoplasms that occur exclusively in the region of the sella turcica and suprasellar cistern or in the third ventricle. Craniopharyngiomas account for approximately 3% of all intracranial tumors and show no gender predominance. Craniopharyngiomas are hormonally inactive lesions. They have a bimodal age distribution; more than half occur in childhood or adolescence, with a peak incidence between 5 and 10 years of age; there is a second smaller peak in adults in the sixth decade. The tumors vary greatly in size, from a few millimeters to several centimeters in diameter. The epicenter of most is in the suprasellar

cistern. Infrequently, the lesions are entirely within the sella or in the third ventricle. Most discussions of craniopharyngiomas in the literature are confined to the most frequent form, the classic *adamantinomatous* type, but a distinct squamous or *papillary* type is becoming recognized with increasing frequency. The classic form of craniopharyngioma is the adamantinomatous type, which is the most frequently encountered form of the lesion. Typically, cases are identified as suprasellar masses during the first two decades of life. These children most often present with symptoms and signs of increased intracranial pressure: headache, nausea, vomiting, and papilledema. Visual disturbances due to compression of the optic apparatus are also frequent but difficult to detect in young children. Others present with pituitary hypofunction because of compression of the pituitary gland, pituitary stalk, or hypothalamus. Occasionally, lesions rupture into the subarachnoid space and evoke a chemical meningitis. Rarely, adamantinomatous craniopharyngiomas are found outside the suprasellar cistern, including the posterior fossa, pineal region, third ventricle, and nasal cavity. Adamantinomatous tumors are almost always grossly cystic and usually have both solid and cystic components. Calcification is seen in the vast majority of these tumors. Extensive fibrosis and signs of inflammation are often found with these lesions, particularly when they are recurrent, so that they adhere to adjacent structures, including the vasculature at the base of the brain. Optic tract edema on T2-weighted images is a common associated finding that is not commonly seen with other suprasellar masses. The inflammatory and fibrotic nature of the lesions makes recurrence a not uncommon event, typically occurring within the first 5 years after surgery. The most characteristic MRI finding is a suprasellar mass that is itself heterogeneous but contains a cystic component that is well defined, internally uniform, and hyperintense on both T1- and T2-weighted images. The lesions often encase nearby cerebral vasculature. The solid portion, which is frequently partially calcified, is represented as the heterogeneous region. On rare occasions the cyst is absent and the solid component is completely calcified. These calcified types of tumors can be entirely overlooked on MRI unless close scrutiny is paid to subtle distortion of the normal suprasellar anatomy. Contrast medium administration causes a moderate degree of enhancement of the solid portion of the tumor, which otherwise may be difficult to see.

Papillary craniopharyngiomas are typically found in the adult patient. These lesions are solid, without calcification, and often found within the third ventricle. Although surgery remains the definitive mode of therapy for all craniopharyngiomas, papillary variants are encapsulated and are readily separable from nearby structures and adjacent brain, so they are generally thought to recur much less frequently than the adamantinomatous type. On pathologic examination, papillary lesions do not show the features characteristic of the adamantinomatous variant. In papillary lesions, there is extensive squamous differentiation. In distinction from their adamantinomatous counterpart, MRI shows papillary craniopharyngiomas as solid lesions. As noted previously, they are often situated within the third ventricle. These lesions demonstrate a non-specific signal intensity pattern, without the characteristic hyperintensity on T1-weighted images of the cystic component of adamantinomatous tumors. Like all craniopharyngiomas, papillary lesions typically enhance.

Rathke's Cleft Cyst

Symptomatic cysts of Rathke's cleft are much less frequent than craniopharyngiomas, although they are a common incidental finding at autopsy. In a recent evaluation of 1000 nonselected autopsy specimens, 113 pituitary glands (11.3%) harbored incidental Rathke's cleft cysts. These cysts are predominantly intrasellar in location. Of incidental Rathke's cysts larger than 2 mm in a large autopsy series, 89% were localized to the center of the gland, whereas the remaining 11% extended to show predominant lateral lesions. In that series, of all incidental pituitary lesions localized to the central part of the gland, 87% were Rathke's cysts. Others may be centered in the suprasellar cistern, usually midline and anterior to the stalk. Rathke's cysts are found in all age groups. They share a common origin with some craniopharyngiomas in that they are thought to originate from remnants of squamous epithelium from Rathke's cleft. The cyst wall is composed of a single cell layer of columnar, cuboidal, or squamous epithelium on a basement membrane. The epithelium is often ciliated and may contain goblet cells. The cyst contents are typically mucoid, less commonly filled with serous fluid or desquamated cellular debris. Calcification in the cyst wall is rare.

Most Rathke's cleft cysts are small, asymptomatic, and discovered only at autopsy. Symptoms occur if the cyst enlarges sufficiently to compress the pituitary gland or optic chiasm and rarely, secondary to hemorrhage. The cysts with mucoid fluid are indistinguishable from cystic craniopharyngiomas on MRI: both are hyperintense on T1- and T2-weighted images. The serous cysts match the signal intensity of cerebrospinal fluid (CSF) and is the only subtype that has the typical imaging features of benign cysts. Those containing cellular debris pose the greatest difficulty in differential diagnosis for they resemble solid nodules. The surgical approaches to Rathke's cleft cyst and craniopharyngioma differ. Because of infrequent postoperative recurrences, partial removal or aspiration is sufficient. Rathke's cleft cysts do not typically enhance. However, occasionally there may be thin marginal enhancement of the cyst wall. This feature can be used to advantage to separate these cysts from craniopharyngiomas in difficult cases. CT may reveal calcification, frequently found in craniopharyngiomas, helping to distinguish the mass from a Rathke's cleft cyst.

Meningioma

Approximately 10% of meningiomas occur in the parasellar region. These tumors arise from a variety of locations around the sella including the tuberculum sellae, clinoid processes, medial sphenoid wing, and cavernous sinus. Meningiomas are usually slow-growing lesions that present because of compression of vital structures. Patients may suffer visual loss because of ophthalmoplegia due to cranial nerve involvement, proptosis due to venous congestion at the orbital apex, or compression of the optic nerves, chiasm, or optic tracts. Accurate differentiation between meningioma and pituitary adenoma is important because meningioma requires craniotomy, whereas a trans-sphenoidal route is preferred for removing most pituitary macroadenomas. Meningiomas are most frequently isointense relative to gray matter on unenhanced T1-weighted sequences, and less commonly hypointense. Approximately 50% remain isointense on the T2-weighted sequence, whereas 40% are hyperintense. Since there is little image contrast to distinguish meningiomas from brain parenchyma, indirect signs such as a mass effect, thickening of the dura, buckling of adjacent white matter, white matter edema, and hyperostosis are important diagnostic features. Other diagnostic signs include visualization of a cleft of CSF separating the tumor from the brain (thus denoting that the tumor has an extra-axial location) and a clear separation of the tumor from the pituitary gland (thus indicating that the tumor is not of pituitary gland origin). The latter sign is particularly well assessed on sagittal views of planum sphenoidale meningiomas. A peripheral black rim has been described on the edges of these meningiomas. This is thought to be related to surrounding veins. Hyperostosis and calcification are features that may be apparent on MRI but are better assessed with CT. Vascular encasement is not uncommon, particularly with meningiomas in the cavernous sinus. The pattern of encasement is of diagnostic value. Meningiomas commonly constrict the lumen of the encased vessel. This is rare with other tumors. As on CT, the intravenous administration of contrast medium markedly improves the visualization of basal meningiomas. They enhance intensely and homogeneously, often with a trailing edge of thick surrounding dura (the "dural tail sign").

Chiasmatic and Hypothalamic Gliomas

The distinction between chiasmatic and hypothalamic gliomas often depends on the predominant position of the lesion. In many cases the origin of large gliomas cannot be definitively determined as the hypothalamus and chiasm are inseparable; therefore, hypothalamic and chiasmatic gliomas are discussed as a single entity. These tumors are for the most part tumors of childhood: 75% occur in the first decade of life. There is an equal prevalence in males and females. There is a definite association of optic nerve and chiasmatic gliomas with neurofibromatosis, more so for tumors that arise from the optic nerve rather than from the chiasm or hypothalamus. Tumors of chiasmal origin are also more aggressive than those originating from the optic nerves and tend to invade the hypothalamus and floor of the third ventricle and cause hydrocephalus. Patients suffer from monocular or binocular visual disturbances, hydrocephalus, or hypothalamic dysfunction. The appearance of the tumor depends on its position and direction of growth. It can be confined to either the chiasm or the hypothalamus; however, because of its slow growth, the tumor has usually attained a considerable size by the time of presentation and the site of origin is frequently conjectural. Smaller nerve and chiasmal tumors are visually distinct from the hypothalamus and their site of origin is more clear-cut. From the point of view of differential diagnosis, these smaller tumors can be difficult to distinguish from optic neuritis, which can also cause optic nerve enlargement. The clinical history is important in these cases (neuritis is painful, tumor is not) and, if necessary, interval follow-up of neuritis will demonstrate resolution of optic nerve swelling. On T1-weighted images, the tumors are most often isointense while on T2-weighted images they are moderately hyperintense. Calcification and hemorrhage are not features of these gliomas but cysts are seen, particularly in the larger hypothalamic tumors. Contrast enhancement occurs in about half of all cases. Because of the tumor's known propensity to invade the brain along the optic radiations, T2-weighted images of the entire brain are necessary. This pattern of tumor extension is readily evident as hyperintensity on the T2-weighted image; however, patients with neurofibromatosis (NF) present a problem in differential diagnosis. This relates to a high incidence of benign cerebral hamartomas and atypical glial cell rests in NF that can exactly mimic glioma. These both appear as areas of high signal intensity on T2-weighted images within the optic radiations. Lack of interval growth and possibly the absence of contrast enhancement are more supportive of a diagnosis of hamartoma while enhancement suggests glioma.

Metastases

Symptomatic metastases to the pituitary gland are found in 1%-5% of cancer patients. These are primarily patients with advanced, disseminated malignancy, particularly breast and bronchogenic carcinoma. The vast majority die of their underlying disease before becoming symptomatic of pituitary disease. Autopsy series have demonstrated a much higher incidence, but these by and large are small and asymptomatic lesions. Intrasellar and juxtasellar metastases arise via hematogenous seeding to the pituitary gland and stalk, by CSF seeding, and by direct extension from head and neck neoplasms. There are no distinctive MRI characteristics of metastases, although bone destruction is a prominent feature of lesions that involve skull base.

Infections

Infection in the suprasellar cistern and cavernous sinuses is usually part of a disseminated process, or occurs by means of intracranial extension of an extracranial infection. The basal meninges in and around the suprasellar cistern are susceptible to tuberculous and other forms of granulomatous meningitis. The cistern may also be the site of parasitic cysts, in particular cysticercosis. In infections of the cavernous sinus, many of which are accompanied by thrombophlebitis, the imaging findings on CT and MRI consist of a convex lateral contour to the affected cavernous sinus with evidence of a filling defect after contrast administration. The intracavernous portion of the internal carotid artery may also be narrowed secondary to surrounding inflammatory change. Infections of the actual pituitary gland are uncommon. Direct viral infection of the hypophysis has never been established and bacterial infections are unusual. There has been speculation that cases of acquired diabetes insipidus may be the result of a select viral infection of the hypothalamic supraoptic and paraventricular nuclei. Tuberculosis and syphilis, previously encountered in this region because of the higher general prevalence of these diseases in the population, are now rare. Gram-positive cocci are the most frequently identified organisms in pituitary abscesses. Pituitary abscesses usually occur in the presence of other sellar masses such as pituitary adenomas, Rathke's cleft cysts, and craniopharyngiomas, indicating that these mass lesions function as predisposing factors to infection. There are a few reports on CT of pituitary abscesses. These indicate that the lesion is similar in appearance to an adenoma. As a result of the frequent coincidental occurrence of abscesses with adenomas, and because of their common clinical presentations, the correct preoperative diagnosis of abscess is difficult and rarely made. Noncontrast MRI demonstrates a sellar mass indistinguishable from an adenoma. With intravenous administration of contrast medium, there is rim enhancement of the mass with persistence of low intensity in the center.

Noninfectious Inflammatory Lesions

Lymphocytic hypophysitis is a rare, noninfectious inflammatory disorder of the pituitary gland. It occurs almost exclusively in women and particularly during late pregnancy or in the post-partum period. The diagnosis should be considered in a female patient who is in the peripartum period with a pituitary mass, particularly when the degree of hypopituitarism is greater than that expected from the size of the mass. It is believed that, if untreated, the disease results in panhypopituitarism. Clinically the patient complains of headache, visual loss, failure to resume menses, inability to lactate, or some combination thereof. Pituitary hormone levels are depressed. CT and MRI demonstrate diffuse enlargement of the anterior lobe without evidence of any focal abnormality or change in internal characteristics of the gland. The distinction between simple pituitary hyperplasia and lymphocytic hypophysitis may be difficult on MRI alone, so clinical correlation is required in this setting.

Sarcoid afflicting the hypothalamic-pituitary axis usually manifests itself clinically as diabetes insipidus, or occasionally as a deficiency of one or more anterior lobe hormones. Low signal intensity on T2-weighted images is one finding that occurs in sarcoid with some frequency, but rarely in other diseases, with few exceptions (other granulomatous inflammatory diseases, lymphoma, some meningiomas). This low signal finding may aid in differential diagnosis. Also, the presence of multiple, scattered intraparenchymal brain lesions should raise the possibility of the diagnosis, as should diffuse or multifocal lesions of the basal meninges. The latter are best defined on coronal contrast-enhanced T1-weighted images.

Tolosa-Hunt syndrome (THS) refers to a painful ophthalmoplegia caused by an inflammatory lesion of the cavernous sinus that is responsive to steroid therapy. Pathologically, the process is similar to orbital pseudotumor. Imaging in this disorder is often normal, or may show subtle findings such as asymmetric enlargement of the cavernous sinus, enhancement of the prepontine cistern, or abnormal soft tissue density in the orbital apex. The lesion resolves promptly with steroid therapy. Hypointensity on T2-weighted images may be observed; since this observation is uncommon in all but a few other diseases (e.g. meningioma, lymphoma, and sarcoid), it may be helpful in diagnosis. Clinical history allows further precision in differential diagnosis: meningioma does not respond to steroids while lymphoma and sarcoid have evidence of a primary disease elsewhere in almost all cases.

Vascular Lesions

Saccular aneurysms in the sella turcica and parasellar area arise from either the cavernous sinus portion of the carotid artery or its supraclinoid segment. These are extremely important lesions to identify correctly. Confusion with a solid tumor can lead to surgical catastrophes. Fortunately, their MRI appearance is distinctive and easily appreciated. Aneurysms are well defined and lack any internal signal on spin echo (SE) images, the so-called signal void created by rapidly flowing blood. This blood flow may also cause substantial artifacts on the image, usually manifest as multiple ghosts in the phase-encoding direction, and in itself is a useful diagnostic sign. Thrombus in the aneurysm lumen fundamentally alters these characteristics, the clot usually appearing as multilamellated high signal on T1-weighted SE images, partially or completely filling the lumen. Hemosiderin may be visible in the adjacent brain, evident as a rim of low signal intensity on T2-weighted SE images, or on gradient echo (GE) images. If confusion exists as to the vascular nature of these lesions, MR angiography is used to confirm the diagnosis, define the neck of the aneurysm and establish the relationship of the aneurysm to the major vessels.

Carotid cavernous fistulas are abnormal communications between the carotid artery and cavernous sinus. Most cases are due to trauma; less frequently they are "spontaneous". These spontaneous cases are due to a variety of abnormalities, including atherosclerotic degeneration of the arterial wall, congenital defects in the media, or rupture of an internal carotid aneurysm within the cavernous sinus. Dural arteriovenous malformations (AVMs) of the cavernous sinus are another form of abnormal arteriovenous (AV) communication in this region. On MRI the dilatation of the venous structures, in particular the ophthalmic vein and cavernous sinus, is usually clearly visible. The intercavernous venous channels dilate in carotid cavernous fistulas and may also be seen on MR images. Furthermore, the internal character of the cavernous sinus is altered; definite flow channels become evident secondary to the arterial rates of flow within the sinus. The fistulous communication itself is most often occult on MRI. The pituitary gland has been noted to be prominent in cases of dural arteriovenous fistula without evidence of endocrine dysfunction. The exact mechanism of pituitary enlargement is not known, however venous congestion is a postulated cause.

Cavernous hemangiomas are acquired lesions and not true malformations. However, there have been a few reports of extra-axial cavernous hemangiomas occurring in the suprasellar cistern. Of importance is that one of these hemangiomas did not have the features usually associated with, and so highly characteristic of, cavernous hemangiomas in the brain. The atypical appearance of extra-axial cavernous hemangiomas indicates that some caution must be exercised in the differential diagnosis of parasellar masses, because even though cavernous hemangiomas in this location are rare, failure of the surgeon to appreciate their vascular nature can lead to unanticipated hemorrhage. Cavernous hemangiomas should at least be considered in the differential diagnosis of solid, suprasellar masses that do not have the classic features of more common lesions, in particular craniopharyngiomas or meningiomas. Furthermore, T2-weighted images should be a routine part of the MRI protocol for suprasellar masses because visualization of a peripheral dark rim may be the only sign of the nature of the lesion.

Other Conditions

Many other lesions may involve the sella turcica and parasellar region. These include mass lesions such as germinoma, epidermoid, dermoid, teratoma, schwannoma, chordoma, ecchordosis, choristoma, arachnoid cyst, hamartoma, and Langerhans cell histiocytosis. Also, there are several important metabolic conditions that may cause pituitary dysfunction or MRI-observable abnormalities in and around the sella. These include diabetes insipidus, growth hormone deficiency, hemochromatosis, hypermagnesemia and hypothyroidism. Space limitations preclude their further discussion in this synopsis.

Suggested Reading

Ahmadi J, Destian S, Apuzzo MLJ, Segall HD, Zee CS (1992) Cystic fluid in craniopharyngiomas: MR imaging and quantitative analysis. Radiology 1812:783-785

Bonneville JF, Cattin F, Gorczyca W, Hardy J (1993) Pituitary micro-adenomas: early enhancement with dynamic CT-implications of arterial blood supply and potential importance. Radiology 187:857-861

Colombo N, Loli P, Vignati F, Scialfa G (1994) MR of corticotropin-secreting pituitary microadenomas. AJNR Am J Neuroradiol 15:1591-1595

Davis PC, Gokhale KA, Josep GJ (1983) Pituitary adenoma: correlation of half dose gadolinium enhanced MRI with surgical findings in 26 patients. Radiology 180:779–784

Dietemann JL, Portha C, Cattin F, Mollet E, Bonneville JF (1983) CT follow-up of microprolactinomas during bromocriptine-induced pregnancy. Neuroradiology 25:133

Doppman JL, Frank JA, Dwyer AJ et al (1988) Gadolinium DTPA enhanced MR imaging of ACTH-secreting microadenomas of the pituitary gland. J Comput Assist Tomogr 12:728-735

Kucharczyk W, Bishop JE, Plewes DB et al (1993) Dynamic MR imaging of pituitary microadenomas with FSE T1-weighted shared view MR1. SMRM Annual Meeting, New York

Kucharczyk W, Bishop JE, Plewes DB, Keller MA, George S (1994) Detection of pituitary microadenomas: comparaison of dynamic keyhole fast spin-echo, unenhanced, and conventional contrast-enhanced MR imaging. AJNR Am J Neuroradiol 163:671-679

Kucharczyk W, Davis DO, Kelly WM, Sze G, Norman D, Newton TH (1986) Pituitary adenomas: high-resolution MR imaging at 1.5 T. Radiology 161:761-765

Kucharczyk W, Montanera WJ, Becker LE (1996) The sella turcica and parasellar region. In: Atlas SW (ed) Magnetic resonance imaging of the brain and spine, 2nd edn. Lippincott-Raven, Philadelphia

Kucharczyk W, Peck WW, Kelly WM, Norman D, Newton TH (1987) Rathke cleft cysts: CT, MR imaging and pathologic features. Radiology 165:491-495

Lundin P, Bergström K, Nyman R, Lundberg PO, Muhr C (1992) Macroprolactinomas: serial MR imaging in long term bromocriptine therapy. AJNR Am J Neuroradiol 13:1279-1291

Lundin P (1997) Long-term octreotide therapy in growth hormone-secreting pituitary adenomas: evaluation with serial MR. AJNR Am J Neuroradiol 18:765-772

Nagahata M, Hosoya T, Kayama T, Yamaguchi K (1998) Edema along the optic tract: a useful MR finding for the diagnosis of craniopharyngiomas. AJNR Am J Neuroradiol 19:1753–1757

Naylor MF, Scheithauer BW, Forbes GS, Tomlinson FH, Young WF (1995) Rathke cleft cyst: CT, MR, and pathology of 23 cases. J Comput Assist Tomogr 19(6):853-859

Oka H, Kawano N, Suwa T, Yada K, Kan S, Kameya T (1994) Radiological study of symptomatic Rathke's cleft cysts. Neurosurgery 35(4):632-636

Steiner E, Knosp E, Herold CJ et al (1992) Pituitary adenomas: findings of postoperative MR imaging. Radiology 185:521-527

Teramoto A, Hirakawa K, Sanno N, Osamura Y (1994) Incidental pituitary lesions in 1,000 unselected autopsy specimens. Radiology 193:161-164

Voelker J, Campbell R, Muller J (1991) Clinical, radiographic, and pathological features of symptomatic Rathke's cleft cysts. J Neurosurgery 74:535-544

Neuroimaging Diagnosis of Primary Brain Neoplasms in Childhood

W.S. Ball

Imaging Research Center, Cincinnati Children's Hospital Medical Center, and Department of Biomedical Engineering, University of Cincinnati, Cincinnati, OH, USA

Introduction

While not as frequent as in the adult population, primary neoplasm of the brain still constitutes the most frequently encountered solid tumor arising in the pediatric age group [1, 2]. Tumors may be encountered in all age groups during childhood [3]. Supratentorial tumors predominate in the first year of life, whereas infratentorial tumors are more frequent in the age range of 1-8 years [3-5]. In the second decade of life, the proportions of infratentorial vs. supratentorial tumors are similar to what is encountered in the adult population, with a predominance of tumors in the supratentorial space. In general, there is a tendency toward less aggressive glial tumors in children than in adults; however, primary brain tumors still account for significant morbidity and mortality in the pediatric age group. More aggressive therapies have also had a greater negative impact on brain development especially when used in the first decade of life. Early diagnosis is still the key to aggressive management and outcome, and other than increased clinical surveillance, imaging plays the most important role of all of the laboratory modalities both in diagnosis and in follow-up.

We generally divide primary brain neoplasms in children into two compartments; those arising in the infratentorial space and those involving the supratentorial space. Further compartmentalization in the supratentorial space includes those tumors involving the sella and suprasellar regions, those involving the pineal region, tumors of the cerebral hemispheres and finally tumors of the cerebrospinal fluid (CSF) spaces and meninges.

Infratentorial Neoplasms in Children

The majority of childhood posterior fossa neoplasms [6-10] originate from brain parenchyma, arising from either brain stem or cerebellum. These are followed in frequency by tumors that are primarily intraventricular in origin, and then by extra-axial neoplasms originating from the surrounding leptomeninges, skull base, cranial nerves, or primitive embryonic rests of tissue. Histologically, gliomas, primarily consisting of astrocytomas of the brain stem and cerebellum and benign ependymomas, are the most common infratentorial tumors in the pediatric age group. These are followed in frequency by the primitive neuroectodermal tumors (PNET) of childhood (e.g. medulloblastoma, ependymoblastoma, primary intracerebral neuroblastoma), tumors arising from the choroid plexus (e.g. papillomas, carcinomas), metastatic disease (e.g. lymphoma, leukemia, small cell tumors, sarcomas) and neoplasms arising from the region of the skull base (e.g. rhabdomyosarcoma, chordoma, chondrosarcoma).

Since it is clear that magnetic resonance imaging (MRI) is the imaging modality of choice in the evaluation of infratentorial neoplasms in all ages of childhood, it is important for radiologists to be familiar with the general clinical signs and symptoms of their presentation in order to appropriately select MRI as the first examination. In children, the signs and symptoms of most infratentorial tumors depend on the site of origin and relationship to surrounding structures, the presence or absence of complications such as hydrocephalus and the extent of disease. For example, a mass arising from the brain stem commonly presents with cranial neuropathies or motor deficits, but rarely obstructs the fourth ventricle, and only as a late manifestation. Hydrocephalus is common, however, with intraventricular tumors such as ependymoma, choroid plexus papilloma/carcinoma or PNET.

Brain Stem Glioma

On computed tomography (CT) and MRI, brain stem gliomas are best identified according to alterations they produce in the size, shape, and density of the brain stem. Enlargement of the brain stem leads to compression of the surrounding cisterns including the perimesencephalic, prepontine, cerebellopontine, and circum-medullary cisternal CSF spaces. The fourth ventricle appears flattened, anterior to posterior, and is displaced posteriorly by the mass. Midbrain tumors commonly extend into the interpeduncular and posterior suprasellar cisterns, or will indent the inferior and posterior aspects of the third ventricle. Cervicomedullary tumors typically involve the medulla from the level of the pons to the upper or middle cervical cord. Except when there is predominant exophytic neoplasm, the brain stem appears expanded, but often maintains its ovoid shape. As a result of tethering of the basilar artery by short perforating arteries supplying the surface of the brain stem, anterior exophytic growth of the tumor will appear to envelop the basilar artery rather than displace this structure anteriorly. Despite what appears to be significant compression of the basilar artery by surrounding tumor, vertebrobasilar arterial insufficiency is quite rare.

MRI is most useful in the detection of small brain stem gliomas, to determine the extent of the tumor, and to reveal the presence or absence of exophytic growth from a primary intra-axial tumor. In this capacity, there is considerably more benefit to performing MRI compared to CT. Sagittal T1-weighted images are essential in defining the extent of the tumor, whereas axial sections permit the evaluation of tumor signal characteristics with the least interference from artifact. On T1-weighted images, tumor appears hypointense, rarely isointense, compared to the normal surrounding brain. The margins of the tumor, as they interface with surrounding CSF, are typically sharp; however, tumor margins with the brain stem or cerebellum are often irregular and poorly defined as the tumor infiltrates the normal surrounding brain. Despite its infiltrating nature, the bulk of the tumor remains relatively homogeneous. Most true tumor cysts, if present, are lower in signal on both T1- and T2-weighted sequences than are solid portions of the tumor, but are typically higher in signal when compared to normal CSF. Necrotic cysts may actually remain isointense on the T1-weighted sections, but are hyperintense on T2-weighted images or enhance with gadolinium. On intermediate and T2-weighted images, the tumor is moderately to markedly hyperintense in signal, and remains relatively homogeneous in appearance. Tumor margins are better defined on T2-weighted images than on T1-weighted sequences. Contrast enhancement with gadolinium is seen as frequently as that on CT with iodinated contrast material. We have observed frequent enhancement in exophytic tumor, compared to the enhancement in the brain stem itself.

Cerebellar Astrocytomas

On MRI, both solid and macrocystic tumors are easily identified on axial and coronal images as originating from the inferior and medial portions of the cerebellar hemisphere adjacent to the cerebellar tonsils, from the lateral cerebellar hemisphere, or from the vermis. The cyst contents appear low in signal intensity on T1-weighted images except for the cyst margin which is typically isointense. The cyst fluid remains high in signal on T1-weighted images when compared to CSF, due to its high-

er protein content. Separation of cyst wall from surrounding brain may be difficult without the addition of contrast medium; however, in most cases, identification of the wall is easier with MRI than with CT. Mural nodules within the cyst wall often give it a lumpy, nodular or plaque-like appearance. Tumor nodules lying outside the cyst wall in surrounding brain parenchyma, however, are more difficult to recognize; they can appear mixed in signal intensity (isointense and hypointense) on T1-weighted images compared to normal cerebellum. On T2-weighted images, the cyst contents are hyperintense compared to CSF, also from their elevated protein content. Exophytic tumor outside the cyst wall may also appear mixed in signal intensity (hypointense and hyperintense) on T2-weighted images, whereas the bulk of tumor within the cyst wall is typically hyperintense. White matter tracts lying adjacent to the tumor appear hyperintense due to diffuse edema; this is a common finding in astrocytomas arising from the cerebellar hemisphere and vermis. Reactive edema in surrounding white matter is less common with intraventricular neoplasms such as medulloblastoma (PNET) or ependymoma, except when these tumors invade or infiltrate the cerebellar hemisphere.

Predominantly solid cerebellar astrocytomas often contain small, more peripheral cysts, which have similar signal characteristics to the larger macrocyst. Solid tumor is usually slightly inhomogeneous in appearance, is isointense or minimally hypointense on T1-weighted images, and is moderately to markedly hyperintense on T2-weighted sequences. With the addition of contrast medium, both solid tumor and the rim of smaller cysts moderately enhance. On delayed images, contrast medium will often leach into the cyst itself, thus shortening its T1 relaxation over time.

Primitive Neuroectodermal Tumors of Childhood

Sagittal midline T1-weighted images are important in determining the likely site of origin of the tumor. An indistinct interface of the tumor with the region of the inferior or superior medullary velum, combined with a relatively sharply defined margin with the brain stem and cerebellum, provide excellent clues as to the most likely site of tumor origin. The intraventricular extension of the tumor is easiest to identify in the sagittal projection as capping of the superior tumor surface by fourth ventricle.

The appearance of the medulloblastoma on MRI is, in large part, due to the dense cellularity of the tumor. I believe that MRI correlates better with the pathologic appearance of this tumor, compared to CT. A typical appearance for medulloblastoma on T1-weighted images is that of a relatively homogeneous mass which is minimally or moderately hypointense compared to cerebellar grey matter. On T2-weighted images, the tumor is only minimally to moderately hyperintense, and remains relatively homogeneous. Prominent vessels are common central to the tumor, appearing as serpiginous areas of signal void on T2-weighted spin echo or gradient acquisition images.

A pattern such as this on MRI most closely correlates with the "classic" pattern on CT, but is frequently found with both CT patterns. Homogeneity on MRI correlates closely with the homogeneous histologic cellular characteristics of the tumor, despite a diverse cellular histology within the same tumor.

Hemorrhage, calcification, and areas of necrosis can give this tumor an inhomogeneous appearance on MRI, which can be confused with ependymoma or cerebellar astrocytoma. Therefore, homogeneity alone cannot be used to indicate the diagnosis of a primitive neuroectodermal tumor. In my experience, heterogeneity in PNET most closely correlates with zones of ependymal or oligodendroglial differentiation in the tumor.

Ependymoma

The margins of the ependymal tumor are typically ill-defined and irregular. Tumor often originates or extends into the lateral recesses of the fourth ventricle, from where it may involve the cerebellopontine angle or grow through the foramen of Magendie into the cisterna magna. Minimal to moderate patchy enhancement is common, compared to the marked enhancement found in the cerebellar pilocytic astrocytoma or hemangioblastoma. Solid ependymomas tend to enhance in a more nonuniform fashion; however, the pattern of enhancement alone is not a reliable sign to distinguish this tumor from other tumors involving the posterior fossa. Enhancement within the margin of necrosis may appear ring-like, and thus be confused with macrocystic rim enhancement of an astrocytoma or an abscess.

The intraventricular location of most ependymomas is best appreciated in the sagittal projection on T1-weighted MR images, in which the fourth ventricle appears draped over the top of the mass. Due to its frequent origin from the floor or lateral recesses of the fourth ventricle, the interface of tumor with the brain stem surface is often indistinct, whereas the interface of the mass with the inferior or superior medullary velum (the most frequent site of origin for medulloblastoma) remains distinct. On T1-weighted images, the tumor is typically inhomogeneous in signal, with areas that appear hypo-, iso-, or hyperintense. Hypointense regions most frequently represent cystic or necrotic degeneration within the tumor. Hyperintense signal is most commonly a result of hemorrhage within tumor parenchyma or true tumoral cysts. Heterogeneity on T2-weighted images is also typical of this tumor. Cystic regions appear especially hyperintense on the second echo of a T2-weighted sequence. Solid tumor may be either isointense or minimally to moderately hyperintense in appearance on T2-weighted images. Areas of signal void within the tumor represent either calcification or prominent blood vessels draining this highly vascular neoplasm. The detection of calcification can be enhanced by the use of gradient acquisition imaging by taking advantage of the susceptibility effect produced by the calcium salts.

Supratentorial Neoplasms

Supratentorial neoplasms [11, 12] in children can be divided based on anatomic location into those involving the sella and suprasellar regions, the pineal region, the cerebral hemispheres, and CSF spaces and meninges.

Sellar and Suprasellar Regions

The sella-suprasellar space is home for a variety of tumors such as astrocytoma (hypothalamic, optic pathway), craniopharyngioma, germinoma, adenoma, teratoma, epidermoid, hamartoma, histiocytoma, and metastases. Astrocytomas are most common, and arise either from the optic chiasm and optic nerves (optic pathway glioma) or from the floor of the third ventricle (hypothalamic glioma). The majority of these tumors are histologically benign, but lie in an unfavorable location. Because it is difficult to distinguish the two, they are often considered together. They are generally solid, enhance moderately, and appear hypointense on T1-weighted and hyperintense on T2-weighted images. Calcification and primary cysts are uncommon, but may appear following radiation therapy. Complications include hydrocephalus by obstructing the third and lateral ventricles, spontaneous hemorrhage and blindness.

Craniopharyngiomas are benign tumors arising from remnants of Rathke's pouch; 95%-98% involve the suprasellar cistern, 85% are cystic, and 85%-90% contain calcification. The appearance of the cyst on MRI depends on the relative amount of protein and keratin debris (hypointense on T1-weighted images, hyperintense on T2-weighted images), hemorrhage (iso- or hyperintense on T1-weighted images, hypo- or hyperintense on T2-weighted images) or cholesterol (hyperintense on T1-weighted images, hypointense on T2-weighted images) secreted by the wall into the cyst. Solid tumor is typically isointense on T1-weighted images and only minimally hyperintense on the T2-weighted images. The cyst may become quit large and extend into the anterior or middle cranial fossa, or into the posterior fossa. CT is best at identifying calcification; however, similar results can be obtained using gradient acquisition sequences with short repetition time (TR) and echo time (TE) and a small flip angle.

Germinomas commonly present with diabetes insipidus. The clinical onset of the diabetes may actually precede the physical evidence of tumor by months. The tumor is a rapidly growing neoplasm that will invade the floor of the third ventricle, infundibulum and suprasellar cistern. The mass is typically slightly hypointense on T1-weighted images, and isointense to minimally hyperintense on T2-weighted images. Marked enhancement is also a characteristic of this tumor. Germinomas are extremely radiosensitive, such that a positive response to radiation therapy is virtually diagnostic of this disorder. Imaging cannot differentiate benign from malignant tumors within this heterogeneous group.

Pineal Region

Tumors of the pineal region include astrocytomas of the midbrain and surrounding cortex, PNETs (pinealoblastoma), tumors of pineal cell origin, germ cell tumors, and tumors of neural origin (ganglioglioma). Tumors arising in the posterior aspect of the third ventricle (choroid plexus tumors, papillary ependymomas) can sometimes be confused with an extra-axial tumor in the pineal region, posterior to the third ventricle. Midbrain astrocytomas may be solid or cystic (20%-30%), and may be calcified (30%). They are generally slow-growing tumors that frequently obstruct the posterior third ventricle. A small tectal "glioma" may be confused with primary stenosis of the aqueduct of Sylvius, especially when there is a late onset of presentation. Tectal gliomas are actually low-grade gliomas or hamartomas with a slow growth potential that may or may not be associated with neurofibromatosis (NF)-1. Appropriate therapy is to treat the hydrocephalus, and simply follow this lesion for evidence of growth.

PNETs of the pineal region are common in young children. They are predominantly solid, but may contain a cystic component that is often hemorrhagic. Signal characteristics vary considerably, however the solid tumor is usually isointense on T1-weighted images and minimally to moderately hyperintense on T2-weighted images. Enhancement is common. The classic association of bilateral retinoblastomas with a mass in the pineal region (trilateral retinoblastoma) represents a secondary locus for PNET (pinealoblastoma). Germinomas and teratomas in the pineal region can appear similar to those located in the suprasellar region.

Both ependymomas and choroid plexus neoplasms may arise in the posterior aspect of the third ventricle. In this location they may be confused with an extra-axial lesion arising from the pineal region, or an intra-axial lesion arising from the midbrain. Both generally appear as inhomogeneous irregular masses that are hypointense or isointense on T1-weighted images and only minimally to moderately hyperintense on T2-weighted images. In general, the anterior interface of a pineal region mass will remain distinct as it pushes the posterior wall of the third ventricle forward, whereas the anterior surface of the third ventricular tumor is usually irregular as it grows unrestrained into the ventricular lumen.

Cerebral Hemispheres

The incidence of cerebral hemispheric tumors in children is less than that found in adults. Low-grade tumors are more common among childhood hemispheric gliomas, whereas higher grade malignancies predominate in adults. Childhood hemispheric gliomas include astrocytomas, oligodendrogliomas and ependymomas. Additional hemispheric tumors in children are PNETs, neural tumors (ganglioglioma, gangliocytoma), and intraparenchymal meningiomas or menigosarcomas. The appearance of most astrocytomas in children is similar to that in adults, with the exception of pilocytic astrocytomas that are often cystic and well defined and that enhance intensely compared to low-grade tumors in adults. Grade three or four astrocytomas and glioblastoma multiforme appear similar in children to their adult counterparts. The childhood oligodendroglioma also differs somewhat in appearance from its adult counterpart. In children, these tumors are generally benign, large and hemorrhagic, contain dense lamellar calcifications, and are often associated with a prominent cyst. Their appearance on MRI is generally that of a heterogeneous tumor with mixed signal characteristics on both T1- and T2-weighted images.

Gangliogliomas have a propensity for the middle cranial fossa and posterior deep parietal lobe. They appear as inhomogeneous solid masses with dense calcification, minimal enhancement, and indistinct margins. Unlike the oligodendroglioma, they generally lack a cystic component. The more cellular gangliocytoma can be difficult to diagnose and to see on imaging. As described by Altman [11], the lesion is hyperdense on CT and does not enhance. On MRI, the lesions are best seen on T1-weighted images or with the first echo of T2-weighted images as having mixed signal, and may disappear or actually decrease in signal on the second echo of T2-weighted images.

CSF Spaces and Meninges

Extra-axial tumors in children comprise meningiomas, meningosarcomas, primary bone tumors, and metastases, often from small round cell tumors such as neuroblastoma. Childhood meningiomas have a high incidence for intraparenchymal involvement compared to those in adults. These lesions are typically isointense on T1-weighted images and low in signal on T2-weighted images. Enhancement is moderate to marked. Metastatic tumors with extra-axial involvement (e.g. neuroblastoma, Ewing's sarcoma) typically include adjacent bony erosion, which must be carefully sought for on CT with bone windows. Intraventricular tumors may arise from a variety of structures and represent several different histologies. Most common are the tumors arising from the choroid plexus, which represent either papillomas or carcinomas, or have mixed histology for both. These are the most common intraventricular tumor to be encountered in the first several years of life. These tumors may result in hydrocephalus, which at times may be severe. The etiology of the hydrocephalus may be secondary to overproduction of CSF by a papillomatous tumor, but is most often obstructive in nature. These tumors are typically isointense to hyperintense on T1-weighted images, and are often isointense or even hypointense on T2-weighted images. Enhancement is common and is typically marked. Imaging differentiation of papilloma from carcinoma is generally not possible, as these tumors are often histologically mixed [9]. Other intraventricular tumors arising in childhood include ependymoma, meningioma, oligodendroglioma and astrocytoma. This group of intra-ventricular tumors typically arise in the older age group of 5-18 years of age. All tend to have similar appearances, and also resemble the papilloma-carcinoma making a specific imaging diagnosis difficult.

References

1. Naidich TP, Zimmerman RA (1984) Primary brain tumors in children. Semin Reontgenol 19(2):100
2. Schoenberg BS, Schoenberg DC, Christine BW et al (1976) The epidemiology of primary intracranial neoplasms of childhood. Mayo Clin Proc 51:51
3. Childhood Brain Tumor Consortium (1988) A study of childhood brain tumors based on surgical biopsies from ten North American institutions: sample description. J Neurooncol 6:9-21
4. Rorke LB, Schut L (1989) Introductory survey of pediatric brain tumors. In: McLaurin RL, Schut L, Venes JL, Epstein F (eds) Pediatric neurosurgery: surgery of the developing nervous system. WB Saunders, Philadelphia, pp 335-337
5. Ambrosino MM, Hernanz-Schulmann M, Genieser NB, Wisoff J, Epstein F (1988) Brain tumors in infants less than a year of age. Pediatr Radiol 19:6-8
6. Segal HD, Zee CS, Naidich TP et al (1982) Computed tomography of neoplasms of the posterior fossa in children. Radiol Clin North Am 20:23
7. Gusnard D (1990) Cerebellar neoplasms in children. Semin Roentgenol 25:264-278
8. Lee BCP, Kneeland JB, Walker RW et al (1985) MR imaging of brain stem tumors. Am J Neuroradiol 6:159-163
9. Vasquez E, Ball WS, Prenger EC, Castellote A, Crone KR (1992) Magnetic resonance imaging of fourth ventricular choroid plexus neoplasms in childhood: a report of two cases. Pediatr Neurosurg 17:48-52
10. Ball WS (1997) Infratentorial tumors. In Ball WS (ed) Pediatric neuroradiology. Lippincott-Raven, Philadelphia, pp ???
11. Altman NR (1988) MR and CT characteristics of gangliocytomas: a rare cause of epilepsy in children. AJNR Am J Neuroradiol 9:917
12. Jones B, Patterson R (1997) Supratentorial feoplasms. In: Ball WS (ed) Pediatric neuroradiology. Lippincott-Raven, Philadelphia, pp ???

Central Nervous System Diseases in Children

C. Raybaud

CHU Timone, Université de la Méditerranée, Marseille, France

Introduction

Central nervous system (CNS) diseases in children are significantly different from those in adults. They are related to age-specific processes (e.g. hypoxic-ischaemic encephalopathies), pathologies (e.g. acute encephalomyelitis), maturation (e.g. age-related epileptic syndromes, age-specific tumours), developmental processes (e.g. brain malformations) and genetic disorders (e.g. metabolic diseases). Technically, at least in very young children, the conditions of investigation – mostly with magnetic resonance imaging (MRI) – are quite different also. This paper provides an overview of what is specific to children in the way of investigating CNS diseases.

Imaging Tools

Ultrasonography (US) is the simplest tool for investigating infants at the bedside. NeuroUS, however, has its own constraints: there are no acoustic windows in the spine of newborn infants after a few days nor in the skull of infants older than a few months. On the other hand, US can be used in utero for satisfactory depiction of brain and spine as early as the third month of gestation. Limitations of US are its relative lack of definition and specificity. Transcranial Doppler sonography may be used after the closure of the sutures in the same conditions as in adults; the technique has a specific role in cases of sickle cell disease.

Computed tomography (CT) is still useful, not only for evaluating the craniospinal skeleton, but also the brain. Its sensitivity is not as good as that of MRI, but it has considerably improved over the years. Its environment is simpler, volume acquisition is possible, and sedation is rarely needed anymore. In some pathologies, CNS examination may be part of a more general body study. Since ionizing radiation has potential noxious effects, especially in infants, CT should be limited to reasonable indications.

Magnetic resonance imaging (MRI) has neuropaediatric peculiarities. Of course, it has unequalled anatomical definition, sensitivity to tissue alterations and specificity (even with conventional sequences). A single machine provides conventional imaging, water imaging (diffusion), chemical imaging (MR spectroscopy), functional imaging (fMRI), vascular imaging (perfusion, MR angiography) and tractography (DTI), in a way compatible with integrated data post-processing (morphometry, signal averaging, multimodality integration, stereotactic surgical neuronavigation, etc.).

Imaging sequences should be adapted to the maturing brain. The repetition time (TR) of a conventional spin echo (SE) sequence has to be three-times longer than the T1, which at 1.0-1.5 T is about 700 ms in adults but 3000 ms in neonates (personal data). A TR close to 10 000 ms is acceptable only with fast SE sequences, which on the other hand "look" more mature than the conventional SE images. In neonates, FLAIR images (T2 images with the free water signal cancelled) show a low white matter signal because the white matter is composed of 90% water. Then as myelin precursors accumulate, the signal looks more like that of conventional T2 images, but the adult pattern is not reached before 3-4 years of age (compared to 2 years on conventional T2-weighted images).

MRI has no known noxious effect on the maturing organism, even foetal. But because of the acquisition times, full cooperation of the child is needed. In very small infants, feeding and simple contention are usually enough. In young or uncooperative children, sedation or anaesthesia is necessary and, therefore, MRI is not completely noninvasive. Simple sedation, whichever drug is used, needs experienced radiologists and nursing personnel and specific care (for monitoring, temperature, freedom of airways) before, during and after the procedure. The sensitive environment of MRI (high magnetic field, radiofrequencies) makes things more difficult for neonates; MRI-compatible incubators have been recently developed.

Conventional digital angiography still has indications in paediatric neuroradiology, for optimal visualization of the vascular tree (in cases of vasculitis, thrombophlebitis, arteriovenous malformations) and for endovascular treatments.

Conventional *myelography* or CT myelography may be considered when the morphology of the spine or the presence of metals makes MRI useless or impossible.

Imaging Strategies

Detailed Imaging of the Foetal CNS

There is no clinical expression of foetal CNS disease. Progression of pregnancy can be watched routinely with US from the early foetal period to term. CT is avoided because of the noxious effect of X-rays. MRI complements the US data in three main instances: abnormal familial context (potential genetic disorder), abnormal maternofoetal context (abnormal pregnancy, infection, anoxia) and abnormal foetal context (abnormal US screening). MRI is not performed before weeks 17-18 of gestation because of the small size of the brain. At 20 weeks (mid-pregnancy), the brain is essentially complete as neuronal migration is achieved. Further growth is due to the multiplication of the fibers, with their supporting astroglia and myelination. The changes in morphology of the brain (sulci and gyri) and the ongoing maturation (proceeding radiologically for at least two more years) are precisely timed. In the foetus, the normal layered pattern of the cerebral mantle, usually not apparent at US, is well demonstrated on MRI; from inside out, these layers are the periventricular germinal matrix, an intermediate glial cell layer (until week 28), the transient sub-plate (until birth), and the cortical ribbon. The pericerebral cerebrospinal fluid (CSF) space is prominent until week 32. The ventricular trigone measures 7-8 mm, and should not be larger than 10 mm. Any radiological diagnosis should take this evolving anatomy into account.

Brain malformations, mostly commissural agenesis, form about one-third of the diagnoses. The group of the ventriculomegalies (above 10 mm) forms the most common indication (40%); their prognosis is worse if MRI uncovers associated abnormalities (e.g. cortex malformations, loss of the tissular layered pattern, necrosis, haemorrhage) often not seen at US. Foetal hydrocephalus may develop without the skull being enlarged.

Better Prognostic Assessment of Neonatal Disease with MRI

The expression of CNS disease in the neonate is poor: failure to thrive, convulsions. US is the first, often the sole investigation of the neonatal brain. Operator-dependent, it should be performed according to a strict protocol so that the images can be read by any concerned physician; this protocol does not exclude focussing on specific abnormalities also, as they are discovered during the study.

The typical features of anoxic-ischaemic encephalopathies (AIE) are well correlated with the gestational age. In the *premature infant*, MRI shows:
- various degrees of subependymal haemorrhages (SEH) with germinal matrix clots, ventricular clots, and paraventricular haemorrhagic venous infarctions, and
- periventricular leucomalacia (PVL) with diffuse periventricular abnormalities.

In the *term baby*, MRI shows necrosis of the central nuclei (short T1, short or long T2) and cortex (loss of contrast, abnormal cortical T1/T2 signal, especially in the depth of the sulci), global brain swelling and venous thrombosis. The T1/T2 shortening should not be confused with normal early myelination. A diffuse, thin subdural haematoma over the tentorium cerebelli due to delivery is common even in normal neonates, and a few punctiform parenchymal haemorrhages along the ventricular wall and in the parenchyma may be observed.

CT can be used in AIE as it has fewer constraints than MRI. However, the prognosis is best approached with MRI: severity and extent of the lesions, and metabolic approach with proton spectroscopy (abnormal lactate peak). On CT, the relatively low density of the parenchyma as compared with the blood in the dural sinuses should not be misread as venous thrombosis.

Other neonatal disorders include malformations, infections, perinatal trauma and breathing failure. A nearly normal-looking brain in a severely ill neonate points to a metabolic disease.

MRI Is the Primary Tool for Assessing Increased Intracranial Pressure

Increased intracranial pressure (ICP) is expressed in the young infant by enlargement of the head with bulging fontanel, sometimes with a "sunset gaze" (Parinaud's syndrome), and in older children by headaches, lethargy and vomiting. The most common causes of increased ICP in children are hydrocephalus or lesions associated with hydrocephalus, and less commonly, mass lesions without hydrocephalus and diverse pathologies such as venous thrombosis.

Hydrocephalus Should Be Evaluated with MRI

The skull contains CSF, blood and brain tissue. Hydrocephalus is due to increased resistance to circulation or decreased resorption of CSF. The CSF compartment expands actively against the blood (acutely) and or the cellular compartments (subacutely or chronically). The CSF and extracellular spaces are in continuity, so the latter tends to expand also in case of hydrocephalus. The periventricular hyperhydration observed in hydrocephalus is a superadded brain oedema rather than a useful resorption process. In the young infant, hydrocephalus can be detected with US but, like in older patients, it should be assessed by MRI to:
- *Ascertain the hydrocephalus*: increased head circumference, enlarged ventricles with rounded temporal horns and compressed hippocampi (never observed in atrophy).
- *Locate the obstacle*: uni-, bi-, tri- or quadriventricular hydrocephalus; cisternal block; peripheral block. Triventricular hydrocephalus is not necessarily an aqueductal stenosis, which should be documented. When a ventricular block is downstream of the anteri-

or third ventricle, ventriculocisternostomy may be performed, avoiding insertion of a shunting device. Documenting the freedom of the extracerebral CSF pathways is possible using flow-sensitive sequences and high definition T2-weighted imaging.
- *Look for complications*: circulatory arrest in acute block (loss of gray-white matter contrast, usually with small, rounded ventricles); herniations; periventricular oedema; loss of brain substance (only in the first months of life has the brain the capacity to recover its full thickness); demyelination, etc.
- *Identify the cause* (together with the clinical context), and prepare for treatment. Overall, 80% of paediatric brain tumours develop in or around the ventricles. Brain malformations, cavitations and cysts within and around the brain may accumulate fluid. Trauma, infections and haemorrhages may reduce the resorption capabilities.

Some infants, especially former premature infants, present *benign idiopathic external hydrocephalus*, an accumulation of fluid over the anterior frontotemporal convexities, with mild anterior ventricular enlargement, and macrocephaly. As a rule, it disappears spontaneously after 18 months. The assumed pathogenesis is immaturity of the arachnoid granulations. Similar features may express an increased venous pressure in infants.

Mass Effects: Tumours and Other Lesions

Any mass effect may induce features of increased ICP, even without producing hydrocephalus. The most common causes in children are pericerebral haematomas (mainly subdural), hemispheric tumours, intracerebral bleeding, expanding extracerebral arachnoid cysts, and septic abscesses and empyemas. In cerebral thrombophlebitis, brain oedema may develop as the sole symptom (so-called pseudotumour cerebri).

Peculiar aspects of brain tumours in children are their frequency (second only to leukaemias), diversity, frequent dissemination along the CSF spaces (spine imaging is mandatory to complement brain imaging) and positive correlation between age and topography and histology (e.g. juvenile pilocytic astrocytoma (JPA), medulloblastomas, choroid plexus papillomas, fibrillary astrocytoma of the pons). Further information on this topic should be looked for in specialized textbooks.

Some tumours are special as they are cortical, developmental and highly epileptogenic. In children, the most common is ganglioglioma, the most specific is infantile dysplastic neurocytoma, and the most typical is dysembryoplastic neuroepithelial tumour (DNET).

Craniocerebral Trauma May Produce Specific Lesions in Children

In grown children, trauma is not different from what it is in adults. In young infants it is different because of the different physical properties of the infantile skull and brain and of the different circumstances. The elasticity of the squamous vault explains the special appearance of the "table-tennis ball fracture". The malleability of the calvarium, without rigid sutures, favours the development of shearing lesions, within the meninges (acute subdural are more common than acute epidural hematomas) and within the brain. The delivery itself is a specific process with specific lesions.

Above all, young children may be victims of nonaccidental trauma. The most common mechanism is shaking that causes brain lesions aggravated by the lack of tonus of the neck muscles. The main clinical features are decreased consciousness and convulsions; fundoscopic examination typically discloses retinal haemorrhages (shaking-related tractions on the optic nerves). Intracranial examination may demonstrate multiple subdural haematomas of different signals (MRI) or intensities (CT), explained either by different dilutions with CSF or by different times of occurrence. A thin lining of acute subdural bleed along the falx is especially suggestive. These bleeds are explained by the rupture of bridging veins; they are accompanied by areas of ischaemia (areas of low signal with loss of the gray-white matter contrast, commonly bilateral in the frontal or temporo-occipital areas, and oedema). Further investigation may disclose multiple fractures (skull, ribs, long bones) at various stages of consolidation. The haematomas may be drained, but the bilateral cerebral lesions are usually devastating with subsequent encephalomalacia and cerebral atrophy.

Acute Neurological Deficits

Intracerebral Haemorrhage Needs an Emergency Diagnosis

Intracerebral haemorrhages in children are *absolute emergencies*. A child may be playing at school, complain of a sudden headache, go into coma, and die in a few hours. There is absolutely no spontaneous brain haemorrhage in children and, except in rare cases of coagulation disorders, causes to be looked for are AVMs (in children, 80% are revealed by bleeding) and cavernomas (usually less severe). The diagnosis should be made as quickly as possible, as surgery is the only way to alleviate the intracranial pressure; it is then better to remove the causal AVM together with the blood collection. The nidus of the AVM may be well seen on conventional imaging, especially MRI. The vasculature of the AVM may be well depicted by MR angiography. Conventional intra-arterial angiography is needed when endovascular treatment is considered.

Arterial Ischaemia of the Brain Is Not Rare in Children

Brain arterial ichaemia is different in children and adults, because the vascular pathologies are different, the metabolic needs and cerebral blood flow are higher in children, and the haemodynamic protection (cerebral autoregulation and collateral anastomoses) is usually higher in children. In cases of profound and prolonged drop of the central perfusion pressure, ischaemic lesions affect primarily the structures with high metabolism (central nuclei, cortex), with a watershed distribution.

Arterial occlusions in children occur mainly at the terminal portion of the carotid siphons and the proximal segments of the cerebral arteries: clots stop there because they cannot go beyond the bifurcations. This segment is the one involved in virus-related vasculitis. It is directly affected by the inflammatory process of septic meningitis. As a common result, the lenticulostriate perforators become occluded at their origin, with necrosis of the basal ganglia and deep paraventricular white matter, while the widely efficient corticopial anastomoses protect the cortical territories downstream of the occlusion. So, typical cerebral ischaemia in children affects the striatum only, sparing the cortex; functional recovery is usually good and recurrences are uncommon. However, when the occlusive process is extensive, several arteries (e.g. anterior choroidal, anterior cerebral) may be occluded, affecting the internal capsule also and compromising the sources of the collateral flow.

The spectrum of aetiologies is extremely large in children: embolic occlusion, usually from heart disease; septic infections adjacent to the arterial tree (cervical adenoiditis, tonsillitis, septic meningitis); virus-related arterial vasculitis (chickenpox, herpes); trauma (cervical, pharyngeal); haemopathies (sickle cell disease); and metabolic diseases (homocystinuria).

One arterial dysplasia, *moyamoya*, is quite specific and is characterized by stenosis of the carotid siphons and of the proximal segments of the middle and anterior cerebral arteries, sparing the posterior circulation. As the stenosis is *slowly progressive*, collateral networks develop and may compensate the occlusion temporarily. They use the small pial arteries, the deep anastomoses between the lenticulostriate and the cortical perforators (aspect of "puff of smoke", *moyamoya* in Japanese), and the dural-pial anastomoses. With progression of the disease, infarctions occur repeatedly. On imaging, multiple lesions of different ages and global atrophy may be observed. Medical and surgical treatments are proposed. Moyamoya *disease* is an idiopathic, maybe genetic disorder. Moyamoya *syndromes* present with similar images and may be observed in different clinical contexts such as sickle cell disease, neurofibromatosis type I, and as a complication of radiotherapy to the sellar region.

CNS Infections

Septic Infections May Present Severe Complications

Septic infections of the CNS are not essentially different in children and adults. However, the immature brain is particularly vulnerable (massive abscesses with tissue destruction) and infants present special complications such as subdural "effusions" that become secondarily infected and form subdural empyemas (meningeal abscesses). In neonates, specific vaginal germs are involved (*Proteus* and *Citrobacter*); these may produce giant abscesses with massive destruction of brain tissue. In all children, ventriculitis, meningeal fibrosis and subsequent hydrocephalus are common.

Viral Infections Can Be Devastating

Viral lymphocytic meningitides are common in children, and usually benign. Encephalitides are clinically impressive but usually benign, with sometimes ill-defined areas of long T1/T2 affecting both the gray matter and white matter. They may be severe when they are due to a herpesvirus, or when they develop in immunodeficient children. Two types of herpes encephalitis occur in children:
- *Herpes type I* encephalitis, not different from what it is in adults, concerns older children, presumably due to infestation from the trigeminal nerve. The necroticohaemorrhagic destructions affect mostly the mesial temporal lobes and adjacent fronto-orbital cortex (possibly having special tropism for the limbic structures). Untreated or treated late, the lesions are devastating, particularly when vasculitis develops in addition.
- *Herpes type II* concerns the neonate contaminated during the birth process by a mother with genital herpes. The viremic diffusion results in a massive destruction of the parenchyma. It can be avoided by systematic use of caesarean section in affected mothers.

Worldwide, the most deadly encephalitides are due to arboviruses, such as the Japanese B encephalitis virus. In Europe, mumps, measles, rubella, and infections with Epstein-Barr virus and coxsakie viruses are common. Varicella-zoster (chickenpox) affects mostly the cerebellum, but also the arteries. Subacute sclerosing panencephalitides rarely may develop after measles or rubella.

Acute Disseminated Encephalomyelitis Is a Common Immune-related Disorder

Acute disseminated encephalomyelitis (ADEM) is a postinfectious, acute, immuno-allergic demyelination that affects mostly children and young adults. It develops within a few days after a febrile episode, typically viral but possibly bacterial, or after an immunisation. It is expressed on imaging by areas of oedematous demyelination, sometimes extensive, affecting both gray matter and white matter, in the brain and spinal cord. The lesions are not symmetrical, and may or may not enhance with contrast agents. Histologically, only the myelin sheath is affected, not the oligodendrocyte, and recovery usually occurs in a few weeks or months. Relapsing forms exist, causing borderline to chronic demyelination such as multiple sclerosis (MS). Schilder's disease is controversial and has been classified both as a form of MS and a form of ADEM. The prognosis depends on the causal virus: smallpox ADEM used to result in significant mortality; measles ADEM leaves neurologic sequelae in about 15% of cases. Idiopathic ADEMs are commonly benign. Acute disseminated haemorrhagic myelitis (AHEM) is an especially severe form of ADEM. Transverse myelitis is likely to be a predominantly spinal form of ADEM.

Degenerative, Progressive Encephalopathies Are Fairly Common

There is no room to fully describe the degenerative encephalopathies. These are metabolic disorders, classified according to the clinical picture correlated with the enzymatic defect (e.g. mitochondriopathies, peroxisomal or lysosomal defects, disorders of intermediate metabolism, aminoacidopathies). Each is rare, but the causal multiplicity is such that, as a group, they are common and probably underdiagnosed. They affect predominantly the white matter (leucodystrophies) or the gray matter (poliodystrophies), or both. Their clinical course is typically progressive. A familial history of similar disorders, or of consanguinity, is common. Some have typical features on MR images, with a specific organisation of the anomalies (adrenoleucodystrophies, metachromatic leucodystrophies, Alexander's disease, Canavan's disease, Wilson disease's, etc.). Others present with different patterns in different patients (most mitochondriopathies). The anomalies (posterior or anterior; central or subcortical; affecting or not the corpus callosum, basal ganglia, brain stem or cerebellum; with or without craniomegaly, cysts, calcification, enhancement; mode of progression, etc.) typically are symmetrical, while the inflammatory lesions typically are not. When the images are not specific, MR spectroscopy may be useful, but the diagnosis fundamentally rests upon the clinical picture, familial history and biological data.

Malformations

Cord and Spine

The processes leading to formation of the spine and cord start with the development of the midline mesodermal structure that induces the transformation of the midline dorsal ectoderm into a neural ectoderm. The vertebral centrum is organised around the notochord independently from the cord, and the neural arches develop around the cord independently from the vertebral centrum. The malformations may be classified into disorders of the notochord, cord (with or without the neural arches) and vertebral centrum, and disorders of segmentation.

1. ***Notochord anomalies***. The persisting *neurenteric canal or cysts* are cysts anterior to the cord in the spinal canal, the spine itself, the mesenterium or the mediastinum (bronchogenic cysts). Exceptional, they represent the abnormal persistence, typically in the

cervicodorsal or dorsolumbar segments of the spine, of the normally transient neurenteric canal. *Diastematomyelia* and *diplomyelia* are presumably related to a duplication of the notochord with duplication of the cord and attempted duplication of the spine.

2. ***Cord anomalies***. The most common cord anomaly worldwide is *myelomeningocele*, in which the neural tube fails to close and remains exposed on the back of the child, with an open spinal canal. As a rule, it is associated with brain stem and cerebellum displaced into the cervical canal, a small posterior fossa, and hydrocephalus, forming the *Chiari II deformity*. *Dermal sinuses and cysts* develop when the skin remains attached to the cord, forming a fistula behind and below the cord that tends to become infected. A *lipomeningocele* is a dysplastic lipoma developing through a spinal hiatus between the cord and the subcutaneous fat. *Sacral agenesis* is a missing distal segment of the spine, together with a lack of the corresponding segment of the cord. *Chiari I "malformation"* and *hydrosyringomyelia* are likely to be related to disturbances of CSF dynamics. All these diseases associate anomalies of the neural arches with anomalies of the cord.

3. ***Vertebral center anomalies***. As a rule, vertebral center anomalies are not associated with cord anomalies. Examples of vertebral center anomalies include complete or partial agenesis and butterfly vertebra with persisting notochordal remnants.

4. ***Segmentation disorders*** (hemivertebrae) are probably mesodermal (somitic) and are not associated with cord anomalies.

Gross Brain Malformations

The most common gross brain malformation worldwide is the *Chiari II malformation* that associates a closure defect of the neural tube with (probably subsequent) deformity of the hindbrain in a small posterior fossa, and other dysplasias of the neural tube. A failure of the forebrain vesicles to differentiate properly results in various degrees of interhemispheric fusion with missing septum pellucidum, the *holoprosencephalies*, sometimes with facial anomalies. Several gene defects may be involved.

Septo-optic dysplasia is characterized by the absence of septum pellucidum, dysplasia of the anterior optic pathways, and a pituitary deficit.

Commissural agenesis (so-called callosal agenesis) is when one or several commissures (anterior, hippocampal, callosal) fail to develop, totally or partially, between the hemispheres, usually together with other white matter tracts. It may be associated with cystic or lipomatous dysplasia of the inter-hemispheric meninges.

In the hindbrain, developmental anomalies of the roof of the fourth ventricle result in cystic malformations of the posterior fossa, with an elevated tentorium, with or without vermian agenesis. These conditions form, as a group, the spectrum of *Dandy-Walker malformations*.

Malformations of Cortical Development (Brain and Cerebellum)

The development of the mantle and cortex proceeds in subsequent steps, and cortical malformations correspond to the failure of any of these. The first step is proliferation; its failure results in *micrencephaly with simplified gyral pattern*. The second step is differentiation into neurons and glia; its failure results in *focal cortical dysplasias (FCD)*, *microdysgenesis* or *hemimegalencephaly*, all characterized by poor cellular differentiation, migration and a poor organisation. *Tuberous sclerosis* is a syndromic, genetic form of cortical dysplasia. If normal neurons fail to migrate properly, they form heterotopias, either *nodular heterotopias* (periventricular or subcortical) or *laminar heterotopias* (also called "double-cortex" and band heterotopias). Depending on the gene defect, they can be mostly anterior (chromosome X) or posterior (chromosome 17). *Agyrias-pachygyrias* are more complete forms of double-cortex, with an absent or simplified gyral pattern. If the migration is adequate but the cortical organisation is not, *polymicrogyria* develops, uni- or bilateral, with an aberrant sulcal pattern. The rare *schizencephaly* is a trans-mantle cleft lined with polymicrogyric cortex, either uni- or bilateral.

Most of these disorders are epiletogenic, with or without neurologic deficits. For some, *developmental tumours* may be classified as cortical dysplasias.

Neuroectodermal Syndromes of Brain, Skin and Other Organs

Neurofibromatosis type I, the most common genetic disorder, is characterised by multiple cutaneous lesions, especially café-au-lait spots. CNS anomalies, when they occur, develop in the young child. The most spectacular is juvenile pilocytic astrocytoma of the optic pathways and of the anterior third ventricle, which may be severe but may also be dormant and even regress spontaneously. The most typical is the presence of multiple areas of high T2/FLAIR signal intensity distributed in the globi pallidi, posterior thalami, brain stem and cerebellar white matter. They exert no or little mass effect, and do not enhance. They disappear at adulthood. Other masses may develop – and regress – elsewhere, especially in the brain stem. Malignant degeneration may occur. Arterial dysplasia with giant cervical aneurysms or moyamoya may be present. In the peripheral nervous system (PNS), neurofibromas may develop, often plexiform, with potential transformation into neurofibrosarcomas. Agenesis of the greater wing of the sphenoid, vertebral scalloping and dural ectasias may be observed.

Neurofibromatosis type II is much less common; it may develop during the second and third decades of life or about the fifth. The disease is characterised by the development of multiple schwannomas (especially acoustic, but also trigeminal, spinal or others), multiple meningiomas and cervical cord ependymoma. The unrelenting development of these tumours makes the disease devastating.

Tuberous sclerosis may affect the skin, heart, kidney, pancreas, lung and brain. The cerebral lesions usually include multiple cortical tubers, subependymal nodules and trans-mantle abnormalities. All are characterised by the presence of so-called giant astrocytes, which are actually undifferentiated neuronoglial cells. The disease is genetic and highly epileptogenic. Subcortical nodules in the vicinity of the interventricular foramen of Monro may develop into slow-growing tumours and need removal.

In Stürge-Weber disease, there are pial angiomas of the posterior part of the hemisphere, metamerically associated with retinal angioma, enlarged choroid plexus, facial port-wine angioma in the territory of the ophthalmic branch of the trigeminal nerve, and abnormal draining veins of the affected hemisphere. Pial calcifications develop. The disease is usually epileptogenic and causes progressive atrophy of the hemisphere.

Childhood Epilepsy Develops According to Age-specific Patterns and Syndromes

Epilepsy is a chronic disease, and it must be differentiated from the acute, symptomatic seizure. In children, its clinical expression is age-related; it usually presents as specific syndromes with specific treatments and specific prognoses. Epilepsy is grossly classified into an idiopathic benign form (familial, often transient) with normal brain, and a symptomatic form when the brain is abnormal. Any chronic brain alteration, either acquired (e.g. after anoxic-ischaemic insults, infections, traumatic scarring) or inborn (e.g. malformations, developmental disorders), may cause epilepsy.

Imaging is necessary to illustrate the potential cause of the disease, as well as its effects on the brain. It may also demonstrate surgically accessible lesions such as developmental tumours or focal cortical dysplasia (FCD). When no abnormality is found at imaging, the epilepsy is said to be cryptogenic.

Chronic Encephalopathies

Mental retardation, associated or not with cerebral palsy or epilepsy, is probably the most common indication for brain imaging in children. The clinical context and the personal and familial histories are diverse. As for epilepsy, any lesion usually affecting the brain diffusely, either acquired or developmental, may be observed. Some are peculiar, such as subtle dysmorphism of the corpus callosum or cerebellar cortical dysplasias. Others are non-specific, such as diffuse atrophy or incomplete myelination.

Orbit and Visual Pathways

M.F. Mafee[1], D.M. Yousem[2]

[1] Department of Radiology, University of Illinois, Chicago, IL, USA

[2] Department of Neuroradiology, The Russell H. Morgan Department of Radiology and Radiological Sciences, The Johns Hopkins Medical Institution, Baltimore, MD, USA

Introduction

The various compartments of the orbit lend themselves to a geographical analysis of lesions involving the orbit. Thus one often finds classifications of orbital diseases describing ocular abnormalities involving the globe vs. intraconal non-ocular abnormalities involving the soft tissues within the muscular cone, conal abnormalities involving the extraocular muscles, and extraconal abnormalities involving those lesions outside the muscular cone. In addition there are specific diseases that affect the orbital "appendages", which include the lacrimal glands, lacrimal sac, and conjunctivae.

Within each of these categories one might use the mnemonic of VITAMIN C AND D to evaluate lesions classified into vascular, inflammatory, traumatic, acquired, metabolic, idiopathic, neoplastic, congenital, and drug-related entities.

Anatomic Considerations

The orbital recesses contain the globes, cranial nerves II, III, IV, V and VI, muscles, blood vessels, connective tissue, and most of the lacrimal apparatus. The bony orbit is bordered by the periosteum (the periorbita or orbital fascia), which is loosely adherent to the surrounding bones except at the trochlear fossa, lacrimal crests and margins of the fissures and canals where it is more tightly bound. Anteriorly, at the margins of the orbit, the periorbita is continuous with the orbital septum, a membranous sheet forming the fibrous layer of the eyelids. Tenon's capsule (fascia bulbi) is a fibroelastic membrane that envelops the eyeball from the optic nerve to the level of the ciliary muscle. The inner surface of Tenon's capsule is separated from the outer surface of the sclera by a potential space, the episcleral or Tenon's space. The intraorbital structures are embedded in a fatty reticulum. This is divided into: (1) peripheral orbital fat outside the muscle cone, and its intermuscular membranes, and (2) the central orbital fat, which is within the muscle cone. The fibroelastic tissue comprising the reticulum divides the fat into lobes and lobules. The four recti and two oblique muscles control eye movement. The recti muscles arise from the annulus of Zinn, a funnel-shaped tendinous ring, which encloses the optic foramen and medial end of the superior orbital fissure.

Ocular Imaging

The eye consists of three primary layers: (1) the sclera, or outer layer; (2) the uvea, or middle layer; and (3) the retina, or inner layer which is the neural, sensory stratum of the eye. The retina has two layers: the inner layer is the sensory retina and the outer layer is the retinal pigment epithelium (RPE), a single lamina of cells whose nuclei are adjacent to the basal lamina (Bruch's membrane) of the choroid. The vitreous body occupies the space between the lens and retina and represents about two-thirds of the volume of the eye. There are basically three potential spaces that can accumulate fluid, resulting in detachment of various coats of the globe:

1. Posterior hyaloid space, the potential space between the base (posterior hyaloid membrane) of hyaloid and sensory retina. Separation of posterior hyaloid membrane from the sensory retina is referred to as posterior hyaloid detachment;

2. Subretinal space, the potential space between the sensory retina and RPE. Separation of sensory retina from RPE is referred to as retinal detachment;

3. Suprachoroidal space, the potential space between the choroid and the sclera. The RPE and Bruch's membrane are tightly adherent to the choroid and become separated when both layers are torn; however, the choroid is loosely attached to the sclera and can be separated resulting in choroidal detachment.

Blood within the anterior chamber of the globe causes a density difference between the affected globe and the unaffected globe, which is visible on computed tomography. This has been termed anterior hyphema and is readily apparent on ophthalmologic evaluation. It is rare to see isolated blood in the posterior chamber since this is a relatively small space intimately associated with the ciliary apparatus. After trauma, one may see rupture of either the anterior chamber (where there is flattening of the globe anterior to the lens) or of the vitreous humor. The latter, more commonly diagnosed by radiologists, appears as a globe that is subtly or grossly abnormal in shape rather than spherical. Hemorrhage may be identified by the difference in density in the two globes within the vitreous humor.

Choroidal or retinal detachments may be associated with globe trauma or rupture and with some neoplasms. Most retinal detachments have an elliptical V-shaped appearance in which the most posterior margin of the detachment is intimately associated with the optic nerve insertion and extends anteriorly to the ora serrata. Choroidal detachments extend farther anteriorly to the ciliary appa-

ratus and may not be restricted by the optic nerve insertion. They are anchored by the vortex veins or ciliary arteries.

Leukocoria refers to a white reflex when a light is shined in the patient's eyes. This is a finding that clinically elicits a wide differential diagnosis, however on imaging one should consider disease entities such as retinoblastoma (Fig. 1), persistent hyperplastic primary vitreous (PHPV), and Coats' disease in children. PHPV is due to persistence of primary vitreous along Cloquet's canal; one can see a fine thread of this residual hyaloid vascular system extending from the (small, anteriorly located) lens to the optic nerve. The globe often is small and noncalcified (distinguishing it from retinoblastoma) and may have variable signal intensity on magnetic resonance imaging (MRI). Coats' disease is due to retinal vascular malformation with associated exuda-

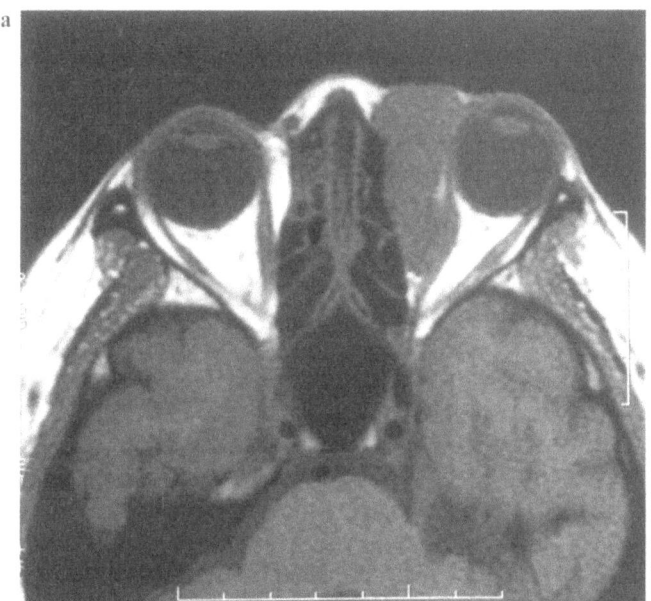
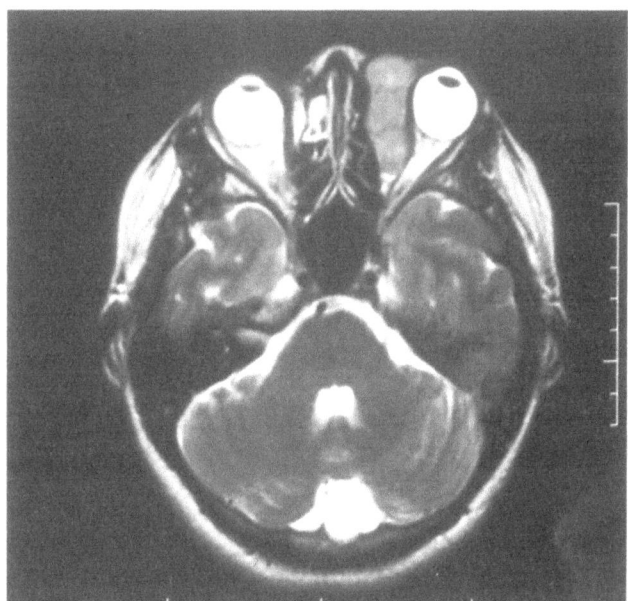
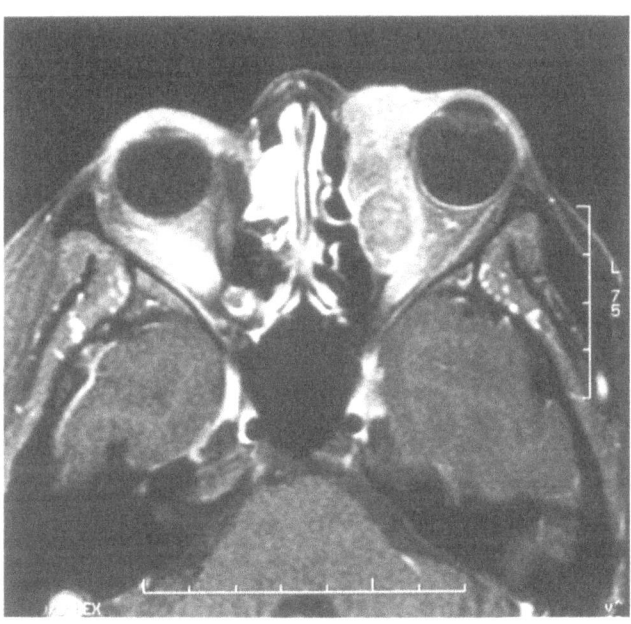

Fig. 1a-c. *Retinoblastoma with involvement of optic nerve.* **a** Axial unenhanced T1-weighted MR image. **b** Axial T2-weighted MR image. **c** Enhanced fat-suppressed T1-weighted MR image

tive retinal detachment. *Toxocara canis* infection may also cause leukocoria in a child. Once again, retinal detachment, increased ocular density, and absence of calcification characterize this entity. Retinopathy of prematurity may lead to noncalcified microphthalmic globes and leukocoria. High oxygen saturation exposure because of bronchopulmonary disease in a premature infant is likely the etiology.

Colobomas are congenital lesions of the globe in which there is an outpouching, usually at the optic nerve insertion, where the optic fissure vesicle closes. Colobomas may appear as two globe-like structures in the orbit; the classic clinical finding is "morning glory syndrome" in which there is a "black eye" reflex. The coloboma may lead to focal expansion of the optic nerve head insertion itself. It is important to look for central nervous system midline anomalies in patients with coloboma.

By the same token, cyclopia may be associated with holoprosencephaly intracranially. Even when there are two globes associated with holoprosencephaly, one should survey for the presence of optic nerve hypoplasia, which is found in all forms of the spectrum of holoprosencephaly, including septo-optic dysplasia. In the latter entity, the septum pellucidum is absent and there is a high rate of schizencephaly.

In a patient infected with human immunodeficiency virus (HIV), a common cause of ocular infection is cytomegalovirus (CMV) retinitis. This may lead to retinal detachment as well as to choroidal abnormalities and abnormalities of the ciliary body.

The most common primary ocular malignancy in adults is melanoma. This usually affects the choroid of the globe. Spread of uveal melanoma within the globe or along the optic nerve sheath into the subarachnoid space must be considered. Melanoma may be hyperdense on noncontrast computed tomography (CT) and have unusual MRI signal intensity characteristics (bright on T1 and dark on T2-weighted images) because of the melanin content. It will usually enhance.

Metastatic disease to the globes should also be considered in adult patients with ocular masses. Breast, lung and kidney primary tumors should be suspected. Often they are clinically silent and found only at the time of eye donation. The tumor is deposited in the choroid or retina and is bilateral in one-third of cases.

Orbital Appendages

Non-neoplastic abnormalities of the lacrimal glands are usually divided into those related to granulomatous disease, lymphoid lesions, and germ-line lesions. Granulomatous diseases include infectious etiologies such as tuberculosis and fungal disease as well as sarcoidosis. Additionally, pseudotumor of the orbit may affect the lacrimal gland as an idiopathic granulomatous inflammatory condition.

One should also consider epidermoid lesions as well as dermoids. Both result from the inclusion of ectodermal elements during closure of the neural tube. Both have a fibrous capsule of varying degrees of thickness. The epidermoid cyst has a lining of keratinizing, stratified epithelium. The dermoid cyst contains one or more dermal adnexal structures such as sebaceous glands and hair follicles. Dermoid cysts are found laterally in the orbit and 85% present with bony changes, usually remodeling. Low density (46%), calcification (14%), and purely cystic nature (80%) characterize these lesions.

In general, epithelial tumors represent 50% of masses involving the lacrimal gland. The remaining 50% of lacrimal gland masses are the lymphoid-inflammatory type. The excellent prognosis for benign mixed tumor, provided it is completely excised at first surgery, necessitates that these lesions should not undergo incisional biopsy, but require en bloc excision along with adjacent tissues.

Less commonly, neoplasms associated with adenocarcinomas and adenoid cystic carcinoma can arise in the lacrimal glands. Lymphoma, post-transplant lymphoproliferative disorders, and Sjogren's disease may affect the lacrimal gland. Most orbital lymphomas are composed of monoclonal B cells. Roughly 10% of non-Hodgkin's lymphomas present in the head and neck region. Lymphoid tumors account for 10%-15% of orbital masses.

The lacrimal sac and lacrimal duct are potential areas of congenital pathology as well. Congenital lesions include dacryocystoceles in which there is marked bulbous enlargement of the descending portion of the lacrimal duct, most commonly from maldevelopment of the valves that produce the appropriate downward flow of tears into the inferior meatus of the nasal cavity. These may present as medial orbital lesions or as sinonasal lesions. Obstruction of the ductal system may occur due to inflammatory condition of the paranasal sinuses or a direct infection of the duct itself. In these cases the patient may present with epiphora (excessive tearing). A number of articles have been written concerning the benefit of balloon angioplasty and stenting of the ducts to improve the flow of tears. This may also be a complication of paranasal sinus or orbital surgery and of radiation therapy.

Skin cancers such as squamous cell carcinoma and basal cell carcinoma may affect the lacrimal sac. Traditionally, transitional cell carcinoma may affect the lacrimal sac as the lining cells of the ductal system leading to the sac or leading from the sac. The lacrimal sac may also be affected by lymphoma. Inflammatory conditions of the lacrimal sac include pseudotumor of the orbit and dacryocystitis secondary to any number of the infectious lesions that affect the conjunctivae or from retrograde spread from sinus infection. The agger nasi cell of the anterior ethmoid complex has a particular propensity for eliciting epiphora as the sac and proximal duct are exposed in this location of sinus infection.

Intraconal Lesions

The most common benign intraconal mass is the hemangioma. This may in fact be a venous vascular malformation (VVF), and it has been reclassified recently in most head and neck treatises. If one finds phleboliths within a mass in the intraconal compartment, one should consider a venous vascular malformation vs. venous varix. These enhance avidly and are usually quite bright on a T2-weighted scan. The differential diagnosis with VVF in the intraconal compartment includes a schwannoma of trigeminal or oculomotor nerve origin or a metastasis.

An orbital varix may be diagnosed through various manipulations that can be performed while the patient is in the scanner. In many cases, a simple Valsalva's maneuver while performing the CT scan through the orbit will show the marked enlargement of the varix as the pressure changes lead to its dilatation from a resting state. Alternatively, one may place the patient in a head-back supine position, which may also increase the intraconal pressure sufficiently to change the size of the varix, which makes the diagnosis. Benign hemangiomas may also enlarge with such a maneuver, however, but the varix usually takes the form of the superior ophthalmic vein with its characteristic course.

Optic nerve sheath meningiomas and optic nerve lesions are also found in the intraconal compartment. Classically the optic nerve sheath meningioma appears as enhancement of the lining of the optic nerve without direct optic nerve enlargement. Sometimes, however, when the lesion is quite large it is difficult to distinguish from an intrinsic optic nerve lesion. Intrinsic optic nerve lesions include the optic nerve glioma, which is often associated with neurofibromatosis. In this instance the optic nerve is diffusely enlarged and may show extension along the entire optic pathway even into the occipital lobes. Optic nerve glioma in children is a benign, well-differentiated, and slow growing tumor. Bilateral optic nerve gliomas are characteristic of type 1 neurofibromatosis (NF1). The natural history of childhood optic glioma does not involve malignant transformation or systemic metastasis. Local invasion into the extraocular muscles (EOMs) rarely occurs. Malignant optic glioma is primarily seen in adults. It is a rare, fatal disease (glioblastoma multiforme) that usually extends from intracranial glioma. CT shows an enlarged fusiform and kinked optic nerves, along with marked to moderate enhancement.

These two neoplasms of the optic nerve and sheath should be distinguished from inflammatory conditions such as pseudotumor and demyelinating conditions such as optic neuritis. The latter is seen as abnormal signal intensity within the orbit on coronal, fat-saturated, T2-weighted scans or as enhancement of the optic nerve on fat-saturated post-gadolinium-enhanced scans. One can also see infectious inflammatory lesions affecting the optic nerve and sheath, particularly herpes infection with herpes zoster ophthalmicus, sarcoidosis, tuberculosis, and toxoplasmosis. Finally, neoplastic spread along the subarachnoid space of the optic nerve sheath should be considered in any patient with ocular melanoma, retinoblastoma, leukemia, lymphoma or metastases to the orbit.

Ischemic optic neuropathy (ION) is an entity seen in the elderly who present with painless visual loss. One may see high signal intensity in the optic nerve on T2-weighted images in the acute phase, followed by optic atrophy in the chronic phase. Vasculitides can cause ION.

Conal Lesions

Conal abnormalities include, most commonly, thyroid eye disease (TED). Grave's ophthalmopathy is another name for this entity. The muscles may be edematous, infiltrated by lymphocytes, mucopolysaccharide, or fat. There may be exophthalmos, unilateral proptosis, increased orbital fat, injection of the fat, and exposed cornea. In TED, the inferior and medial recti are the most commonly enlarged muscles with sparing of the tendinous insertion. This finding is contrasted with the stereotypical findings of pseudotumor of the orbit, which tends to affect the tendinous insertion of the muscles to the globe. Orbital pseudotumor is defined as a non-specific, idiopathic inflammatory condition for which no local identifiable cause or systemic disease can be found. Pain is an important feature of orbital pseudotumor. The histopathology can vary from polymorphous in inflammatory cells and fibrosis, with a matrix of granulation tissue, eosinophils, plasma cells, histiocytes, germinal follicles and lymphocytes, to a predominantly lymphocytic form. Pseudotumor may be classified as: (1) acute and subacute idiopathic anterior orbital inflammation; (2) acute and subacute idiopathic diffuse orbital inflammation; (3) acute and subacute idiopathic myositic orbital inflammation; (4) acute and subacute idiopathic apical orbital inflammation; (5) idiopathic dacryoadenitis; and (6) perineuritis (optic nerve).

The extraocular muscles, however, can also be affected by adjacent inflammatory sinusitis or by lesions, which may cause venous congestion within the orbit. The latter may be seen in patients who have dural vascular malformations, cavernous carotid fistulae, orbital apex obstructions, or veno-occlusive disease. In this case, all of the extraocular muscles may be affected and there is usually injection of the fat due to the widespread edema.

The extraocular muscles are striated muscle or of striated muscle origin. Therefore, primary neoplasms of the muscle include rhabdomyosarcoma (Rh). Orbital Rh is the most common primary orbital malignancy in children. Clinically, its occurrence involves the differential diagnosis of acute and subacute proptosis of childhood. Rapidly progressive unilateral proptosis is the hallmark of orbital Rh. These tumors are capable of rapid growth and they have the potential to destroy orbital bones. The MRI features of these tumors are characteristic of long T1 and long T2 lesions (Fig. 2). There is significant contrast enhancement on enhanced CT and MRI scans (Fig. 2c). Rarely one sees lymphoma or metastases directly to the extraocular muscles.

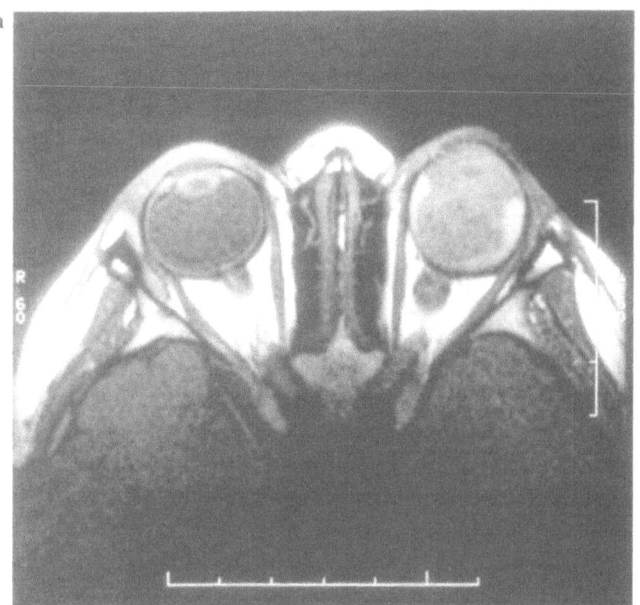

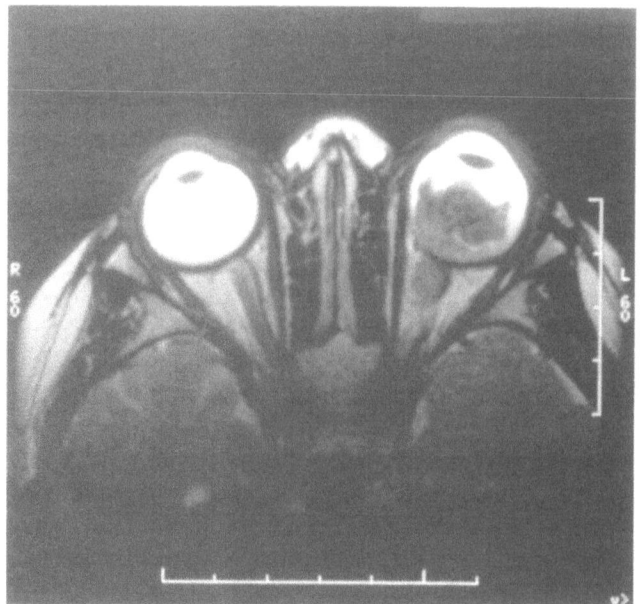

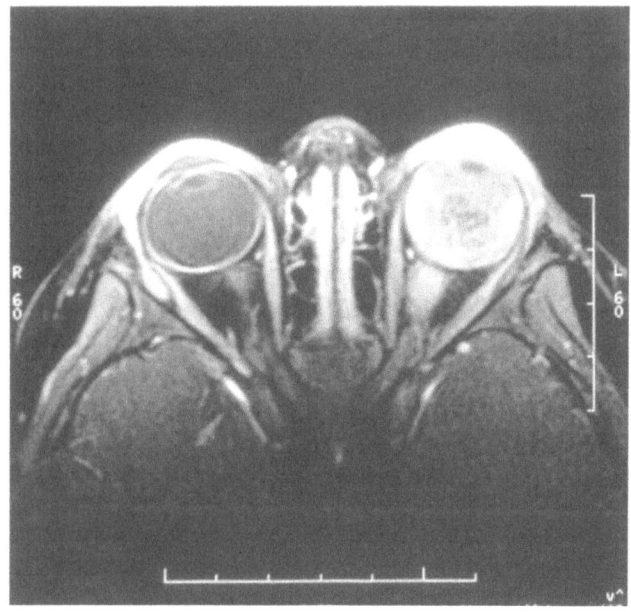

Fig. 2a-c. *Rhabdomyosarcoma*. **a** Axial T1-weighted MR image. **b** Axial T2-weighted MR image. **c** Post-contrast fat-suppressed T1-weighted MR image

Brown's syndrome is a tenosynovitis of the tendon of the superior oblique muscle. This is identified on imaging as thickening of this muscular tendon. Clinically, the patients have restricted eye movement.

Extraconal Space

The majority of lesions in the extraconal space fall in the category of infectious and neoplastic etiologies. Lymphangiomas tend to populate the extraconal space. These are often multilocular cystic lesions that have a tendency to bleed. Orbital lymphangiomas occur in children and young adults. In contrast to rapid, self-limited growth of infantile capillary hemangiomas, lymphangiomas gradually and progressively enlarge during the growing years. On MRI, lymphangiomas are hypointense or relatively hyperintense on T1-weighted images and are usually very hyperintense on T2-weighted images. Fluid-fluid levels due to hemorrhage may be present. The lesions do not enhance unless they also contain a hemangiomatous component.

The most common infectious source of extraconal pathology is sinusitis. Sinusitis is also the most common cause of orbital cellulitis. The classification of orbital cellulitis includes five categories or stages of orbital involvement from sinusitis. These are: (1) inflammatory edema; (2) subperiosteal phlegmon and abscess; (3) orbital cellulitis; (4) orbital abscess; (5) ophthalmic vein and cavernous sinus thrombosis. Distinguishing between a phlegmon and a periosteal abscess is difficult, since rim enhancement of the periosteal abscess is rare in this location. What one sees is a low-density collection running parallel to the medial wall of the orbit, which displaces the extraocular muscles laterally. This is less commonly due to frontal sinusitis. Rarely one may see a small collection of air within the larger periosteal collection. There may also be injection of the fat and extraocular muscle enlargement as the infection proceeds through the orbit. The most dangerous of the infections to involve the orbit are those from *Mucorales* or *Aspergillus*, which can invade the vascular structures of the orbit leading to the cavernous sinus and internal carotid artery and consequent intracranial vascular complications (stroke, vasculitis, sinus thrombosis).

Traumatic lesions of the orbital wall also may form extraconal collections. These are usually hematomas that occur along the roof or the floor and medial orbital walls in association with blowout fractures. The muscles again are displaced inward by the extraconal collection. There may be associated swelling of the muscle or intraconal compartment.

The bony orbit is also included in the extraconal tissue. Therefore, primary lesions of the bone such as multiple myeloma, fibrous dysplasia, Paget's disease and other fibrochondroosseous lesions of the surrounding bone may present with orbital symptomatology. One classic finding is dysplasia of the greater wing of the sphenoid, which is found as a primary criterion for neurofibromatosis type 1. Often these patients present with pulsatile exophthalmos secondary to transmitted cerebrospinal fluid (CFS) pulsations and intracranial pressure to the orbit since the bony protection is missing in the greater wing of the sphenoid. On plain films this may appear as an "empty orbit".

Another example of how the orbits may be affected by extraconal pathology is given by meningoencephalocele. Once again there is a defect in the orbital bony confines and CSF, meninges or brain may show mass effect on the orbital structures.

References

1. Adler IN, James CA, Glasier CM (2001) Ophthalmologic disease in children. Magn Reson Imaging Clin N Am 9(1):191-206
2. Castillo M, Mukherji SK, Wagle NS (2000) Imaging of the pediatric orbit. Neuroimaging Clin N Am 10(1):95-116
3. Chawda SJ, Moseley IF (1999) Computed tomography of orbital dermoids: a 20-year review. Clin Radiol 54(12):821-825
4. Chong VF, Fan YF, Chan LL (1999) Radiology of the orbital apex. Australas Radiol 43(3):294-302
5. de Keizer R (2003) Carotid-cavernous and orbital arteriovenous fistulas: ocular features, diagnostic and hemodynamic considerations in relation to visual impairment and morbidity. Orbit 22(2):121-142
6. Escott EJ (2001) A variety of appearances of malignant melanoma in the head: a review. Radiographics 21(3):625-639
7. Go JL et al (2002) Orbital trauma. Neuroimaging Clin N Am 12(2):311-324
8. Hayashi N et al (1999) Congenital cystic eye: report of two cases and review of the literature. Surv Ophthalmol 44(2):173-179
9. Hullar TE, Lustig LR (2003) Paget's disease and fibrous dysplasia. Otolaryngol Clin North Am 36(4):707-732
10. Kulkarni V, Rajshekhar V, Chandi SM (2000) Orbital apex leiomyoma with intracranial extension. Surg Neurol 54(4):327-330
11. Lapointe A, Peloquin L (2002) Wegener's granulomatosis of the orbit. J Otolaryngol 31(6):390-392
12. Mafee MF, Pai E, Philip B (1998) Rhabdomyosarcoma of the orbit: evaluation with MR imaging and CT. Radiol Clin N Am 36:1215-1227
13. Mafee MF, Edward DP, Koeller KK et al (1999) Lacrimal gland tumors and simulating lesions: clinicopathological and MR imaging features. Radiol Clin N Am 37:219-239
14. Mafee MF, Peyman GA (1984) Choroidal detachment and ocular hypotony: CT evaluation. Radiology 153:697-703
15. Mafee MF, Peyman GA, Grisolano JE et al (1986) Malignant uveal melanoma and simulating lesions: MR imaging evaluation. Radiology 160:773-780
16. Mafee MF (1998) Uveal melanoma, choroidal hemangioma, and simulating lesions: role of MR imaging. Radiol Clin N Am 36:1083-1099
17. Mafee M F, Haik BG (1987) Lacrimal gland and fossa lesions: role of computed tomography. Radiol Clin N Am 25(4):767-779
18. Mafee MF, Pruzansky S et al (1986) CT in the evaluation of the orbit and the bony interorbital distance. AJNR Am J Neuroradiol 7(2):265-259
19. Mafee MF, Putterman A et al (1987) Orbital space-occupying lesions: role of computed tomography and magnetic resonance imaging. An analysis of 145 cases. Radiol Clin N Am 25(3):529-559
20. Maus M (2001) Update on orbital trauma. Curr Opin Ophthalmol 12(5):329-334
21. Narla LD et al (2003) Inflammatory pseudotumor. Radiographics 23(3):719-729
22. Potter BO, Sturgis EM (2003) Sarcomas of the head and neck. Surg Oncol Clin N Am 12(2):379-417
23. Rootman J (2003) Vascular malformations of the orbit: hemodynamic concepts. Orbit 22(2):103-120
24. Tovilla-Canales JL, Nava A, Tovilla y Pomar JL (2001) Orbital and periorbital infections. Curr Opin Ophthalmol 12(5):335-341
25. Yousem DM (1993) Imaging of sinonasal inflammatory disease. Radiology 188(2):303-314
26. Yousem DM, Atlas SW et al (1989) MR imaging of Tolosa-Hunt syndrome. AJNR Am J Neuroradiol 10(6):1181-1184
27. Yousem DM, Galetta SL et al (1989) MR findings in rhinocerebral mucormycosis. J Comp Assisted Tomogr 13(5):878-882

Temporal Bone and Auditory Pathways

J.W. Casselman

Algemeen Ziekenhuis St. Jan Brugge, Brugge, Belgium

Introduction

Today the anatomy of the temporal bone can be evaluated in detail. Computed tomography (CT) is the method of choice to look at the external ear and middle ear. But CT also provides much information about the inner ear. New CT equipment, using helical scanning and multidetector technology, enables us to scan the temporal bone in detail. Once the images are made, one can recalculate them even every 0.1 mm. On these very thin images, partial volume is no longer a problem and hence every tiny structure can be seen. Moreover, excellent multiplanar reconstructions can be made. Structures like the branches and footplate of the stapes and chorda tympani can now be evaluated in a reliable way.

Magnetic resonance imaging (MRI) is used to look at the inner ear. Especially T2-weighted gradient echo (CISS) and turbo spin echo (DRIVE, FSE, FIESTA) sequences can be used. These images show the intralabyrinthine fluid in detail and enable us to see the scala tympani and vestibuli separately inside the cochlea. Another advantage is that the facial nerve and the cochlear, inferior vestibular and superior vestibular branches of the eighth cranial nerve can all be distinguished on these images. Even the posterior ampullar nerve and the ganglion of Scarpa can today be seen on 0.7-mm images made every 0.35 mm, using a 1024 matrix (Fig. 1).

MRI is also the only technique that can visualise lesions along the auditory pathway. Selective images through the cochlear nuclei, trapezoid body, lateral lemniscus, inferior colliculus, medial geniculate body and auditory cortex often detect the cause of deafness when the selective CT and MRI studies of the temporal bone are negative.

As a general rule one can say that patients with conductive hearing loss (CHL) should be examined with CT, while patients presenting with sensorineural hearing loss (SNHL), vertigo or tinnitus should immediately get an MRI study. There are of course exceptions and in many cases both CT and MRI can be useful. In the following paragraphs, I discuss the most frequent indications to perform imaging of the temporal bone. For each indication, the choice between CT and MRI is discussed.

Otosclerosis

In otosclerosis, the dense ivory-like endochondral bone layer around the labyrinthine capsule is replaced by foci of spongy, vascular, irregular new bone. The cause of this replacement is still under discussion. Patients with otosclerosis present with mixed hearing loss. However, the conductive component is most often predominant and the lesions are often only visible on CT. Hence CT is the method of choice. Otosclerosis (and otospongiosis) can be fenestral or retrofenestral.

In fenestral otosclerosis, the promontory, facial nerve canal and oval and round windows are involved. The most frequent lesion is a hypodense area or even mass at the fissula ante fenestrum. These lesions can also occur on the promontory or at the round window. At the level of the oval window, otospongiosis can block the anterior branch of the stapes so that they can no longer move freely, causing conductive hearing loss. Thickening of the footplate can also occur and has the same result. Lesions near the footplate are difficult to visualise, and a double oblique technique is needed to visualise both branches of the stapes and the footplate in one plane (Fig. 2). To achieve this, helical acquired images should be reconstructed every 0.1 mm so that double oblique images with sufficient quality are ob-

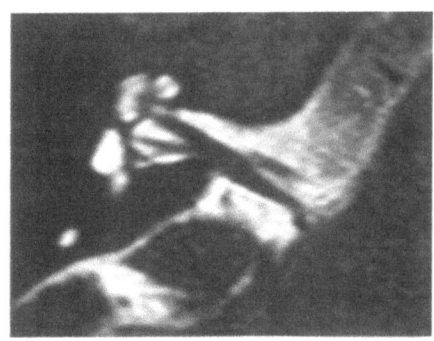

Fig. 1. 1024 matrix, 0.7-mm DRIVE image shows the posterior ampullar nerve, originating from the posterior wall of the inferior vestibular nerve, and the separation in scala vestibuli and tympani inside the cochlea

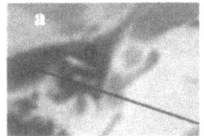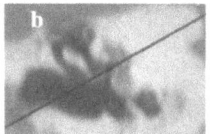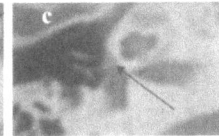

Fig. 2a-c. *The only reliable way to evaluate fenestral otosclerosis is the double oblique technique.* **a** Paracoronal images are made on the axial plane through the stapes. **b** Then, double oblique images are made when a reconstruction parallel to the incudostapedial junction on the paracoronal images is made. **c** The resulting double oblique image clearly shows otospongiosis (arrows) at the fissula antefenestrum, encasing the anterior branch of the stapes

tained. The round window should always be checked, as some studies have shown that surgery of the stapes and oval window is less successful when the round window is obliterated.

Retrofenestral otosclerosis involves the cochlea or the bone around the membranous labyrinth (with the exception of the lateral wall of the labyrinth). A hypodense ring can develop around the complete cochlea and is then called "the fourth ring of Valvassori". However, the lesions can also be more subtle and frequently a small hypodense spur can be seen anterior to the antero-inferior wall of the fundus of the internal auditory canal.

Trauma

Fractures of the temporal bone can best be seen on CT. Both longitudinal and transverse fractures can be distinguished. Longitudinal fractures follow the long axis of the temporal bone, from the surface of the petrous-mastoid bone to the middle ear cavity and geniculate ganglion area and even petrous apex. Transverse fractures run perpendicularly on the long axis of the petrous bone and petrous apex and, hence, nearly always involves the inner ear. Post-traumatic CHL is most often explained by the CT findings. Post-traumatic obliteration of the middle ear cavity and fractures or luxation of the ossicles can easily be recognized on CT today. However, CT sometimes does not provide an explanation for post-traumatic SNHL and facial nerve palsy. In these cases, MRI of the temporal bone can often provide the answer, but CT is and remains the most important and first study in case of trauma.

Unenhanced T1-weighted images must be used to recognize post-traumatic intralabyrinthine haemorrhage which represents inner ear concussion. Cloth or fibrosis formation in the labyrinth can be excluded using thin T2-weighted images (DRIVE, CISS, FIESTA). The high signal intensity of the fluid disappears in case of fibrosis or cloth formation; the fluid however keeps its normal high signal intensity when it is mixed with fresh blood. Post-traumatic intralabyrinthine enhancement can also occur. When the trauma causes a leak of intralabyrinthine fluid towards the middle ear, the inner

ear reacts with a higher fluid production to compensate the loss. This results in hyperaemia of the labyrinth and can, during the acute phase, sometimes be seen as enhancement.

Fractures through the tegmen can result in formation of meningocele or encephalocele. Blood or inflammation in the middle ear can only be distinguished from meningo- or encephalocele formation in a reliable way when MRI is performed.

Finally, the cause of hearing loss can also be located along the auditory pathways. The most frequent structures involved in trauma are the inferior colliculi (concussion when they are hit by the free edge of the tentorium during trauma) and the auditory cortex (hit by overlying bone or damaged by concussion or bleeding caused by the contrecoup). Again, these lesions are often only visible or their full extent is only visible on MRI.

Facial nerve palsy is not always caused by a fracture running through the facial nerve canal (e.g. tympanic segment). Therefore, sometimes CT shows normal results in patients with post-traumatic facial nerve palsy. The labyrinthine segment of the nerve is vulnerable because it occupies 95% of the available space of the canal. Hence, retrograde oedema can easily cause compression and secondary necrosis of this facial nerve segment. This can be seen as enhancement of the labyrinthine segment and enhancement near the fundus of the internal auditory canal, which is always abnormal. In such a case, decompression of the nerve should be considered in order to save the facial nerve.

Chronic Middle Ear Inflammation

In chronic middle ear inflammation, middle ear aeration is often disturbed and hence the drum is frequently retracted and thickened. Moreover, mucosal thickening or even obliteration of the middle ear cavity by fluid and or thickened glue-like material can be present. Chronic infection can cause demineralisation of the ossicles; traction on the ossicle can even cause luxation of the ossicles. However, clear destruction or displacement of the ossicles is not seen. Middle ear inflammation often follows pre-existing structures like the plicae and ligaments forming the tympanic diaphragm. Therefore, when middle ear obliteration suddenly stops at these structures, forming a straight barrier with the aerated part of the rest of the middle ear, then one is nearly always dealing with inflammation. The diagnosis is more difficult if the complete middle ear and mastoid are obliterated. In this case, a small cholesteatoma can be hidden somewhere in the inflammation. In these patients, one should carefully check whether the bony septa between the mastoid and antral aerated cells are intact. If they are, one is probably dealing with inflammation; if they are not, cholesteatoma is suspected. Comparison of the bony septa of both ears helps to detect an underlying cholesteatoma. When the thickened drum or inflammatory tissue in the middle ear calcifies, then one is dealing with tympanosclerosis. It is obvious that only CT can depict these middle ear changes in a reliable way.

Cholesteatoma

Cholesteatoma is a sac lined by keratinizing, stratified, squamous epithelium trapped in the middle ear and growing in the middle ear or mastoid. This lesion displaces the ossicles when it becomes large enough and also destroys the ossicles and walls of the middle ear cavity. Typically, the lateral wall of the middle ear cavity is eroded and the scutum is amputated. In the antrum and mastoid, the septa between the different aerated cells are destroyed by the lesion. As cholesteatomas grow and become masses, they develop convex borders; this is however only visible when the surrounding part of the middle ear or mastoid is aerated. So, when a mass has two convex borders, it is likely to be a cholesteatoma; when one border is convex there is suspicion of a cholesteatoma. When only straight or concave borders are seen, one is probably dealing with inflammation. Again, CT is the method of choice to evaluate the walls of the middle ear and the ossicles. The technique is also suited to check whether recurrent cholesteatoma is present and to help the surgeon decide whether to perform a second-look operation or a re-intervention.

When the middle ear is completely obliterated on CT, it is often impossible to distinguish among post-surgery changes, inflammation and recurrent cholesteatoma. Moreover, when surgery has been performed previously, landmarks such as intact ossicles and walls of the middle ear cavity can often not be used, as they may already have been damaged by the original lesion or the previous surgery. In these cases, one often has no clue whether cholesteatoma is present or not. Today MRI plays an important role in these patients.

A cholesteatoma has rather specific signal intensities on MRI: high signal intensity (SI) on T2-weighted images, low SI on unenhanced T1-weighted images, low SI on gadolinium-enhanced T1-weighted images but with a thin rim of enhancement around the lesion, and high SI on diffusion-weighted MR images (b–1000). Hence, MRI can in most cases tell the surgeon which type of lesion will be found, obviating the need for surgery in many cases. The same goes for patients who were already operated and in whom a second-look operation is scheduled.

Today MRI can be used to exclude recurrent cholesteatoma and can therefore avoid the second-look operation in many patients. There is, however, still a problem with partial volume effects as it is difficult to acquire diffusion-weighted MR images thinner than 3 mm. Hence, small recurrences can still be overlooked. On the other hand, there are no false positives on the diffusion-weighted MR images, which means that when high signal intensity is present on b-1000 images, a cholesteatoma will be found (Fig. 3).

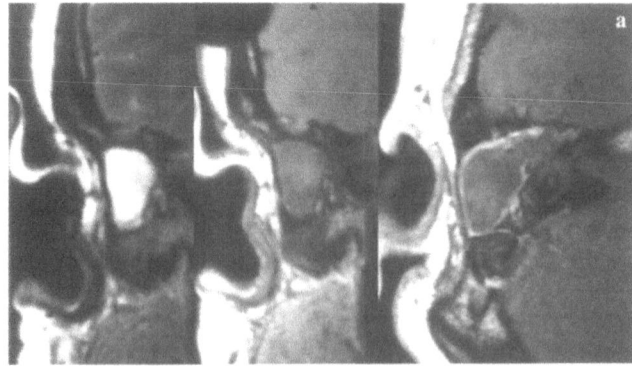

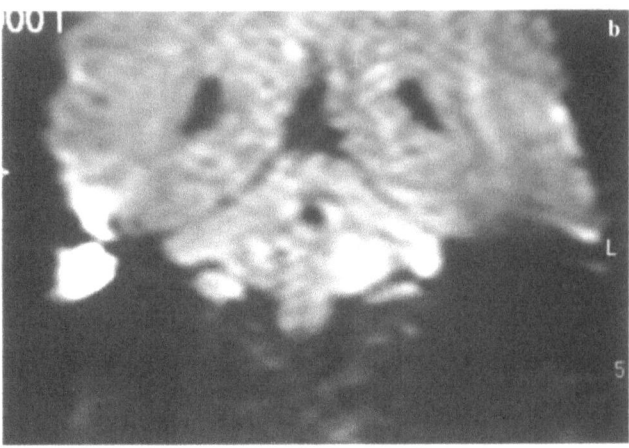

Fig. 3a, b. *Cholesteatoma in right middle ear and mastoid.* **a** High signal intensity (SI) on coronal T2-weighted image (*left*) , low SI on coronal T1-weighted image (*middle*), and low SI on axial gadolinium-enhanced T1-weighted image but with rim enhancement (*right*). **b** High SI on b-1000 diffusion-weighted image

Other lesions, such as a cholesterol granuloma, have specific signal intensities as well (high SI on both T1- and T2-weighted images, low SI on diffusion-weighted images). Middle ear inflammation is typically hyperintense on contrast-enhanced T1-weighted images. If doubt persists, "late-phase" images often show the enhancement better and then confirm that one is dealing with inflammation (cholesteatomas do not enhance at all).

Congenital Middle Ear Malformations

Congenital malformations of the middle ear and external ear are linked embryologically and therefore are often both present in the same patient. CT is the method of choice to look for these congenital malformations, as air and bone are best seen on CT. In the middle ear, the status of the ossicles must be evaluated and described in detail, as surgeons need to know if the hearing loss can be caused by a malformation of the ossicles. If the ossicles are malformed, they want to know if enough ossicles are present to reconstruct a functioning ossicular chain. Moreover, they must know if normal, open round and oval windows are present. Detailed imaging is needed to provide this information, and thin images (0.1-mm reconstructions) are needed to see these often subtle malformations. When the external ear and middle ear are malformed, one must always check the position of the facial nerve. The nerve often shifts anteriorly and runs through the middle ear cavity (Fig. 4); it can even split in 2 or more mastoid branches. Hence, the nerve is at risk and therefore it is the task of the radiologist to warn the surgeon when the nerve has an abnormal course. The middle ear can of course not be evaluated when the external auditory canal is absent or when an atresia plate is present. In these cases, the surgeon is completely dependent on the imaging findings, which indicate whether the external ear and ossicular chain can be reconstructed.

Acoustic Schwannoma

Acoustic schwannomas, the most frequent lesion found inside the internal auditory canal (IAC), can cause SNHL, vertigo and tinnitus. They can be detected on gadolinium-enhanced T1-weighted images, however differentiation from neuritis can be difficult. Gradient echo T2-weighted images are used to distinguish both entities. In schwannoma, a nodular hypointensity is found in the course of the involved nerve, while in neuritis a normal or fusiform, thickened nerve is found. This applies especially to facial nerve neuritis, as enhancement of the vestibulocochlear nerve (eighth nerve neuritis) is rarely seen.

When the schwannoma is small, one can even distinguish on which branch (cochlear, inferior vestibular or superior vestibular) of the eighth nerve it is located. Imaging studies showed that vertigo is more frequently correlated with small and strictly intracanalicular schwannomas. Clinical studies also showed that purely intracanalicular acoustic schwannomas result in earlier onset of vestibular symptoms.

Once the diagnosis of schwannoma is made, the growth potential of the lesion must be assessed. This is best achieved using 1-mm T1-weighted gradient echo images (e.g. 3DFT-MPRAGE) on which volume measurements are performed. In the first year, follow-up studies should be acquired every 6 months and subsequently annually in case the schwannoma is not growing fast.

Once it is decided that a schwannoma must be removed, one must determine if hearing preservation surgery is possible. Here, imaging plays a key role today. First, the presence of fluid between the schwannoma and the fundus of the IAC must be assessed. If fluid is still present, the surgeon can stay away from the base of the cochlea and a suboccipital or middle cranial fossa approach can be used, therefore preserving hearing function. If no fluid is left, the surgeon has to drill in the cochlear canal, and the patient becomes deaf; therefore, the less invasive translabyrinthine approach is chosen in these patients.

Another important sign is the signal intensity of the cerebrospinal fluid (CSF) between the schwannoma and fundus of the IAC, as well as the signal intensity of the intralabyrinthine fluid . Normal signal intensity of these fluid spaces seems to correlate well with good results after hearing preservation surgery. However, when the signal intensity of the fluid is decreased, the success of hearing-preservating surgery is significantly worse (Fig. 5).

Labyrinthitis

Only "end-phase" ossifying labyrinthitis is visible on CT. Acute labyrinthitis (seen with gadolinium enhancement) and subacute labyrinthitis (fibrosis formation, only seen on TSE or GE T2-weighted images) are only detectable on MRI. Therefore, MRI is the method of choice to examine these patients. Moreover these patients present with sensorineural hearing loss, which also directs them

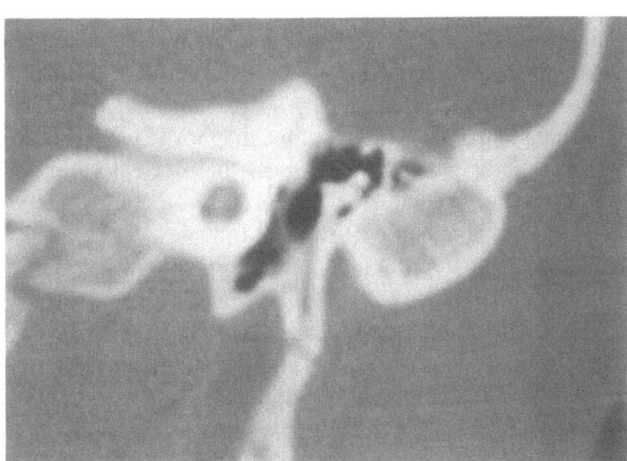

Fig. 4. *Coronal CT image shows aplasia of the external auditory canal and bony atresia plate with fixation of the fused ossicles.* The facial nerve decends in the middle of the middle ear cavity

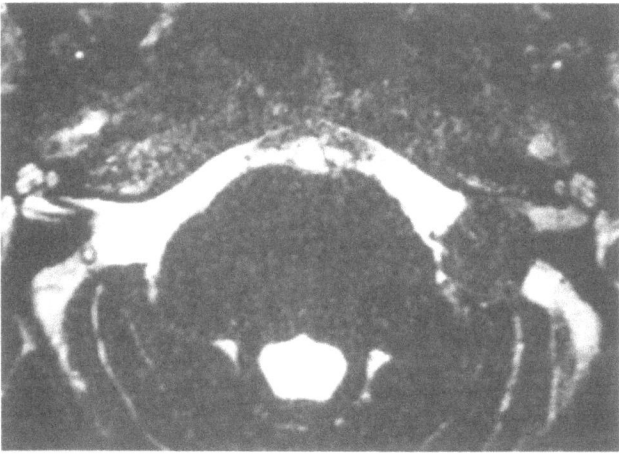

Fig. 5. *Axial 0.7-mm gradient echo T2-weighted MR image.* The signal intensity inside the left labyrinth is decreased, which is a bad predictor for success following hearing preservation surgery

towards an MRI examination. However, when the high signal intensity of fluid is lost on T2-weighted TSE or GE images, one cannot differentiate between fibrosis and ossification. A combination of MRI and CT is needed to get a complete picture of the labyrinthitis.

Labyrinthitis is most often viral. In these cases, gadolinium enhancement is seen but the fibrosis formation and ossification are most often not present. In case of meningococcus or pneumococcus infection (meningitis), it is a different story. Fibrosis develops quickly and calcification can already appear in 3-4 weeks. Meningitis occurs of course most frequently in children; when both ears are affected complete deafness can be the consequence. The only solution for these children is to install a cochlear implant as soon as possible, before labyrinthine fibrosis and ossification occur. As this can happen very fast, CT and MRI have to be performed quickly and this indication must be considered an emergency. Scheduling such a patient 1-2 weeks later can result in permanent deafness. As most of these children are examined under anaesthesia, it is wise to perform CT and MRI at the same time in order to avoid a second anaesthesia, with its associated risks, in case MRI or CT alone cannot give all the answers.

Congenital Inner Ear Malformations

Patients with inner ear malformations present with "congenital" sensorineural hearing loss. The bony inner ear malformations can be seen on CT but these malformations are better seen on MRI. Only MRI can be used to evaluate if fluid is still present inside the malformed labyrinth, and can also distinguish the scala tympani and vestibuli in a reliable way. Moreover MRI can also be used to check whether a normal cochlear nerve is present (Fig. 6). If the vestibulocochlear nerve or cochlear branch of this nerve is absent, then cochlear implant surgery can no longer solve the problem and an unnecessary expensive intervention can be avoided.

More frequent inner ear malformations are an enlarged endolymphatic duct and sac (enlarged vestibular aqueduct) and a saccular lateral semicircular canal. The latter most often has no clinical consequences. An enlarged endolymphatic duct and sac is, however, linked with SNHL and frequently intracochlear changes are present.

The danger of a "gusher ear" is always present when inner ear malformations are detected. The absence of a normal bone barrier between the fundus of the internal auditory canal and the base of the cochlea (very likely) and the presence of a large vestibular aqueduct (less likely) are signs that should warn the surgeon of a potential gusher ear. In a gusher ear, the CSF pressure is transmitted to the intralabyrinthine fluid. When the surgeon operates on the oval window and footplate, the fluid can gush out of the oval window and a completely deaf ear will result. Hence, it is important to warn the surgeon if one of these suspicious signs is seen. Unfortunately, gusher ears can occur in inner ears that are radiologically completely normal.

Pathology Involving the Central Auditory Pathways

When SNHL is present, the pathology is frequently located along the auditory pathways. In these patients, selective CT and MRI studies are normal. Therefore, MRI is the method of choice in these patients and selective inner ear MRI should always be completed by a brain study. The cochlear nuclei, trapezoid body, lateral lemniscus, inferior colliculus, medial geniculate body and auditory cortex can all be affected. Infarctions (in older patients), multiple sclerosis (in younger patients), trauma, tumour and inflammation can affect these structures and cause sensorineural hearing loss. Congenital malformation (pachygyria or polymicrogyria) can even be present in the auditory cortex and should be checked in all cochlear implant candidates.

Tinnitus

Patients with pulsatile tinnitus can today be examined noninvasively with MRI. Patients with subjective and nonpulsatile tinnitus can also be examined using magnetic resonance angiography (MRA) but the diagnostic yield is much lower. Neurovascular conflicts near the root entry zone of the facial and vestibulocochlear nerves can best be recognised on gradient echo T2-weighted images. These images can also be used to provide the surgeon with virtual images of the conflict in the cerebellopontine angle (CPA). Vascular time of flight (TOF) images can be used to identify the vessel causing the conflict or to differentiate between arteries and veins (nonenhanced and gadolinium-enhanced images). However, neurovascular conflict is not the most frequent cause of pulsatile tinnitus at all. Paragangliomas, dural arteriovenous fistulas, idiopathic venous tinnitus and benign intracranial hypertension are the most frequent causes, and only the first two pathologies can be shown on MRI.

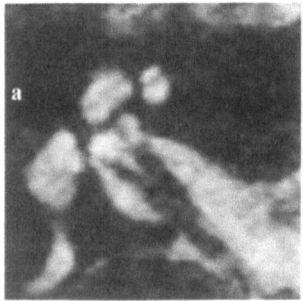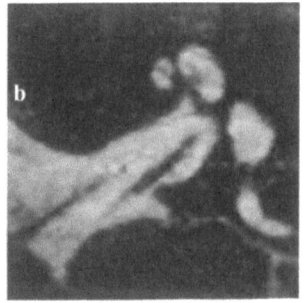

Fig. 6a, b. *Congenital deafness on the left side due to absence of the cochlear branch of the eighth cranial nerve in an otherwise normal left inner ear.* **a** Both the cochlear and inferior vestibular branch of the VIIIth nerve can be seen in the right internal auditory canal. **b** On the left side the cochlear branch is absent and hence no nerve can be seen near the base of the cochlea

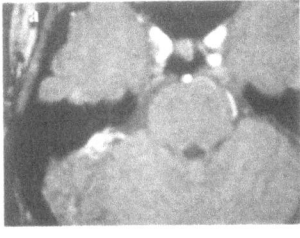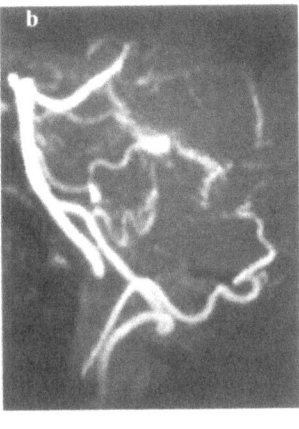

Fig. 7a,b. *Dural fistula.* **a** The unenhanced time of flight (TOF) MRA image shows increased flow velocity in the area of the superior petrosal sinus. **b** Selective reconstructed maximum intensity projection (MIP) image shows that an occipital artery branch, PICA, AICA and branches from the superior cerebellar and posterior cerebral arteries are feeding the fistula

Dural fistulas (Fig. 7) causing early venous drainage can be detected on nonenhanced images. Glomus tumours, arteriovenous malformations, aberrant vessels running through the middle ear, high or dehiscent jugular bulbs, tortuous carotid arteries near the skull base, fibromuscular dysplasia and carotid dissection can be detected on both unenhanced and gadolinium-enhanced MRA images. Vascularised tumours such as meningiomas cause higher arterial and venous flows in their surroundings and therefore can cause tinnitus. This is why tumours in the neighbourhood of the temporal bone must be excluded in these patients. Finally, CT is sometimes necessary to find the cause of tinnitus, for example in the case of Paget's disease. However, MRA has become the method of choice because it is more successful than CT in detecting the causes of tinnitus. Angiography is only used in treatment (e.g. embolisation) or for diagnosis when pulsatile tinnitus renders a normal life impossible and MRI and CT remain negative.

Suggested Reading

Alexander AE, Caldemeyer KS, Rigby P (1998) Clinical and surgical application of reformatted high-resolution CT of the temporal bone. Neuroimaging Clin N Am 8:31-50

Bradley WG (1991) MR of the brain stem: a practical approach. Radiology 179:319-332

Casselman JW (2002) Diagnostic imaging in clinical neuro-otology. Curr Opin Neurol 15:23-30

Casselman JW, Kuhweide R, Ampe W, et al. (1996) Inner ear malformations in patients with sensorineural hearing loss: detection with gradient-echo (3DFT-CISS) MR imaging. Neuroradiology 38:278-286

Casselman JW (1996) Temporal bone imaging, Neuroimaging Clin N Am 6:265-289

Casselman JW, Offeciers EF, De Foer B, et al. (2001) CT and MR imaging of congenital abnormalities of the inner ear and internal auditory canal. Eur J Radiol 40:94-104

Casselman JW, Offeciers FE, Govaerts PJ, Kuhweide R, Geldof H, Somers T, D'Hont G (1997) Aplasia and hypoplasia of the vestibulocochlear nerve: diagnosis with MR imaging. Radiology 202:773-781

Dietz RR, Davis WL, Harnsberger HR, Jacobs JM, Blatter DD

(1994) MR imaging and MR angiography in the evaluation of pulsatile tinnitus. AJNR Am J Neuroradiol 15:890-892

Deplanque D, Godefroy O, Guerouaou D, Laureau E, Desaulty A (1998) Sudden bilateral deafness: lateral inferior pontine infarction. J Neurol Neurosurg Psychiatry 64:817-818

Dubrulle F, Ernst O, Vincent C, Vaneecloo FM, Lejeune JP, Lemaitre L (2000) Enhancement of the cochlear fossa in the MR evaluation of vestibular schwannoma: correlation with success at hearing preservation surgery. Radiology 215458:462

Lo WWM, Solti-Bohman LG (1996) Vascular tinnitus. In: Som PM, Curtin HD (eds) Head and neck imaging. Mosby-Year Book, St. Louis, pp 1535-1549

Lo WWM, Solti-Bohman LG (1996) Tumors of the temporal bone and the cerebellopontine angle. In: Som PM, Curtin ND (eds) Head and neck imaging. Mosby-Year Book, St. Louis, pp 1449-1534

Maheshwari S, Mukherji SK (2002) Diffusion-weighted imaging for differentiating recurrent cholesteatoma tissue after mastoidectomy: case report. AJNR Am J Neuroradiol 23:847-849

Mark AS, Casselman JW (2002) Anatomy and diseases of the temporal bone. In: Atlas SW (ed) Magnetic resonance imaging of the brain and spine, 3rd edn. Lippincott Williams Wilkins, Philadelphia, pp 1363-1432

Mark AS (1994) Contrast-enhanced magnetic resonance imaging of the temporal bone. Neuroimaging Clin N Am 4:561-578

Nayak S (2001) Segmental anatomy of the temporal bone. Semin Ultrasound CT MR 22:184-218

Nair SB, Abou-Elhamd KA, Hawtorne M (2000) A retrospective analysis of high resolution computed tomography in the assessment of cochlear implant patients. Clin Otolaryngol 25:55-61

Phelps PD, Reardon W, Pembrey M (1991) X-linked deafness, stapes gushers and a distinctive defect of the inner ear. Neuroradiology 33:326-330

Sartoretti-Schefer S, Kollias S, Wichmann W, Valavanis AS (1998) T2-weighted three-dimensional fast spin-echo MR in inflammatory peripheral facial nerve palsy. AJNR Am J Neuroradiol 19:491-495

Sartoretti-Schefer S, Wichmann W, Valavanis A (1997) Contrast-enhanced MR of the facial nerve in patients with posttraumatic peripheral facial nerve palsy. AJNR Am J Neuroradiol 18:1115-1125

Sasaki O, Ootsuka K, Taguchi K, Kikukawa M (1994) Multiple sclerosis presented acute hearing loss and vertigo. ORL J Otorhinolaryngol Relat Spec 56:55-59

Somers T, Casselman J, de Ceulaer G, Govaerts P, Offeciers FE (2001) Prognostic value of MRI findings in hearing preservation surgery for vestibular schwannoma. Am J Otology 22:87-94

Swartz JD, Harnsberger HR (1998) Temporal bone vascular anatomy, anomalies, and diseases, emphasizing the clinical-radiological problem of pulsatile tinnitus. In: Swartz JD, Harnsberger HR (eds) Imaging of the temporal bone. Thieme, New York, pp 170-239

Swartz JD, Harnsberger HR (1998) The otic capsule and otodystrophies. In: Swartz JD, Harnsberger HR (eds) Imaging of the temporal bone. Thieme, New York, pp 240-317

Van den Brink JS, Watanabe Y, Kuhl CK, et al. (2003) Implications of SENSE MR in routine clinical practice. Eur J Radiol 46:3-27

Veillon F, Riehm S, Emachescu B, et al. (2001) Imaging of the windows of the temporal bone. Semin Ultrasound CT MR 22:271-280

Veillon F, Baur P, Dasch JC, Braun M, Pharaboz C (1991) Traumatismes de l'os temporal. In: Veillon F (ed) Imagerie de l'oreille. Médecine-Sciences Flammarion, Paris, pp 243-281

Williams MT, Ayache D, Alberti C, Heran F, Laffite F, Elmaleh-Berges M, Piekarski JD (2003) Detection of residual cholesteatoma with delayed contrast-enhanced MR imaging: initial findings. Eur Radiol 13:169-174

Imaging the Temporal Bone

F. Veillon, S. Riehm

Service de Radiologie 1, University of Strasbourg, Strasbourg, France

Anatomy, How Reading Imaging

Imaging of the temporal bone must be integrated into the clinical context because the information provided by otologists is of great interest. The temporal bone contains three cavities: two are filled with air (external ear and middle ear) and one contains fluid (inner ear, or labyrinth, connected to the brain by the eighth cranial nerve). The aims of imaging are, in all pathologies, to avoid surprises during surgery of the middle ear and to provide information about the morphology of the cavities, in particular the inner ear and internal auditory meatus. The procedures for analyzing the different structures of the temporal bone on diagnostic images are the same, and regard both the content and the walls of the cavities.

Regarding the *external ear*, the content of the external auditory meatus is easily analyzed at otoscopy. However, the adjacent regions, including the temporomandibular joint (TMJ), lateral pharyngeal area, and third portion of the facial nerve, have to be shown by imaging.

The *middle ear* contains mucosa, the auditory ossicles, tendons, ligaments and, in pathological cases, also soft tissue. The radiologist must analyze the different walls of the middle ear:
- The bony roof, separating the middle ear from the dura, the cerebrospinal fluid (CSF) and the brain;
- The floor, with the passage of the jugular vein;
- The external wall, made of the tympanic membrane (drum) and the squamous bone;
- The posterior wall, with the facial nerve and the posterior petrous cells;
- The anterior wall, bordered by the internal carotid artery, the eustachian tube below and the middle cranial fossa above;
- The inner wall, containing the round and oval windows and abutting on the lateral semicircular canal and the second part of the facial nerve.

Imaging analysis of the *inner ear* considers the size, shape and structure of the otic capsule, as well as the nature of the fluid contents of the cavity. Furthermore, we must evaluate the walls of the *internal auditory meatus*, its contents (fluid and the seventh and eighth cranial nerves), and the nature of the canals in its fundus.

Imaging Techniques

The radiologist has two techniques for analyzing the different cavities of the temporal bone: spiral computed tomography (CT) and magnetic resonance imaging (MRI). Both techniques are useful for imaging the external, middle and inner ears, and the internal auditory meatus, depending on the clinical context.

Spiral CT with a 16-row detector provides good images of the cavities and canals of the temporal bone. In our experience, the slices should be 0.6-mm thick, with an overlap of 0.2, 0.5 or 0.7 mm, depending on the chosen plane. Magnification of the windows is useful. The lateral semicircular canal is parallel to the axial imaging plane. Imaging in the frontal (coronal) plane is always performed; the sagittal plane is used in cases of trauma or malformation, after middle ear surgery, and for all pathologies of the external auditory meatus.

The choice of MRI protocol depends on the cavity to be analyzed:
- *External auditory meatus*. The main pathology for which MRI is needed is external malignant otitis media, an infection of the external ear and its adjacent regions. The best sequence consists of gadolinium-enhanced, fat-saturated T1-weighted images in the horizontal (axial) plane with 1- or 2-mm sections parallel to the roof of the orbit and centered on the temporal bone.
- *Middle ear*. MRI is useful for the evaluation of the soft tissue content. The most appropriate protocols consist of T1-weighted imaging without and with gadolinium enhancement and diffusion-weighted imaging in the axial or frontal plane. Frontal T2-weighted images are useful for analyzing the relationships of the middle ear with the dura mater, CSF and brain. High-resolution T2-weighted images provide further information about the fluid or solid contents of the middle ear. Actual slice thickness (0.5-0.9 mm) depends on the scanner. The field of view must be small (10×10 cm^2), and the matrix is 256×256.
- *Inner ear*. T1-weighted images without and with gadolinium enhancement in the axial plane parallel to the roof of the orbit (1- or 2-mm sections) provide information about the content, size and shape of the

labyrinth. High-resolution T2-weighted images offer more precise information about the shape of the labyrinth and its fluid contents.

- *Internal auditory meatus.* T1-weighted images without and with gadolinium enhancement, possibly with fat saturation, and high-resolution T2-weighted images are appropriate for analyzing the signal of the CSF, and the size and shape of the seventh and eighth cranial nerves.

Temporal Bone Pathologies

Inflammation

In emergency situations of *mastoiditis*, CT is necessary for determining the integrity of the middle ear and inner ear walls, which may be destroyed. CT with contrast medium is always necessary if MRI is not planed for the search for a lateral sinus thrombosis, meningitis, or an abscess outside or inside the adjacent brain.

Tympanosclerosis, a frequent pathology of the middle ear, consists of the calcification of the soft tissue, ligaments or tendons. CT is of particular importance in evaluating the amount of calcification and the possible blockage of the ossicles. The stapes is often highly calcified, with increased thickness of the footplate. As in all chronic forms of otitis media, there may be destruction of the ossicles, particularly the long process of the incus.

Imaging is never requested in the evaluation of *hyperplasia*. Nevertheless, the radiologist must know its CT and MRI presentations, for it is often associated with cholesteatoma. Hyperplasia often appears as an increased thickness of the mucosa of the tympanic cavity. It may fill up the whole middle ear. If a suspicion of cholesteatoma remains doubtful on CT, an MRI examination is necessary for the differential diagnosis: a keratoma appears gray in signal on T1-weighted images, while hyperplasia shows peripheral enhancement on gadolinium-enhanced images.

When visible at otoscopy, *granulomas* appear as blue-red masses. At CT they are bowl-shaped; at MRI, they are white (hyperintense) on T1- and T2-weighted images, and show no enhancement after gadolinium administration.

Fibrosis may totally fill an operated cavity of the temporal bone. It appears as a gray, soft-tissue area on CT images. The diagnosis is only possible with MRI: fibrosis appears gray (isointense to the cerebellum) on unenhanced T1-weighted images and hyperintense on T1-weighted images 45 min after gadolinium administration.

Cholesteatoma complicates a retraction with a perforation of the drum in most cases. It is white at otoscopy but not always completely visible if the extension is located in the attic. At CT, the typical aspect is the one of a rounded mass in the external part of the attic with destruction of the scutum. The extension may be important throughout the tympanic cavity and in the antrum (Fig. 1). In rare cases, it is associated with destruction of the posterior wall of the petrous bone; the dura is never destroyed. The ossicles can be normal or partially or totally destroyed. The labyrinthine

bone is eroded in 5%-10% of cases, and in the majority of cases it is open to the lateral semicircular canal. While the extent of tumor is not so well evaluated by CT, particularly when the keratoma totally fills the cavity, MRI can provide good information. The lesion appears gray on T1-weighted images, does not enhance after gadolinium injection, and morphologically consists of a round or oval mass with a ring of hyperplasia (Fig. 2). When a fistula is

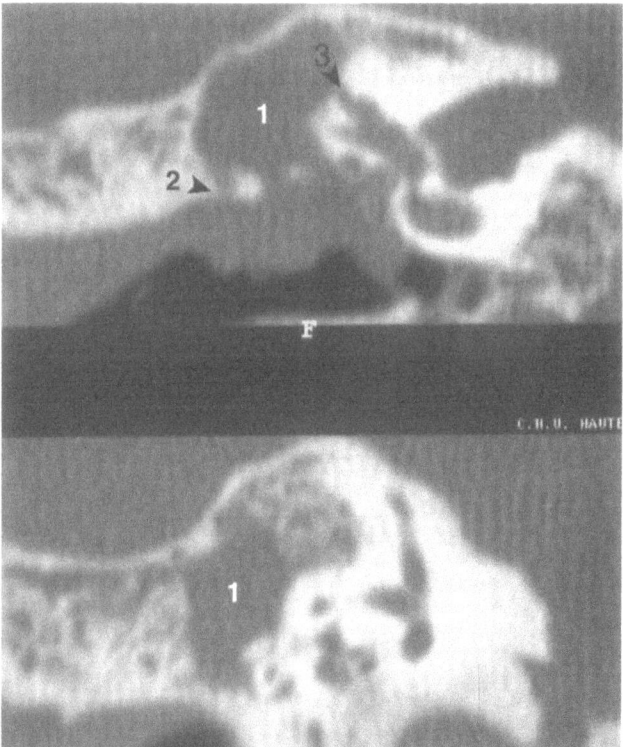

Fig. 1. Frontal view of a cholesteatoma at computed tomography. *1, cholesteatoma; 2,* destruction of the scutum; *3,* fistula of the superior semicircular canal

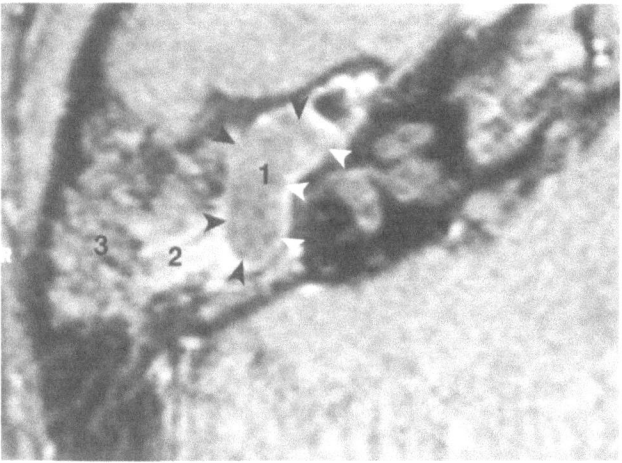

Fig. 2. Axial T1-weighted MR image of cholesteatoma after gadolinium administration. *1,* cholesteatoma; *2,* rim of enhancement in the surrounding hyperplasia; *3,* inflammation in the squamous cells with enhancement

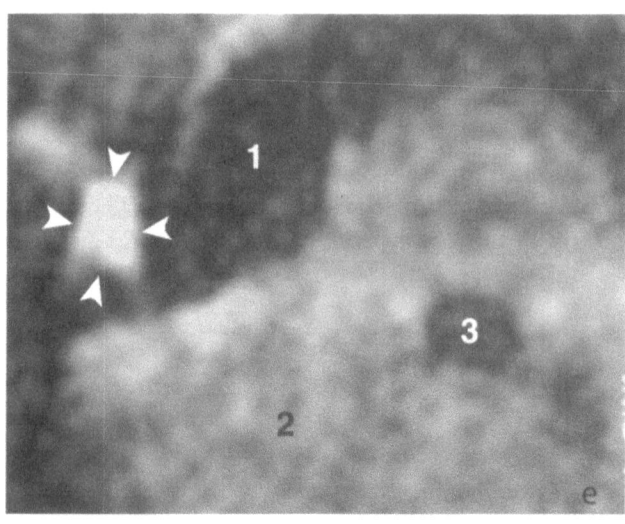

Fig. 3. Axial diffusion-weighted image of cholesteatoma. *1*, petrous bone; *2*, posterior cranial fossa; *3*, fourth ventricle; *arrows*, hyperintense signal of the cholesteatoma

suspected at CT, high-resolution T2-weighted MR images can evaluate the extension to the perilabyrinthine compartment. On diffusion-weighted images, cholesteatoma has a high signal (Fig. 3).

Malformations

The *bony external auditory meatus* may be small or absent, rendering the examination of the middle ear difficult. When imaging the *middle ear* for possible malformations, the main interest regards the careful evaluation of the ossicles, since conductive hearing loss can be successfully treated surgically, provided that the facial nerve is spared. CT can evaluate the presence, absence, fusion or fixation of the ossicles. The anatomy of the windows (normal, small or absent) must always be determined (Fig. 4).

Malformations of the *inner ear* are common. The majority consists of small or more important deformities of

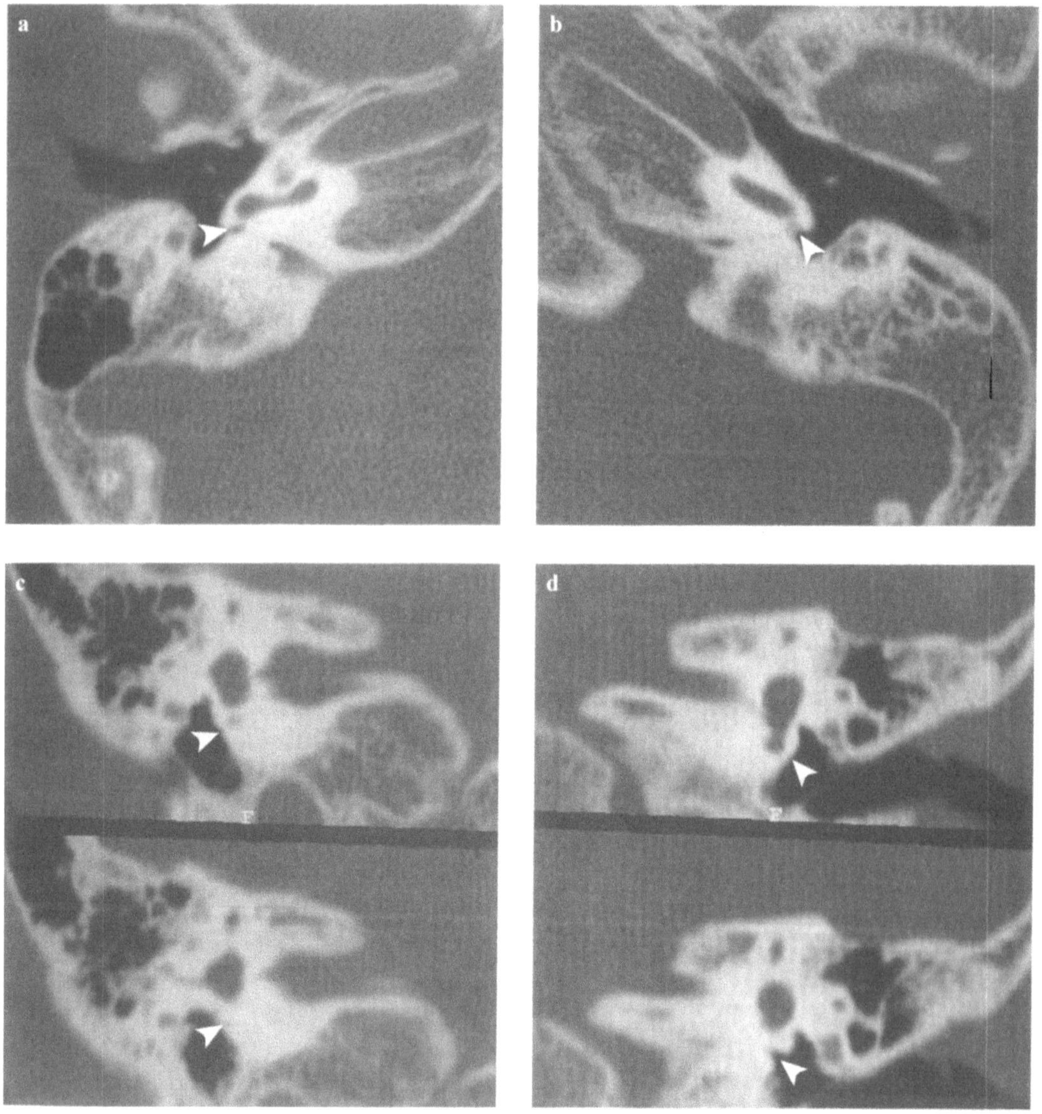

Fig. 4a-d. *Malformation of the round windows.* **a, b** Stenosis of both round windows (*arrows*) in the axial plane. **c, d** Frontal views: absence of access to the membrane of the round windows (*arrows*)

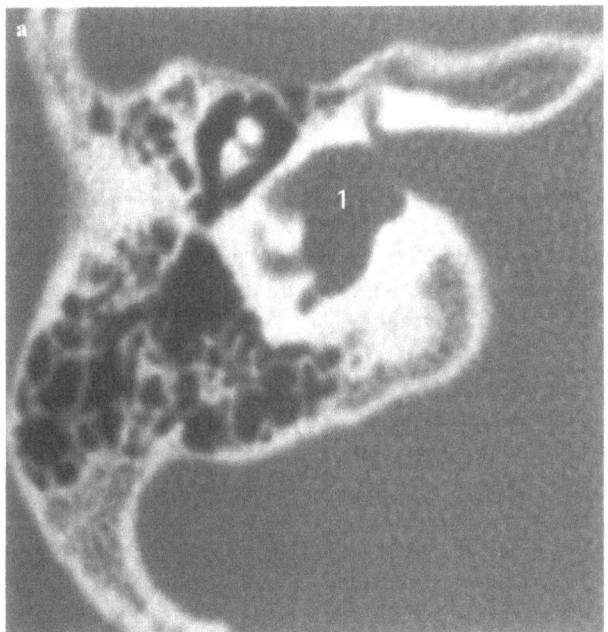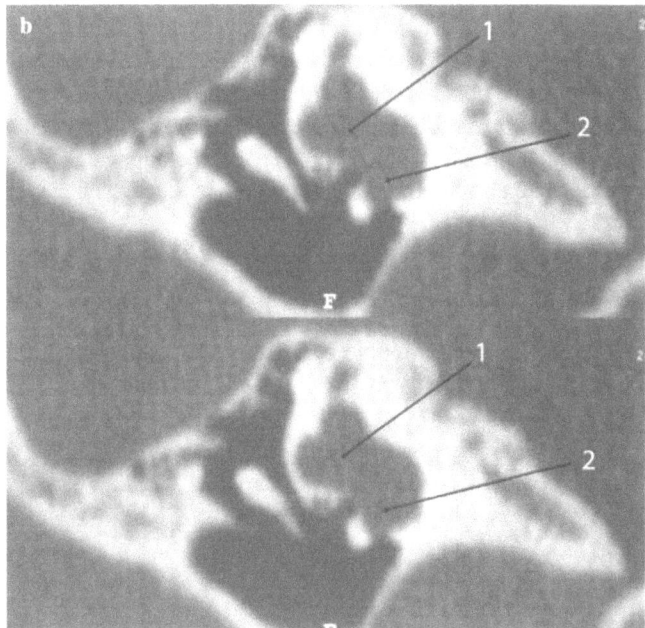

Fig. 5a, b. *Malformation of the inner ear.* **a** Dilatation of the vestibule and lateral and posterior semicircular canals. **b** Dilatation of the lateral semicircular canal (*1*) and of the vestibule (*2*)

the posterior labyrinth (Fig. 5). The second most common abnormality is dilatation of the aqueduct of vestibule, which contains the dilated endolymphatic canal. Dilatation and abnormality of the cochlea, with or without a dilated aqueduct of vestibule, is a third common abnormality. Segmentation of the cochlea may be abnormal; this is better demonstrated by MRI than by CT. Again, analysis of the windows is important. CT and MRI are complementary examinations in the study of the inner ear malformations: the shape of the labyrinth is analyzed by both imaging modalities, the windows are best imaged with CT, and the content of the labyrinth is best studied using MRI.

CT reveals deformities of the canals in the *fundus of the internal auditory meatus,* and demonstrates when the modiolus is absent in cases of suspected gusher syndrome. In other cases, the problem is to analyze the presence and size of the auditory nerve on MRI. Sagittal T1-weighted sections are important for this evaluation.

Imaging is necessary before *cochlear implantation.* CT is used to evaluate the ventilation of the tympanic cavity, the presence of an open round window, and possible calcifications in the labyrinth. MRI helps in the evaluation of the fluid contents of the labyrinth, the size of the auditory nerve, and the nature of the cochlear pathways in the brain. It is important to use both imaging modalities to evaluate the integrity of the labyrinthine lumen.

Otosclerosis

In otosclerosis, a common inner ear pathology, the labyrinthine bone is replaced by areas of spongy bone (otospongiosis). Usually, the small focus of otosclerosis is lo-

cated close to the anterior part of the oval window (Fig. 6). In 10% of cases, the round window is also abnormal. The whole labyrinthine capsule may be involved by the otosclerotic process. Surgery is the usual treatment, with placement of a prosthesis on the oval window. CT confirms the diagnosis and assists in the evaluation of the round window (the surgical results are not so good if the round window is

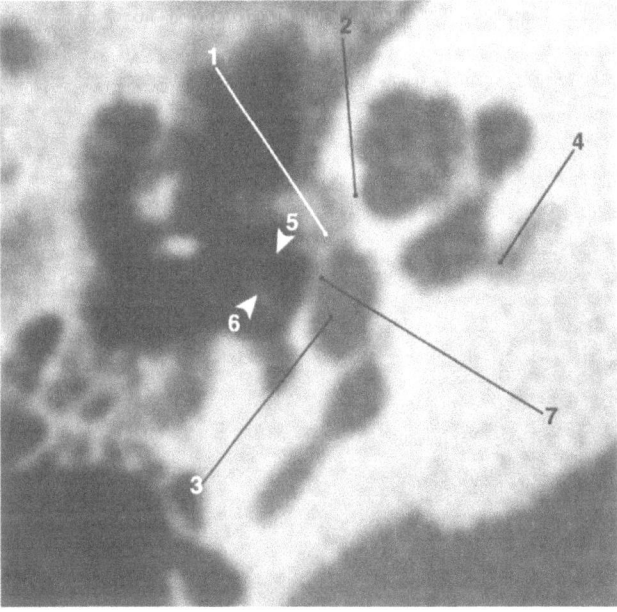

Fig. 6. Otosclerosis. *1,* otosclerosis (hypodensity); *2,* otic capsule; *3,* vestibule; *4,* internal auditory meatus; *5,* anterior crus of the stapes; *6,* posterior crus of the stapes; *7,* footplate

involved), the extension to the labyrinthine capsule, the position of the facial nerve above the oval window, and the length of the long process of the incus. CT allows surgeons to analyze the position and length of the prosthesis after implantation. Rare post-surgical complications, particularly a granuloma of the perilabyrinthine space, may appear; MRI is the best examination to study this process.

Trauma

Trauma to the temporal bone is frequent. In 88% of cases, fractures run in the middle ear through the squamous or petrous bone and may involve the tympanic bone (Fig. 7); the ossicles may be displaced or fractured. CT in the three imaging planes helps analyze the outcome of trauma and the condition of the ossicles. In 7% of cases, trauma involves only the labyrinthine bone, with a fracture running in the inner ear (Fig. 8). Again, CT is useful for this analysis, while high-resolution T2-weighted MR images help evaluate the content of the labyrinthine lumen. This point is quite important if no fracture is visible at CT. In 5% of cases, the fracture is tympanolabyrinthic and involves the middle ear and inner ear, usually through the windows. A fistula of perilabyrinthine space is then common. If no fracture is demonstrated in a patient with post-traumatic vertigo, tinnitus and hearing loss, MRI (particularly T2-weighted imaging) is necessary for evaluating the auditory and vestibular systems in the brain.

Temporal Bone Tumors

In the *external auditory meatus,* the most common pathology is pseudotumoral malignant otitis media; in diabetic patients this condition is usually due to infection with *Pseudomonas aeruginosa.* CT and MRI are performed to evaluate the extension of the inflammatory process. Carcinoma of the external auditory meatus is rare; the destruction and invasion of the adjacent regions are revealed by CT and MRI.

Among tumors affecting the *middle ear,* glomic tumor is a common lesion that originates close to the inner wall of the middle ear along the inferior tympanic nerve (Jacobson's nerve). It appears at otoscopy as a red, rounded mass; on both CT and MRI, the lesion enhances after contrast medium injection. The position of the mass and its extension to the eustachian tube along the carotid canal, in the hypotympanum, are important to evaluate. A jugulotympanic tumor originating in the wall of the jugular vein may invade the tympanic cavity; this tumor

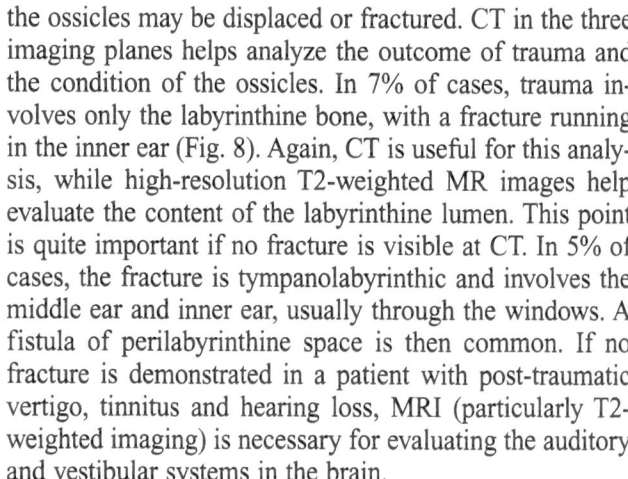

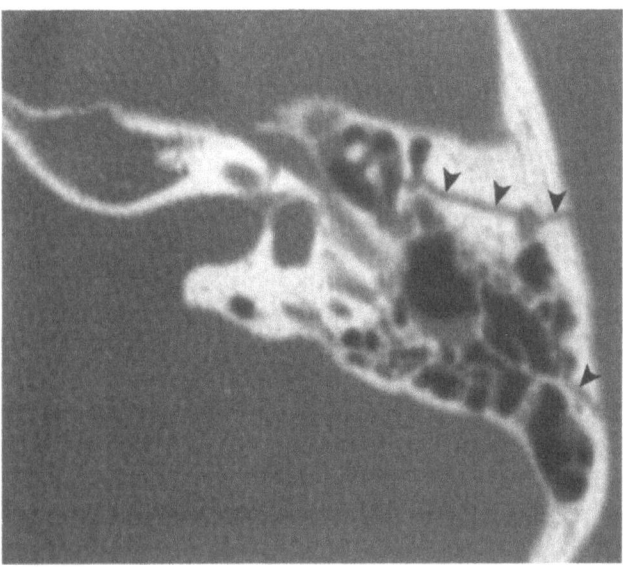

Fig. 7. Trauma of the petrous bone (axial CT section). Longitudinal extralabyrinthine fractures of the squamous bone (*arrows*)

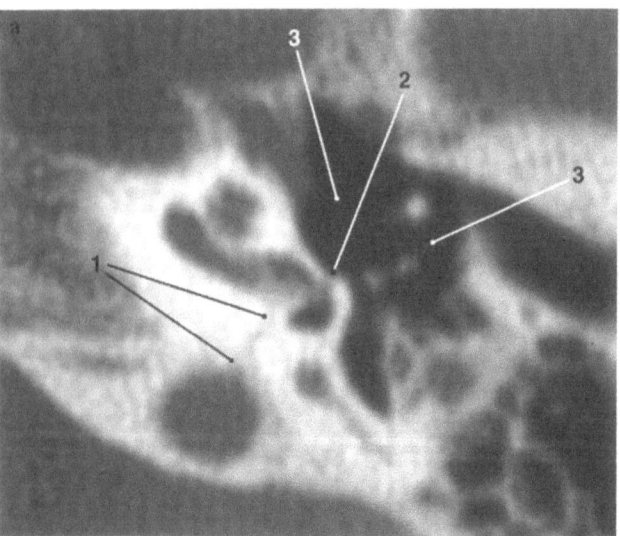

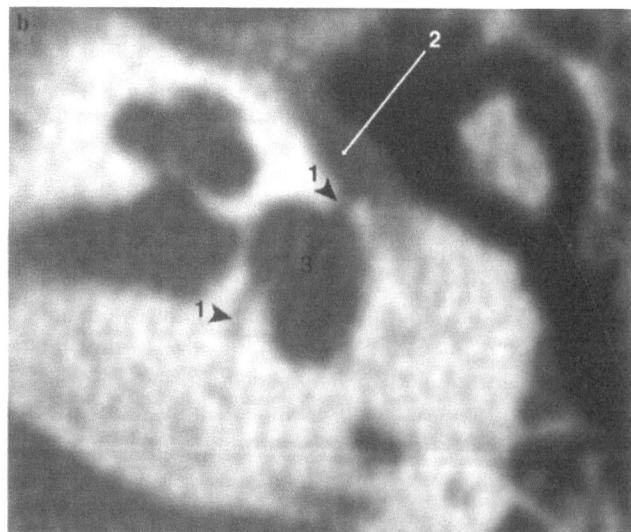

Fig. 8a, b. Trauma of the temporal bone, with translabyrinthine fracture. **a** Axial CT image. *1*, fracture of the otic capsule; *2*, fracture of the promontory; *3*, middle ear without blood effusion. **b** Magnified axial CT image. *1*, translabyrinthine fracture; *2*, tympanic facial nerve; *3*, vestibule

shows strong enhancement on CT and MR images after contrast medium injection. Primitive cholesteatoma is a rare lesion related to some rests of epidermoid tissue left in the middle ear. Usually it is small and located in the mesotympanum, not in the attic, like a secondary keratoma. The mass is white and visible at otoscopy; it appears rounded at CT. There is no need for MRI if the keratoma is small. The destruction is usually limited. Other tumors (adenoma, carcinoid, meningioma, neuroma) are rare in the middle ear.

The *inner ear* may be eroded or destroyed by tumors of the adjacent regions: apex, jugular foramen, internal auditory meatus. One tumor, the papillary tumor of the endolymphatic sac, originates in the inner ear lumen. This mass originates in the aqueduct of vestibule and leads to destruction of the inner wall of the petrous bone, with extension to the cerebellopontine angle and the middle ear. The mass is hyperintense on T1- and T2-weighted images and shows heterogeneous contrast enhancement. It is frequent in patients with von Hippel-Lindau disease. The primitive cholesteatoma of the inner ear is commonly located in the otic capsule or apex, with or without facial palsy. The signal on MR images is not different from that of secondary keratoma of the middle ear.

Conclusions

CT and MRI are of a great importance in imaging the pathology of the temporal bone. These techniques allow the otologist to choose between conservative or surgical treatment. In the case of surgery, imaging helps the surgeon choose the surgical approach to the cavities and discuss the expected clinical results after surgery with the patient.

Suggested Reading

Swartz JD, Harnsberger HR (1998) Imaging of the temporal bone. Thieme, New York Stuttgart

Veillon F, Riehm S, Enachescu B, Haba D, Roedlich MN, Greget M, Tongio J (2001) Imaging of the windows of the temporal bone. Semin Ultrasound CT MR 22:271-280

Imaging the Pharynx and Oral Cavity

B. Schuknecht[1], A.N. Hasso[2]

[1] Department of Neuroradiology, University Hospital, Zurich, Switzerland
[2] University of California, Irvine Medical Center, Orange, CA, USA

Introduction

Both magnetic resonance imaging (MRI) and computed tomography (CT) are commonly used to evaluate the upper aerodigestive tract formed by the pharynx and oral cavity. Spatial anatomical descriptions of the head and neck structures are well suited to the axial and coronal sections provided by MRI and CT. These techniques are helpful for detecting lesions in clinical blind spots such as the submucosal spaces and the skull base and provide a more useful basis for differential diagnosis of pathological entities than the traditional descriptions based upon the triangles of the neck.

MRI Applications in the Head and Neck

Receiver Coils

Because of inherently poor signal-to-noise ratio (SNR) in the head and neck area, dedicated surface or phased-array coils are often needed to boost signal to acceptable levels. In a phased-array coil, data are combined to form a composite image. In general, the smallest possible coil that fits the anatomical region is recommended. Arrays of detection coils have recently been used to encode spatial information as well as to receive the MR signal. Simultaneous detection of spatial harmonics (SENSE) and simultaneous acquisition of spatial harmonics (SMASH) are parallel imaging techniques that take advantage of the geometry of a coil array to encode multiple lines of MR image data simultaneously. In this way, scan time can be reduced by an integral factor up to 6 in both basic and advanced sequences such as contrast-enhanced magnetic resonance angiography (MRA) and echo-planar imaging (EPI).

Gadolinium Contrast Agents

Unlike iodine, gadolinium (Gd) contrast agents do not produce a signal directly. Rather, they shorten both T1 and T2 relaxation times of nearby mobile protons. Since T1 relaxation times are much longer than T2, gadolinium is a preferentially T1-enhancing agent. Gd contrast agents have pharmacokinetics and volumes of distribution similar to iodinated contrast agents. Unlike free Gd, gadolinium chelated with DTPA, DTPA-BMA, HP-DO3A, BOPTA or DOTA is a non-toxic product that allows for rapid renal excretion. MRI contrast agents rarely cause side effects, nephrotoxicity, or anaphylactoid reactions. Dynamic images can be obtained and tissue perfusion can be visualized with fast gradient echo techniques after power injection of the contrast agent. as it sequentially distributes intravascularly and extracellularly [1]. Hypervascularized lesions (e.g. paraganglioma, metastatic thyroid carcinoma) and normal tissue differ in contrast kinetics and therefore may be distinguished from metastatic cervical lymphadenopathy, edema, inflammation, necrosis and fibrosis, which enhance late due to their larger interstitial spaces.

Superparamagnetic Iron Oxide Particles

MR lymphography with gadolinium chelates or novel ultra-small superparamagnetic iron oxide particles (SPIO) is beginning to show promise. Normal lymph nodes take up SPIO and have reduced signal intensity on post-contrast T2- or T2*-weighted sequences due to magnetic susceptibility effects. Nodal metastases do not show signal changes on post-contrast T2- or T2*-weighted scans. Early clinical experience suggests that SPIO-enhanced MR lymphography improves the sensitivity and specificity for the detection of nodal metastases and may be helpful in presurgical planning [2].

CT Applications in the Head and Neck

Multislice spiral CT offers increased temporal and spatial resolutions and thus allows dynamic volume scanning. Collimation is in the range from 0.75 to 1.0 mm, calculated slice thickness varies between 0.75 for a 16-row scanner and 1.25 mm for a 4-row scanner, and the corresponding slice increment is between 0.5 and 0.7

mm. The table feed is 3.5 mm/rotation for a 4-row scanner (rot time, 0.5 s) and 8 mm for a 16-row detector scanner (rot time, 0.75 s), leading to scan times of 30 s and 25 s, respectively, to cover 20-22 cm from the orbital roof to the sternoclavicular junction. This protocol covers the primary locations of head and neck tumors, including potential sites of spread like the skull base and cavernous sinus, and delineates lymph node levels from the skull base to the jugulum.

Variations in the aforementioned protocol primarily affect scan times and therefore require careful adjustment of the amount and flow rate of contrast medium. In a typical protocol, the flow rate is 2 ml/s, the acquisition is started following injection of 80 ml contrast medium, and the remaining 20 ml is injected during the subsequent scan and pushed with 20 ml of saline. With the exception of acute trauma and thyroid carcinoma, administration of nonionic contrast medium (iodine, 300 mg/ml) is virtually always required in head and neck CT.

Imaging of the carotid and vertebrobasilar arteries, either targeted with a limited scan range or from the aortic arch to the circle of Willis, has become feasible using a 4- or 16-row scanner [3]. Delineation of supra-aortic vessels is feasable using 40 ml contrast medium at a higher concentration of iodine (400 mg/ml) with an injection rate of 4 ml/s and a table feed of 18 mm/rotation. Recognition of vessel involvement by the primary tumor or metastatic lymphadenopathy and visualization of particular external carotid artery branches allow precise noninvasive surgical planning of tumor resection as well as reconstruction by microvascular anastomosed flaps.

Imaging of head and neck vessels is based on a volume-rendering technique (VRT). Morphologic imaging uses multiplanar reconstructions (MPR) with 3-mm contiguous slices in the axial and coronal planes [4] Additional sagittal slices are required in lesions derived from the nasopharynx, base of the tongue, and posterior wall of the oro- and hypopharynges, and in cases of levels III-V lymph node involvement. Biplanar (axial and coronal) high-resolution bone window algorithm images are particularly useful in detecting involvement of the skull base and mandible; sagittal images are required to detect infiltration of the prevertebral fascia or vertebral column by neoplasm or inflammation.

MRI of the Upper Aerodigestive Tract

The key to interpreting the structures of the aerodigestive tract is the differences in MR signal intensity on various pulse sequences. T1-weighted images outline the musculofascial anatomy best (Fig. 1a). T2-weighted images readily distinguish between mucosal structures and superficial adenoidal tissues. Mucosal and adenoidal tissues have a slightly prolonged T1 signal and a significantly prolonged T2 signal in comparison with muscle and fibrous tissues. The lingual tonsils are seen as U-

shaped structures with high signal intensity, located at the base of the tongue. Pasavant's ridge is a U-shaped mucosal band formed by the levator and tensor veli palatini muscles that insert laterally on the hard palate. This ridge functions as a sphincter during swallowing. The soft palate, the pharyngeal constrictor muscles, and the levator and tensor veli palatini muscles form a region of low signal intensity surrounding the airway at the level of the soft palate [5, 6].

T1-weighted MR sequences allow good fat-muscle contrast, while T2-weighted sequences afford good differentiation between muscle and lymphoid tissue. The lymphoid tissues of the palatine or lingual tonsils have a slightly more intense signal than muscle on T1-weighted images and a much more intense signal than muscle on T2-weighted images [7]. If the lymphoid tissues are hypertrophic, this signal may be similar to that of surrounding fat. Significant enhancement following contrast medium administration is deemed secondary to capillary permeability resulting from chronic inflammation of the lymphoid tissues (Fig. 1b). The pala-

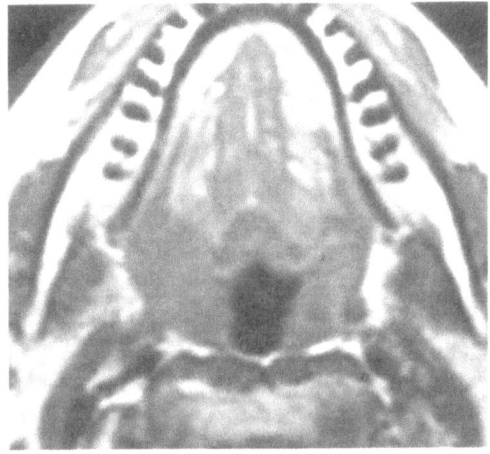

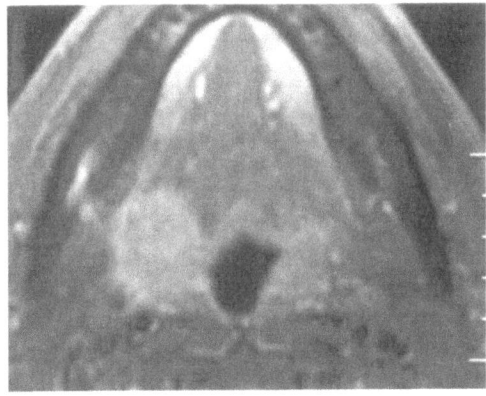

Fig. 1. *Carcinoma of the right tonsil.* **a** Top T1-W image. The signal intensity of the tumor in the right tonsil is incorporated into the signal from the adjacent muscles and lymphoid tissues in Waldeyer's ring. **b** Bottom T1-W image following gadolinium contrast administration. Note that enhancement in the tumor in the right tonsil helps to clearly demarcate its margins from the muscles, but not from the lymphoid tissues.

tine tonsils are the only component of Waldeyer's ring that have a capsule which is low in signal compared to the high signal of parapharyngeal fat on T1-weighted images.

The combination of minor salivary glands mixed with fat results in a heterogeneous appearance of the palate on T1-weighted images and increased signal on T2-weighted images. The median glossoepiglottic fold and the lateral pharyngoepiglottic folds are hyperintense on T1-weighted images, as is the remaining pharyngeal mucosa [8].

T1-weighted images achieve the best contrast between a tumor (intermediate signal) and the loose areolar tissue of the preepiglottic and paraglottic spaces. On T2-weighted images, a tumor may be hyperintense in comparison to the intermediate signal of the surrounding areolar tissues.

Benign Lesions of the Pharynx

Benign lesions of the pharynx may be epithelial (e.g. papilloma, adenoma) or mesenchymal (e.g. hemangioma, angiofibroma, chondroma, chordoma) in origin, or may derive from specialized tissues (e.g. teratoma, craniopharyngioma, paraganglioma) [9-11].

Juvenile Nasopharyngeal Angiofibroma

Angiofibromas are benign, locally aggressive, nonencapsulated vascular tumors that arise in adolescent males. These tumors are typically located in or near the sphenopalatine foramen. In most cases, the tumor expands the pterygopalatine fossa and extends into the sinonasal cavities, nasopharynx, orbital apex and cavernous sinus (Fig. 2). Common presenting symptoms include recurrent spontaneous epistasis and nasal obstruction; more advanced cases may show proptosis or cranial nerve deficits. The histologic makeup of angiofibromas consists of fibrous tissue with many thin-walled vessels that lack contractile tissue. Extensive biopsy is discouraged due to the strong vascularity of these tumors. Surgery is the treatment of choice, with preoperative embolization via the feeding arterial pedicles in order to reduce blood loss. MRI demonstrates a lesion with intermediate signal intensity on T1- and T2-weighted images; multiple flow void channels are characteristic. There is typically prominent enhancement on both CT and T1-weighted images following contrast medium infusion. CT shows a permeative type of bone erosion. Navigation CT may increase the likelihood of radical resection of tumors confined to the nasal cavity and paranasal sinuses.

Chordoma

Cranial chordomas arise near the spheno-occipital synchondrosis of the clivus and typically destroy the adjacent skull base. Large tumors show extensive bony inclusions

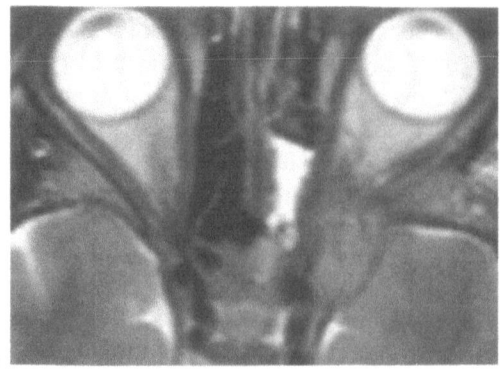

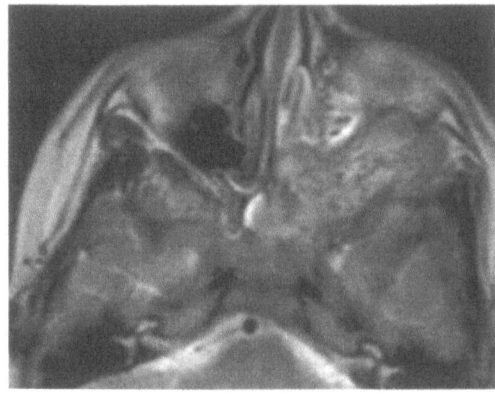

Fig. 2. *Angiofibroma of the pterygopalatine fossa with spread into the left orbital apex and cavernous sinus.* **a** Top and **b** bottom T2-W image. There is marked expansion of the left pterygopalatine fossa by a heterogenous tumor mass showing fine vascular flow voids. **b** The tumor is also seen in the orbital apex with a tongue of tissue extending along the lateral portion of the carotid artery in the cavernous sinus

or calcifications within the soft tissue mass; the soft tissue component of chordomas is frequently disproportionately large. So-called inferoclival chordomas may protrude anteriorly into the nasopharynx. The tumors may occur at any age but most affect men in the third and fourth decades. Chordomas are predominantly hypointense in signal on T1-weighted images and characteristically show high signal intensity on T2-weighted images. A heterogeneous pattern on MRI and CT is due to the presence of bone residue, calcification or hemorrhage. Nearly all chordomas enhance vigorously and nonuniformly following the administration of contrast agents.

Malignant Neoplasms of the Pharynx

Malignant neoplasms of the nasopharynx represent 0.25% of all malignancies in Caucasian patients. There is an incidence of 1 per 100 000 men and 0.4 per 100 000 women. These neoplasms are much more common in patients of southern Chinese origin, with an incidence of 18 per 100 000. There is a strong indication of viral origin in a variety of malignant tumors of the nasopharynx.

Elevated titers of Epstein-Barr virus antibodies are found in almost all patients with advanced nasopharyngeal carcinoma.

Many patients with neoplasms of the nasopharynx present at the age of 40-50 years; however, these cancers can occur during infancy and childhood. The most common presenting symptoms include unilateral or bilateral conductive hearing loss, which is primarily due to obstruction of the eustachian tube with secondary serous otitis media. The second most common symptom is a cervical mass resulting from metastatic lymphadenopathy. Approximately one-third of patients presents with nasal obstruction, congestion, rhinorrhea or epistasis. Direct invasion by the tumor outside the nasopharynx may lead to cranial nerve deficits caused by involvement of the foramen ovale, cavernous sinus, petrous apex or jugular fossa.

Neoplasms of the pharynx may be epithelial (e.g. undifferentiated carcinoma of nasopharyngeal origin, squamous cell carcinoma) or mesenchymal (e.g. lymphoma, lymphosarcoma, adenoid cystic carcinoma, adenocarcinoma) in origin or may derive from specialized tissues (e.g. rhabdomyosarcoma, malignant melanoma) [12-17].

Epithelial Malignant Carcinomas

Epithelial malignant carcinomas represent 80% of all neoplasms of the nasopharynx. The remaining 20% comprise a diverse group that includes tumors of mixed epithelial origin such as lymphoepitheliomas and mucoepitheliomas. The most common site of origin of these tumors is in the lateral recess of the nasopharynx.

MRI is particularly superior to CT in this location. The tumor can spread directly exophytically into the airway and may extend inferiorly to invade the tonsillar pillars and soft palate. MRI depicts disruption of the musculofascial planes around the tensor and levator veli palatini muscles, skull base invasion and submucosal spread along the deep musculofascial planes or neural pathways. Anterior extension into the pterygoid muscles results in invasion of the nasal cavity and destruction of the pterygoid plates; lateral spread involves the parapharyngeal spaces. Retropharyngeal lymph node involvement is common. Lesions greater than 5 mm in diameter are suspicious, while those greater than 8 mm are highly probable for metastatic involvement. The most effective treatment for epithelial nasopharyngeal carcinomas is radiation therapy, both with and without adjunct chemotherapy. Radiation therapy results in a 5-year survival rate of approximately 30%-50%.

Lymphoma

Malignant lymphoid neoplasms of the nasopharynx are usually non-Hodgkin's lymphomas or lymphosarcomas [18]. They constitute approximately 18% of malignant neoplasms of the nasopharynx, the second-most common site after the palatine tonsils. Patients typically present in the fourth through eighth decades. In young adults and children, there is a higher incidence of Hodgkin's disease and Burkitt's lymphoma. The Epstein-Barr virus is strongly associated with the development of lymphoproliferative disorders in post-transplant patients. In immunocompromised individuals, lymphoproliferative disease should therefore be included in the differential diagnosis.

On MRI and CT, there are no specific distinguishing features that unmistakably point to the diagnosis of lymphoma. However, a large mass that presents with little bony erosion points away from the diagnosis of squamous cell carcinoma. Lymphomas typically have intermediate signal intensity on the T1-weighted images and relatively low, homogeneous signal intensity on T2-weighted images; they show moderate enhancement following the administration of contrast medium. Lymphoid hyperplasia in Waldeyer's ring also enhances, but there are internal septations. These fibrous septations help distinguish reactive hypertrophy from neoplasm. The treatment of choice for disseminated lymphoma is chemotherapy.

Rhabdomyosarcoma

Rhabdomyosarcomas of the head and neck are four-times more prevalent in Caucasian children than in children of other races. The disease is associated with a specific chromosomal translocation in 50% of cases. The peak incidence is between 2 and 5 years of age, with 70% of all cases observed in subjects less than 10 years of age [19]. Nearly one-third of head and neck rhabdomyosarcomas involve the pharynx. Most of these pharyngeal tumors affect the nasopharynx and are of the embryonal type. These tumors arise from the rhabdomyoblasts of the nasopharyngeal musculature. Invasion of the eustachian tube orifice and skull base is common and may result in serous otitis media and dysfunction of the cavernous sinus cranial nerves. Large tumors tend to involve the nasal cavity, paranasal sinuses, or orbits. Bulky naso-oropharyngeal masses present with nighttime dyspnea.

Imaging findings in rhabdomyosarcomas are similar to those of malignant epithelial carcinomas; however, since these neoplasms arise from muscle, they may not necessarily involve the mucosal space. The most typical finding is a bulky nasopharyngeal mass with signal intensity intermediate between those of muscle and fat on T1-weighted images. Necrotic areas may be seen producing heterogeneous signal intensities on both T1- and T2-weighted images. Following administration of contrast medium, there is variable, heterogeneous enhancement of both the primary neoplasm and any associated metastatic lymph nodes.

Malignant Melanoma

Primary nasopharyngeal melanomas are rare, accounting for less than 1% of all malignant melanomas [20]. More often, there may be metastasis to the nasopharynx from a primary tumor elsewhere. There are racial differences, with a higher incidence of mucosal melanomas in persons of Japanese origin. The melanocytes in the nasal cavity are located primarily in the nasal septum or in the turbinates. Such tumors enlarge to involve the nasopharynx by direct extension. With MRI, it is possible to determine the extent of tumor. Melanomas have relatively homogeneous signal intensity, unless there is evidence of associated hemorrhage. Non-hemorrhagic lesions tend to be hypointense or isointense on T1-weighted images and isointense or hyperintense on T2-weighted images. Melanomas generally show moderate enhancement following administration of contrast media. Post-contrast T1-weighted fat-suppressed scans are useful in the search for evidence of parapharyngeal, skull base and intracranial involvement.

Squamous Cell Carcinoma of the Oropharynx

Oropharyngeal squamous cell carcinomas, including the lymphoepithelioma variant, are usually poorly differentiated. These tumors are characterized by extensive primary disease with a 50%-70% incidence of cervical lymph node metastasis (Table 1) and a 10%-20% incidence of bilateral lymph node disease if the midline structures are affected. Early disease is rarely recognized since patients usually are asymptomatic. Some early lesions may be detected on discovery of a neck mass. Persistent unilateral sore throat, referred otalgia and difficulty in speech or swallowing are symptoms of advanced disease. Squamous cell carcinomas of the oropharynx have a propensity to spread extensively along the mucosal surfaces of the soft palate, lateral pharyngeal wall and base of the tongue. The three sites of squamous cell carcinoma of the oropharynx are the tonsils, base of the tongue, and oropharyngeal wall.

Carcinoma of the tonsil is prone to spread posteriorly to the lateral pharyngeal wall, inferiorly to the base of the tongue, and superiorly to the soft palate. This tumor can also grow directly into the soft tissues of the neck and posteriorly and laterally to invade the carotid artery. Lymph node metastasis is present in 60%-70% of pa-

tients. Bilateral nodal involvement is seen in 15%-20% of cases in which a large portion of the base of the tongue or soft palate is involved by carcinoma.

Squamous cell carcinomas of the base of the tongue are aggressive, deeply infiltrative, moderately or poorly differentiated neoplasms. There is a 75% incidence of lymph node metastasis at presentation (33%-50% of which are bilateral) due to a rich lymphatic network. The most commonly involved lymph nodes are the jugulodigastric, jugulo-omohyoid and the more cephalad lymph nodes of the internal jugular chain. Of all clinically normal lymph nodes, 10%-20% has occult metastatic disease.

Early disease is rarely detectable since the patient is often asymptomatic. Moderately advanced tumor presents with pain, unilateral sore throat, odynophagia, dysphagia, otalgia and occasionally hemorrhage. Early disease is radiosensitive and curable by radiation alone (with results comparable to those of surgery without mutilation), while late disease requires combined radiation and surgical treatment or chemotherapy.

Sagittal and coronal MR images permit an excellent appreciation of the volume of tumor in the tongue base. Such carcinomas are usually hyperintense on T2-weighted images, may form ulcerative bulky masses, or may present as deeply infiltrative processes along the muscle planes. Carcinoma of the base of the tongue is distinguished from tonsillar hyperplasia by the invasion and disruption of the muscle bundles of the tongue. Following the administration of gadolinium chelates, there is typically fairly intense enhancement.

The lateral and posterior portions of the oropharynx and the posterior tonsillar pillar form the oropharyngeal wall. Squamous cell carcinomas of this region are often ulcerative and may infiltrate inferiorly into the hypopharynx. Such tumors are usually moderately or poorly differentiated. Because of the lack of early symptoms, 75% of patients present with extensive primary disease and lymph node metastasis, frequently bilaterally. The most commonly involved lymph nodes are the jugulodigastric and jugulo-omohyoid nodes of the internal jugular chain and the lateral retropharyngeal lymph nodes.

Squamous Cell Carcinoma of the Hypopharynx

Squamous cell carcinomas of the hypopharynx are predominantly moderately or poorly differentiated tumors. These neoplasms spread with ease from one anatomic site to another as well as from the hypopharynx to the larynx, since there are no fascial boundaries between these structures. Common sites are the piriform sinus (65%), followed by the post-cricoid area (20%) and the posterior pharyngeal wall (15%). The incidence of lymph node metastasis is 50%-70%, with 10%-20% bilateral involvement owing to the rich lymphatic pathways in the hypopharynx.

Early symptoms of hypopharyngeal carcinomas include sore throat, intolerance to hot and cold liquids, dys-

Table 1. Incidence and location of cervical lymph node metastases according to the site of the primary tumor

Site of primary tumor	Incidence of lymph node metastasis, %	Nodal levels involved
Nasopharynx	86-90	II, III, IV
Tongue (base)	50-83	II, III, IV
Tonsillar fossa	58-76	I, II, III, IV
Hypopharynx	52-75	II, III, IV
Oropharynx	50-71	II, III
Tongue (oral portion)	34-65	I, II, III
Floor of mouth	30-59	I, II
Retromolar trigone	39-56	I, II, III
Soft palate	37-56	II
Supraglottic larynx	31-54	II, III, IV

phagia, odynophagia and ipsilateral otalgia. Whenever otalgia is present, the tumor is large and has invaded the superior laryngeal nerve with referred pain via the throat back to the vagus nerve. Involvement of the post-cricoid area leads to dysphagia, while extensive carcinomas of the piriform sinus result in hoarseness, laryngeal stridor and hemoptysis.

Piriform sinus carcinomas are usually unilateral and submucosal in location. Deep extension of the disease and lymph node metastasis are well evaluated with CT and MRI. T1-weighted images maximize contrast between the intermediate signal of the tumor and the bright signal in adjacent loose areolar tissue. Tumors originating from the apex of the piriform sinus are aggressive and infiltrative with extension into the adjacent posterior margin of the thyroid cartilage and infrahyoid muscles. Spread of disease towards the larynx and trachea is common.

Carcinoma of the post-cricoid area is usually well differentiated and thought to represent an "iceberg" presentation of carcinoma of the upper cervical esophagus, especially involving the anterior wall of the esophagus. Despite aggressive surgery, the 5-year survival is 10%-20% owing to extensive spread of disease at the time of initial presentation. This site has the worst prognosis of all three sites of carcinoma of the hypopharynx.

Carcinoma of the posterior pharyngeal wall is the least common carcinoma of the hypopharynx. Such lesions are large and exophytic at presentation, and may extend to the lateral pharyngeal wall or to the cervical esophagus below. The prevertebral muscles and the vertebral bodies may not be involved until late in the disease, owing to the presence of the prevertebral fascia. About 50% of afflicted patients have cervical lymph node metastasis at diagnosis, often bilaterally.

Imaging the Oral Cavity

Anatomy

The oral cavity [14, 15, 21] includes the floor of the mouth, the anterior two-thirds of the tongue, lips, and gingivobuccal (oral vestibule) and buccomasseteric regions. The oral cavity is separated from the oropharynx by the circumvallate papillae of the tongue, the soft palate and palatoglossal arch (anterior tonsillar pillar). The posterior one-third of the tongue belongs to the oropharynx.

The tongue is composed of the intrinsic musculature (superior and inferior longitudinal, transverse and vertical muscle fibers) and extrinsic muscles (genioglossus, styloglossus, hyoglossus and palatoglossus), which originate externally to the tongue but insert into the tongue itself.

The floor of the mouth is composed of the mylohyoid muscles united by a median raphe and the midline geniohyoid muscles located below the genioglossus mus-

cles, and is supported inferiorly by the anterior belly of the digastric muscles. These muscles border the triangular submental space that contains fat and lymph nodes (nodal level IA). At the posterior margin of the mylohyoid muscles, the submandibular gland extends through a gap between the hyoglossus and mylohyoid muscles. Its deep portion is contained in the sublingual space together with the sublingual gland, the submandibular duct (Wharton's duct), the hypoglossal and lingual nerves laterally and the lingual artery and vein medially. Posteriorly the sublingual space communicates with the submandibular space. The submandibular space contains lymph nodes (level IB) and the submandibular gland, with the facial artery medially and the facial vein laterally.

The oral vestibule separates the lips and cheeks from the teeth and alveolar process by a reflection of buccal mucosa onto the maxilla and mandible. Adjacent to the alveolar process, the gingivobuccal sulcus and the glosso-alveolar sulcus are common locations for squamous cell carcinoma of the vestibule and floor of the mouth, respectively. The retromolar trigone between the third molar and the ramus mandibulae is another frequent site. The pterygomandibular raphe is a fascial band extending from the hamulus to the mylohyoid ridge of the mandible and thus provides origin for the buccinator and superior pharyngeal constrictor muscles. Retromolar malignancies may spread along this pathway to the tuber maxillae superiorly and to the retroantral masticator space posteriorly and inferiorly to reach the floor of the mouth. The buccomasseteric region is composed of the buccal space traversed by the parotid duct, the buccinator and masseter muscles and the body of the mandible.

Benign Lesions of the Oral Cavity

Germ Cell Derivatives

Germ layer derivatives embedded during midline closure of the first and second branchial arches lead to formation of developmental lesions that are termed either teratomas or dermoid cysts. These terms are commonly used synonyms that refer to all three types of manifestations: epidermoid, dermoid and teratoid cysts.

Epidermoid cysts (ectodermally derived) are composed of squamous epithelium contained within a fibrous wall. *Dermoids* (ectodermal and mesodermal components) additionally contain hair follicles, sebaceous glands and fatty tissue. *Teratoid cysts* are composed of any kind of ecto-, meso- or entodermal tissue and bear the name teratoma if recognizable organs are found. Dermoids are commonly found along the floor of the mouth (and within the orbit and median nose). Depending on the amount of fatty tissue, they appear less dense on CT and T1-hyperintense compared to epidermoids; the T2 signal is hyperintense in both manifestations. The cyst wall displays mild enhancement. Contrary to epidermoids, dermoid and teratoid cysts bear malignant potential. However, teratoid cysts in the floor of the mouth or nasopharynx are usually composed of well-differentiated tissues.

Vascular Lesions

In infancy and childhood, two types of vascular lesions are encountered: hemangiomas and vascular malformations.

Hemangiomas are tumors characterized by endothelial cell proliferation and formation of vascular channels within a soft tissue stroma. They commonly become apparent within the first months of life, enlarge rapidly during a proliferative phase and subsequently regress by adolescence. Bluish discoloration of the skin and compressibility are encountered as well as subcutaneous and deep locations that affect the pharynx, oral cavity, glandular tissue, or orbits. Hemangiomas require abstention from treatment unless functional compromise (respiration, deglutition, vision) occurs. Hemangiomas are typically hyperintense on T2-weighted MR images, enhance moderately, and may contain flow voids in the proliferative stage, indicating the early high-flow nature of the lesion.

Vascular malformations, unlike hemangiomas, are not tumors but inborn errors of vascular morphogenesis. Based on the predominant type of the vascular component, angiomas or vascular malformations are classified into capillary, arterial, venous and lymphatic malformations. Vascular malformations are present since birth and grow commensurate with the growth of the child, even though endocrine stimuli or trauma including surgery may cause exacerbation. Capillary malformations (port-wine stain, nevus flammeus) are slow-flow lesions that occur in an isolated fashion or as part of several syndromes (e.g. Sturge-Weber, ataxia-telangiectasia, Rendu-Osler-Weber, Wyburn-Mason's, Cobb's). Venous malformations commonly affect the oral cavity or may be entirely intramuscular, most commonly within the masseter muscle. T2 hyperintensity, gadolinium enhancement on MRI, muscle isodensity on CT and rounded phleboliths are characteristic findings. Arteriovenous malformations are high-flow lesions that may attain large size with abundant flow voids affecting the midface, masticator space and oral cavity. Lymphatic malformations or lymphangiomas display increased signal on T1-weighted images and mild hyperdensity due to high protein content. Lymphangiomas represent a continuum of lesions that includes cystic hygromas, cavernous and capillary lymphangiomas, and lymphangiomas with additional vascular elements (hemangiolymphangiomas). Any of these components may be found in a single lesion. Fluid-fluid levels due to hemorrhage may occur. Hemangiomas and lymphangiomas are ill-defined lesions, unlike the cystic hygroma that is preferentially located in the posterior triangle of the neck and within

the sublingual and submandibular spaces. The cavernous type commonly affects the floor of the mouth, tongue or salivary glands in a permeative pattern, but presents with less contrast enhancement than a deeply located hemangioma.

Benign Cystic Lesions

Ranulas are mucous retention cysts due to obstruction of a gland, most commonly the sublingual gland. Simple ranulas are true cysts, while the plunging ranula develops following rupture of the cyst wall (pseudocyst) and presents as a lesion extending posteriorly into the submandibular space. A "cystic" lesion in relationship to the submandibular gland thus may be a ranula (medial), a second *branchial cleft cyst* (posteriorly), a dermoid, cystic hygroma, or lipoma (commonly anteriorly). An extravasation *mucocele* is a pseudocystic lesion in the anterior submandibular space following obstruction and disruption of the submandibular duct caused by trauma, tumor or sialolithiasis.

The *thyroglossal duct cyst* is the most common congenital lesion located in the midline between the foramen cecum and the level of the hyoid. Infrahyoid cysts (50%-65%) frequently extend off midline encased within the infrahyoid muscles along the course of the embryonic thyroglossal duct. Persistent thyroid tissue may occur anywhere along the duct and typically enhances markedly on CT and MRI studies. The possibility of malignancy (usually papillary carcinoma) or infection should be taken into consideration.

Inflammatory and Infectious Lesions

Inflammation of the floor of the mouth, the submental or submandibular space, and the buccomasseteric region may arise from ductal obstruction due to sialolithiasis, strictures or a neoplasm obliterating the orifice of Wharton's (submandibular) duct or Stensen's (parotid) duct. Glandular inflammation (*sialadenitis*) may display swelling and increased contrast medium uptake by the gland and its fascial lining. CT is superior to conventional radiography to depict sialolithiasis in glandular inflammation. This holds true despite advanced techniques like MR sialography. Frank parenchymal *abscess* formation is rare and in the absence of a predisposing condition should imply a search for a specific (tuberculous) etiology. Inflammation within the oral cavity may alternatively arise from infection of a preexisting lesion (ranula, dermoid, thyroglossal duct cyst) or may be of odontogenic origin.

Periapical or periodontal disease that gains access to the subperiosteal space may eventually lead to perimandibular phlegmonous infiltration or abscess formation. Access to cancellous bone and cortical bone via Volkmann's canals results in *mandibular osteomyelitis* [23]. An orthopantomogram supplemented by CT with bone window algorithm is the imaging modality of choice to recognize complications of odontogenic infection. Early signs are cortical bone erosion and periosteal reactions; later signs include sequestration, pathologic fracture and progressive bone sclerosis. MRI, however, is superior to CT in recognition of bone marrow involvement in osteomyelitis or the unusual development of intramuscular or subperiosteal masticator space abscess derived from dentogenic infection.

Benign Tumors

In the oral cavity and buccal space [24], *pleomorphic adenomas* are the most common benign glandular tumors. Lesions may cause pressure erosion at the posterior hard palate, and display cystic changes, hypodensity with little enhancement on CT, and T2 hyperintensity and inhomogeneous enhancement on MRI. Malignant minor salivary gland tumors in the oral cavity and buccal space usually are also well defined [24]. A similar imaging appearance is found in schwannomas. The tongue, floor of the mouth and hard palate are the most common locations in the oral cavity. Oral *neurofibromas* as a manifestation of von Recklinghausen's syndrome are rare (4%-5%). *Rhabdomyomas* are benign, frequently encapsulated tumors of striated muscle that occur in middle-aged men and preferentially affect the base of the tongue, floor of the mouth and pharynx. Granular cell myoblastomas contain neurogenic and muscular elements and most probably are of primitive neuroectodermal origin. As nonencapsulated tumors, they may display a more infiltrating pattern. The lesions are of muscle density and signal intensity. Overall, 50% affect the oral cavity, the dorsum and lateral tip of the tongue in particular.

Malignant Neoplasms of the Oral Cavity

Overall, 90% of malignancies of the oral cavity consist of squamous cell carcinoma (SCC). Other neoplasms are minor salivary gland tumors (e.g. adenocystic carcinoma, adenocarcinoma, mucoepidermoid carcinoma), sarcomas, and lymphomas. The squamous epithelium within the oral cavity originates from ectoderm and thus gives rise to better-differentiated neoplasms than the entodermally derived mucosa of the oropharynx.

The questions answered by imaging [14, 15, 21] relate to precise description of the tumor location, submucosal and potential neurovascular spread, and cortical bone and lymph node involvement. Common sites for SCC are the floor of the mouth, tonsillar pillar, retromolar trigone and lateral tongue, in decreasing order of frequency. SCC of the floor of the mouth is most commonly found in the anterior third and may spread medially to obstruct the submandibular duct, laterally and posteriorly within the glosso-alveolar sulcus along the mylohyoid muscle to affect the lingual and occlussal cortical mandibular surfaces, and along the neurovascular bundle within the

sublingual space. Small tumors may be missed on axial sections both by CT or MRI, unless the coronal images are scrutinized. Lymph node drainage affects the submental (nodal level IA), submandibular (IB) and jugulodigastric (II) lymph nodes. SCCs of the lateral tongue originate from the middle and posterior thirds and tend to invade the intrinsic and extrinsic tongue muscles. Assessment of midline involvement is important as is recognition of extension to the floor of the mouth and to the soft palate via the anterior tonsillar pillar. Carcinomas of the gingiva, the gingivobuccal sulcus and retromolar trigone are prone to cause mandibular erosion, and spread into the buccal space and masticator space [25].

Anterior tonsillar pillar carcinomas may mimic a tumor arising in the retromolar trigone due to extension along the palatoglossus muscle and the pterygomandibular raphe. However, invasion of the tongue base in more advanced tonsillar tumors and superior extension into the soft palate and ipsilateral nasopharynx are distinguishing features. Levels I and II lymph nodes are primarily affected. MRI in most instances excludes dental artifacts and is superior to CT in recognition of the pathways of extension. Early recognition of cortical bone erosion, however, requires high-resolution CT. Obliteration of fat by tumor extension along the nasopalatine nerves into the pterygopalatine fossa and widening of the descending palatine canal are signs indicating perineural tumor spread or recurrence, and have important therapeutic implications.

Staging of Cancer of the Pharynx and Oral Cavity

Accurate staging [26, 27] is the most important factor in assessment, treatment planning, and prognosis in patients with head and neck cancer. The staging system of the American Joint Cancer Committee (AJCC) incorporates three aspects of tumor growth: the extent of primary tumor (T), the involvement of regional lymph nodes (N), and distant metastasis (M).

The primary tumor (T) is scored as follows:

TX   Primary tumor cannot be assessed
T0   No evidence of primary tumor
Tis   Carcinoma in situ
T1-T4 Increasing size or local extent of the primary tumor

The exact definitions of T1-T4 depend on the actual site of the primary tumor (Table 2). T4 lesions are further subdivided into: T4A (resectable), T4B (unresectable), and T4C (advanced distant metastasis).

Nodal involvement (N) is scored with the following system:

NX   Regional lymph nodes cannot be assessed
N0   No regional lymph node metastasis
N1   Metastasis in single ipsilateral lymph node, 3 cm or less in greatest dimension

N2a   Metastasis in single ipsilateral lymph node, more than 3 cm but not more than 6 cm in greatest dimension

N2b   Metastasis in multiple ipsilateral lymph nodes, none more than 6 cm in greatest dimension

N2c   Bilateral or contralateral metastatic lymph nodes, none more than 6 cm in greatest dimension

N3   Metastasis in a lymph node, more than 6 cm in greatest dimension

Finally, distant metastases (M) are scored as follows:

Mx   Distant metastasis cannot be assessed

MO   No known distant metastasis

M1   Distant metastasis present (specify area or structure)

The resulting tumor stages are then defined by the combination of tumor (T), node (N) and metastasis (M) scores:

Stage I	T1	NO	MO
Stage II	T2	NO	MO
Stage III	T3	NO	MO
	T1 or T2 or T3	N1	MO
Stage IV	T4	NO or N1	MO
	Any T	N2 or N3	MO
	Any T	Any N	M1

Table 2. Definitions of T1-T4 for tumors of the pharynx and oral cavity [27]

Primary tumor	Definition
Nasopharynx	
T1	Tumor confined to one site of nasopharynx or no tumor visible (positive biopsy only)
T2	Tumor involving two sites (both posterosuperior and lateral walls)
T3	Extension of tumor into nasal cavity or oropharynx
T4	Tumor invasion of skull base or cranial nerve involvement, or both
Oropharynx and oral cavity	
T1	Tumor 2 cm or less in greatest diameter
T2	Tumor more than 2 cm but not more than 4 cm in greatest diameter
T3	Tumor more than 4 cm in greatest diameter
T4	Massive tumor more than 4 cm in diameter with invasion of contiguous structures
Hypopharynx	
T1	Tumor confined to site of origin
T2	Extension of tumor to adjacent region or site without fixation of hemilarynx
T3	Extension of tumor to adjacent region or site with fixation of hemilarynx
T4	Massive tumor invading bone or soft tissues of the neck

Imaging Cervical Metastasis

Imaging is especially useful in patient management whenever metastatic nodes are found in a clinically negative neck. The main imaging criteria for assessing nodal metastases [28-30] include the size and shape of the node, the presence of necrosis, and the presence of a localized group of nodes in an expected nodal draining area for a specific primary tumor (Table 1).

There is disagreement about the best way to measure nodes, but in the simplest case, nodes are considered abnormal if they are larger than 10 mm in diameter. Exceptions include the larger level II nodes and the smaller retropharyngeal nodes that are considered abnormal if their diameters exceed 15 mm and 8 mm, respectively. Imaging cannot yet identify microscopic tumor foci. Normal lymph nodes are oval or oblong, while metastatic lymph nodes are round or spherical.

Central nodal necrosis is considered a more specific sign of metastasis. Evaluation sensitivity is enhanced significantly when both necrosis and nodal size are used as criteria. On CT, necrosis appears as a rim of irregular enhancement surrounding a hypoattenuated central region. On post-contrast, fat-suppressed, T1-weighted MR images, peripheral enhancement surrounds a central hypointense area. Infection, prior surgery and irradiation can produce similar findings.

Extranodal tumor spread decreases survival by 50% compared to confined tumors. Extranodal extension is seen on CT and MR images as a poorly defined nodal border with variable enhancement. In addition, there may be obliterated fat planes adjacent to the node. Any lymph node with ill-defined margins is abnormal. The combination of nodal capsular penetration and the presence of a nodal mass surrounding at least 75% of an adjacent structure is highly suggestive of fixation to the adjacent structure.

The most common malignant neoplasm of the extracranial head and neck in patients older than 40 years is metastatic disease. In approximately 5% of cancer patients and nearly 15% of head and neck cancer patients, the sole presenting sign is cervical metastasis. Metastasis to the neck soft tissues can take other forms such as direct extension of a neoplasm or perineural spread of tumor.

The primary neoplasms that commonly metastasize to the cervical lymph nodes are the squamous cell carcinomas of the head, neck, esophagus and lung. Metastasis to the neck can also occur by direct extension of a primary or metastatic bone tumor of the mandible or spine. Finally, distal perineural spread may occur along the cranial and spinal nerves, thus gaining access to noncontiguous regions of the neck.

References

1. Fischbein NJ, Noworolski SM, Henry RG et al (2003) Assessment of metastatic cervical adenopathy using dynamic contrast-enhanced MR imaging. AJNR Am J Neuroradiol 24:297

2. Mack MG, Balzer JO, Straub R et al (2002) Superparamagnetic iron oxide-enhanced MR imaging of head and neck lymph nodes. Radiology 222:239-244
3. Schuknecht B (2004) Multislice CT angiography in vascular neuroradiology. In: Claussen CD, Fishman EK, Marincek B, Reiser M (eds) Multislice CT: a practical guide. Springer, Berlin Heidelberg New York, pp 53-59
4. Lenz M, Greess H, Baum U et al (2000) Oropharynx, oral cavity, floor of the mouth: CT and MRI. Eur J Radiol 33:203-215
5. Hasso AN, Nickmeyer CA (1994) Magnetic resonance imaging of soft tissues of the neck. Top Magn Reson Imaging 6:1-21
6. Mukherji SK (2003) Pharynx. In: Som PM, Curtin HD (eds) Head and neck imaging, 5th edn. Mosby Year Book, St Louis, pp 1465-1520
7. Davis WL, Harnsberger HR, Smoker WRK et al (1990) Retropharyngeal space: evaluation of normal anatomy and diseases with CT and MR imaging. Radiology 174:59-64
8. Parker GD, Harnsberger HR, Jacobs JM (1990) The pharyngeal mucosal space. Semin Ultrasound CT MR 11:460-475
9. Dillon WP, Mancuso AA (1988) The oropharynx and nasopharynx. In: Newton TH, Hasso AN, Dillon WP (eds) Computed tomography of the head and neck, vol. 111. Raven, New York, chapt. 10
10. Harnsberger HR (1990) Head and neck imaging. Year Book Medical, Chicago, pp 112-255 (Handbooks of radiology)
11. Schuller DE (1987) Clinical evaluation of tumors of the neck. In: Batsakis JG, Lindberg RD (eds) Comprehensive management of head and neck tumors, vol. 2. Saunders, Philadelphia, pp 1230-1240
12. Vogl T, Dresel S, Bilaniuk LT et al (1990) Tumors of the nasopharynx and adjacent areas: MR imaging with Gd-DTPA. AJNR Am J Neuroradiol 11:187-194
13. King AD, Teo P, Lam WWM et al (2000) Paranasopharyngeal space involvement in nasopharyngeal cancer, detection by CT and MRI. Clin Oncol 2:397-402
14. Kassel EE, Keller MA, Kucharczyk W (1989) MRI of the floor of the mouth, tongue and oropharynx. Radiol Clin North Am 27:331-351
15. McKenna KM, Jabour BA, Lufkin RB, Hanafee WN (1990) Magnetic resonance imaging of the tongue and oropharynx. Top Magn Reson Imaging 2:49-59
16. Thawley SE, Panje WR (eds) Comprehensive management of head and neck tumors. WB Saunders, Philadelphia, p 778
17. Batsakis JG (1979) Tumors of the head and neck. Williams Wilkins, Baltimore, pp 200-228
18. Sakai O, Curtin HD, Romo LV, Som PM (2000) Lymph node pathology: benign proliferative, lymphoma, and metastatic disease. Radiol Clin North Am 8:979-998
19. McGill T (1989) Rhabdomyosarcoma of the head and neck: an update. Radiol Clin North Am 22:631-636
20. Ramos R, Som PM, Solodnik P (1990) Nasopharyngeal melanotic melanoma: MR characteristics. J Comput Assist Tomogr 14(6):997-999
21. Smoker WRK (2003) The oral cavity. In: Som PM, Curtin HD (eds) Head and neck imaging, 5th edn. Mosby Year Book, St Louis, pp 1377-1464
22. Som PM, Smoker WRK, Curtin HD, Reidenberg JS, Laitman J (2003) Congenital lesions. In: Som PM, Curtin HD (eds) Head and neck imaging, 5th edn. Mosby Year Book, St Louis, pp 1828-1864
23. Schuknecht B, Valavanis A (2003) Osteomyelitis of the mandible. Neuroimaging Clin N Am 13:605-618
24. Kurabayashi T, Ida M, Ohbayashi N et al (2002) MR imaging of benign and malignant lesions in the buccal space. Dentomaxillofacial Radiol 31:344-349
25. Kimura Y, Sumi M, Yoshiko A et al (2002) Deep extension from carcinoma arising from the gingiva: CT and MR imaging features. AJNR Am J Neuroradiol 23:468-472
26. Lowe VJ, Stack Jr. BC, Watson RE Jr (2003) Head and neck cancer imaging. In: Ensley JF, Gutkind JS, Jacobs JR, Lippman SM (eds) Head and neck cancer: emerging perspectives. Academic, Amsterdam Boston, pp 23-32
27. American Joint Committee on Cancer (2002) AJCC cancer staging manual, 6th edn. Lippincott-Raven, New York
28. Som PM (1997) Lymph nodes of the neck. Radiology 165:693-600
29. Hillsamer PJ, Schuller DE, McGhee RB et al (1990) Improving diagnostic accuracy of cervical metastases with computed tomography and magnetic resonance imaging. Arch Otolaryngo Head Neck Surg 116:1297-1301
30. Van den Brekel MWM, Castelijns JA (1999) New developments in imaging neck node metastases. In: Mukherji SK, Castelijns JA (eds) Modern head and neck imaging. Springer, Berlin Heidelberg New York, pp 133-156

Imaging of the Larynx

H.D. Curtin

Massachusetts Eye and Ear Infirmary, Harvard Medical School, Boston, MA, USA

Introduction

Imaging of the larynx must be coordinated with the clinical exam. The information acquired at imaging usually emphasizes the deeper tissues, as the superficial assessment is done by direct visualization. The description of anatomy is key to the description of any lesion.

Anatomy

Important Mucosal Landmarks

Several key anatomic structures are important to the radiologist seeking to evaluate the larynx. Perhaps the most important relationship in the larynx is that of the false vocal folds, true vocal folds and ventricle complex. The ventricle is a crucial reference point. Much imaging of tumors is aimed at defining the position of a lesion relative to this key region. Another important landmark is the cricoid cartilage. This cartilage is the only complete ring of the cartilage framework and is key to the integrity of the airway.

A major role in speech generation is played by the glottis or true vocal folds (cords). They stretch across the lower larynx and are in the horizontal or axial plane. There is a small crease just above the true vocal folds called the ventricle. Immediately above the ventricle and again parallel to both the ventricle and true folds is a second pair of folds called the false vocal folds. Above the false folds, the mucosa curves out laterally to the upper edges of the larynx called the aryepiglottic folds which, in turn, curve around and extend up to the margins of the epiglottis.

These structures are the basis for anatomic localization within the larynx. The glottic larynx refers only to the true folds. It has been defined as stretching from the ventricle to a plane approximately one centimeter below the ventricle. Here, the glottis merges with the subglottis (the lower part of the larynx). The subglottis extends from the lower margin of the glottis to the inferior margin of cricoid cartilage. Everything above the ventricle of the larynx is the supraglottis.

Another important anatomic term relating to the mucosa is the anterior commissure. This is the point where the true folds converge anteriorly and insert into the thyroid cartilage.

Cartilage Framework

The cartilages make up the framework of the larynx and give it structure. The cricoid cartilage is the foundation of the larynx and is the only complete ring. It is responsible for keeping the airway open. Above the cricoid cartilage and attached its lateral margins is the thyroid cartilage. This shield-like cartilage provides protection to the inner workings of the larynx. The arytenoid cartilages perch upon the posterior edge of the cricoid cartilage.

In axial imaging, the cartilages can help orient us to the mucosal levels in the larynx. The cricoid is at the level of the glottis and subglottis. The upper posterior edge of the cricoid cartilage is actually at the level of the true folds. The lower edge of the cricoid cartilage represents the lower boundary of the larynx and, therefore, the lower edge of the subglottis.

The arytenoid cartilage spans the ventricle. The upper arytenoid is at the level of the false folds, whereas the vocal process defines the position of the vocal ligament and, therefore, the true folds. The epiglottis is totally within the supraglottic larynx.

Deep Soft Tissues

There are many muscles within the larynx. The key muscle for the radiologist is the thyroarytenoid muscle. This forms the bulk of the true folds and extends from the arytenoid up to the anterior part of the thyroid cartilage at the anterior commissure. The radiologist should be familiar with this muscle because identifying it is helpful in attempting to identify the true folds.

The *paraglottic* space refers to the major part of the soft tissue between the mucosa and the cartilaginous framework of the larynx. At the supraglottic or false fold level, this is predominantly made up of fat, whereas at the level of the true folds, the paraglottic region is filled with the thyroarytenoid muscle. Again, this concept is helpful in orienting oneself to the level within the larynx. The level of the ventricle is identified as the transition between the fat and muscle.

Pathology and Imaging

Imaging of the larynx and upper airway is done in many situations [1-6]. At Massachusetts Eye and Ear Infirmary, most laryngeal imaging studies relate to the evaluation of tumor or trauma.

Tumors of the larynx can be separated into two categories. Most tumors of the larynx are squamous cell carcinomas and arise from the mucosa. A few tumors arise from the cartilaginous skeleton or from the other submucosal tissues.

The endoscopist almost always detects and diagnoses the mucosal lesions. Indeed, imaging should not be used in an attempt to "exclude" squamous cell carcinoma of the larynx. In squamous cell carcinoma, the role of the radiologist is almost always to determine the of depth of spread. Submucosal tumors are, however, somewhat different. These the endoscopist can usually visualize, but since they are covered by mucosa there may be considerable difficulty in making the diagnosis; in these cases the clinician may ask the radiologist to identify the type of tumor.

In *squamous cell carcinoma*, much of imaging concerns the determination of the depth of extension. Radiologists can see submucosal disease, which can make a difference in choice of therapy. It is important to know some of the indications and contraindications of various alternatives to total laryngectomy. Standard classic partial laryngectomies are supraglottic laryngectomy and vertical hemilaryngectomy. In many institutions, similar surgeries are now done via endoscopic approach. If the information needed for these procedures is gathered through imaging, then there is more than enough information for radiotherapists and other clinical specialists as well.

- *Supraglottic laryngectomy* removes everything above the level of the ventricle, and is used for tumors arising in the epiglottis, false folds or aryepiglottic folds. Tumor may obstruct the endoscopist's view of the lower margin of the tumor, or can cross the ventricle by "tunneling" beneath the mucosal surface. Such submucosal spread can travel along the paraglottic pathway around the ventricle, and is a contraindication to supraglottic laryngectomy. Since it can be missed by direct visualization, the radiologist must try to detect this phenomenon. Cartilage involvement is another contraindication, but this is rare in supraglottic cancers unless the lesion has actually crossed the ventricle. Other contraindications include significant extension into the tongue or significant pulmonary problems. These mostly relate to difficulty in relearning how to

swallow once the key part of the laryngeal protective mechanism has been removed.
- *Vertical hemilaryngectomy* is performed for lesions of the true folds. The aim is to remove the tumor but to retain enough of one true fold so that the patient can still create speech using the usual mechanism. Actually, the lesion can extend onto the anterior part of the opposite fold and there can still be a satisfactory removal. In these areas, the radiologist looks most closely at inferior extension. Does the tumor reach the upper margin of the cricoid cartilage? In most institutions, such extension would mean that the patient is not a candidate for vertical hemilaryngectomy but rather should have total laryngectomy or alternative therapies.

Lesions of the *anterior commissure* may extend anteriorly into either the thyroid cartilage or through the cricothyroid membrane into the soft tissues of the neck. This may be invisible to the examining clinician and is again a key point to evaluate.

Involvement of both the arytenoid cartilages is also a contraindication to total laryngectomy, but this is usually evaluated by direct visualization.

Radiotherapy is a speech-conserving treatment. Here the therapist is mostly concerned with cartilage invasion or the thickness of the tumor.

In order to image *laryngeal squamous cell carcinoma*, at Massachusetts Eye and Ear Infirmary, we begin with computed tomography (CT). The new multidetector CT scanners give excellent resolution and good coronal and sagittal plane image reformats. The study can be done in a short time interval. Newer scanners can perform the entire study during a single breath hold. Magnetic resonance imaging (MRI) is reserved for evaluating lesions close to the cartilage or ventricle. A limited study may be done to clarify a particular margin.

Imaging of *cartilage involvement* is controversial. Some clinicians favor CT while others prefer MRI. At CT, sclerosis of the cartilage and obliteration of the low density fat in the medullary space indicate involvement. The negative finding, intact fat in the medullary space with a normal cortex, is considered reliable. On MRI, one begins with the T1-weighted image. If there is high signal intensity in the medullary space, the cartilage is considered normal. If the area is dark, then one examines the T2-weighted image. Nonossified cartilage remains dark while tumor is usually brighter. High signal intensity on T2-weighted images can mean tumor or edema related to tumor; at my institution, the high signal intensity is presumed to represent tumor. More research is needed to determine the relevance of signal changes to prognosis.

Submucosal lesions may arise from the cartilages, minor salivary glands, or other soft tissue structures. CT with intravenous contrast medium administration can be helpful. Chondromatous lesions can arise from any cartilage. Those arising from the cricoid cartilage have a characteristic appearance as they expand cartilage. Hemangiomas enhance intensely as do the rare glomus (paraganglioma) tumors. There are other lesions that arise in the submucosal region but do not enhance nor involve the cartilage. In these cases, the identity cannot be made precisely but it is helpful to the clinician if one can exclude a vascular or chondroid lesion.

Another submucosal lesion that is important is the *laryngocele*. This lesion can present as a submucosal swelling but is actually totally benign and results from obstructive dilatation of the small saccule (appendix) of the ventricle. Although benign, it may be associated with a malignancy at the level of the ventricle. It is important to carefully evaluate this level. Again, we must realize that radiologically we cannot totally exclude small lesions of the mucosa. This must be done endoscopically.

Trauma

Trauma to the airway can obviously be life-threatening. Most patients who have a demonstrable fracture of the larynx undergo endoscopy to identify mucosal tears. If there is a fragment of cartilage exposed to the airway, then chondritis and eventual chondronecrosis can be expected. One should carefully evaluate the integrity of the thyroid cartilage and the cricoid ring. These fractures are associated with edema of the endolarynx; this observation can be helpful especially when the cartilages are not completely calcified, for example in young patients.

Fractures

Fractures of the cricoid cartilage usually cause the ring to collapse. The anterior arch of the cricoid cartilage is pushed posteriorly into the airway. The thyroid cartilage can fracture vertically or horizontally. The vertical fracture is usually easily seen but horizontal fractures are in the plane of the axial image and can be missed. Hemorrhage in the adjacent pre-epiglottic fat may be a clue to this type of fracture. The arytenoid cartilage does not fracture but can be dislocated.

Dislocations

Dislocations can occur at the cricothyroid articulation or at the cricoarytenoid joint. Cricothyroid dislocation is usually associated with significant trauma. There is usually a fracture of the inferior horn of the thyroid cartilage rather than a true dislocation. Cricoarytenoid dislocation may occur with minor trauma. The status of these joints can be difficult to determine at imaging, but the radiologist should indicate if the cartilages appear to be normally aligned.

Conclusions

At Massachusetts Eye and Ear Infirmary, we currently prefer CT for the evaluation of cancer of the larynx. MRI, however, has a slight advantage in evaluating vertical extension, especially relative to the ventricle and in evaluating the cartilage. With newer and faster MRI sequences, this may change. For submucosal lesions, we use an enhanced CT scan to differentiate among chondroid lesions, vascular lesions and laryngocele. For trauma, we use CT to look for fractures and dislocations.

Suggested Reading

Becker M, Zbaren P, Delavelle J et al (1997) Neoplastic invasion of the laryngeal cartilage: reassessment of criteria for diagnosis at CT. Radiology 203:521-532

Becker M (1998) Larynx and hypopharynx. Radiol Clin North Am 36:891-920

Castelijns JA, Becker M, Hermans R (1996) Impact of cartilage invasion on treatment and prognosis of laryngeal cancer. Eur Radiol 6:156-169

Curtin HD (1989) Imaging of the larynx: current concepts. Radiology 173:1-11

Curtin HD (2003) The larynx. In: Som PM, Curtin HD (eds) Head and neck imaging, 4th edn. Mosby, St. Louis, pp 1595-1699

Zbaren P, Becker M, Lang H (1997) Staging of laryngeal cancer: endoscopy, computed tomography and magnetic resonance versus histopathology. Eur Arch Otorhinolaryngol 254[Suppl 1]:S117-122

Imaging the Larynx and Hypopharynx

M. Becker

Department of ENT and Maxillofacial Radiology, Division of Diagnostic and Interventional Radiology, Geneva University Hospital, Geneva, Switzerland

Introduction

The larynx and hypopharynx are imaged with either computed tomography (CT) or magnetic resonance imaging (MRI). A standard CT examination is done in the supine position, and the patient is instructed to resist swallowing or coughing. Axial slices are obtained from the base of the skull to the trachea with a scan orientation parallel to the true vocal cords. Iodinated contrast material (total dose, 35-40 g iodine) is given intravenously with an automated power injector. Images are obtained during quiet breathing rather than during apnea because the abducted position of the true vocal cords facilitates evaluation of the anterior and posterior commissures. Acquisitions with 3-mm collimation at pitch 1 and overlapping reconstruction intervals of 2 mm are the minimum parameters necessary to evaluate the larynx. With multislice CT scanners, a slice thickness of 1.3 mm and overlapping reconstructions every 0.6 mm are used routinely by many investigators, including myself, allowing high quality two-dimensional (2D) reconstructions in the coronal or sagittal plane.

To date, MRI of the larynx and hypopharynx is performed using dedicated surface neck coils in phased-array (multicoil) configuration. Two basic pulse sequences are currently used by most investigators, namely T1-weighted and T2-weighted sequences. Axial T2-weighted fast spin echo (FSE) and T1-weighted SE or FSE images are obtained with a scan orientation parallel to the true vocal cords. Typical image parameters include a slice thickness of 3-4 mm with a 0-1 mm intersection gap, and a field of view of 18×18 cm^2 or less. The acquisition matrix should be 256×512 cm^2 or 512×512 cm^2. Additional axial T1-weighted images after intravenous administration of gadolinium chelates are obtained routinely. Fat-saturated T1-weighted images with or without contrast enhancement and fat-saturated T2-weighted images are optional. Images in the coronal or sagittal plane may be obtained in order to evaluate certain anatomic spaces, such as the preepiglottic space in the sagittal plane, or the paraglottic space and the ventricle in the coronal plane.

The most common indications to perform cross-sectional imaging of the larynx include:
1. Squamous cell carcinoma
2. Non-squamous cell tumors
3. Cysts and laryngoceles
4. Vocal cord paralysis
5. Inflammatory lesions, and
6. Traumatic lesions.

Squamous Cell Carcinoma

Over 90% of laryngeal and hypopharyngeal tumors are squamous cell carcinomas [1-17]. With few exceptions, squamous cell tumors are located at the mucosal surface, and the clinical diagnosis is readily confirmed by endoscopic biopsy. However, submucosal tumor extension cannot be assessed reliably with endoscopy alone. Because the degree of infiltration into the surrounding deep anatomic structures has implications for treatment and prognosis, cross-sectional imaging with either CT or MRI is required for the diagnostic workup of laryngeal and hypopharyngeal tumors. Unusual malignant neoplasms of the laryngohypopharyngeal region, such as chondrosarcomas, lymphomas and lipomas, are often entirely submucosal. The origin and extension of these tumors are difficult to diagnose with endoscopy, and planning of biopsy and treatment usually depends on imaging findings.

Patterns of Tumor Spread

Carcinoma of the larynx arises in the supraglottic region (30%), glottis (65%) or subglottic region (5%) [3, 6].

Supraglottic tumors originating from the epiglottis primarily invade the preepiglottic space. MRI diagnosis of tumor spread to the preepiglottic space is made when the high signal intensity of fat normally seen on the T1-weighted image is replaced by a mass with low signal

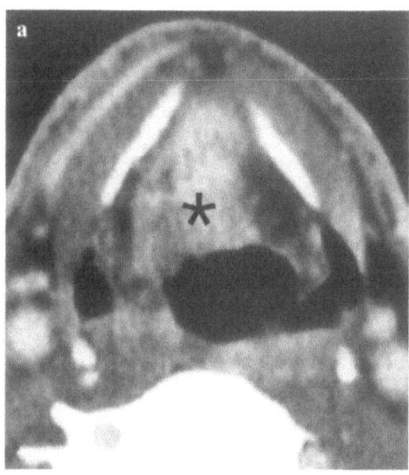
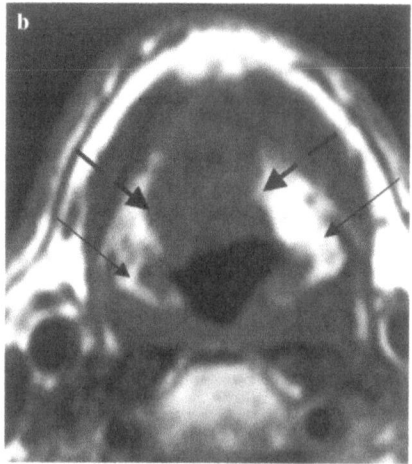
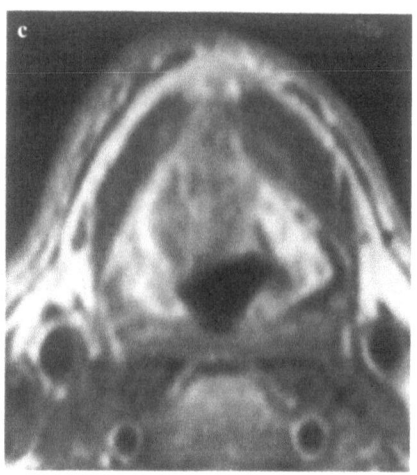

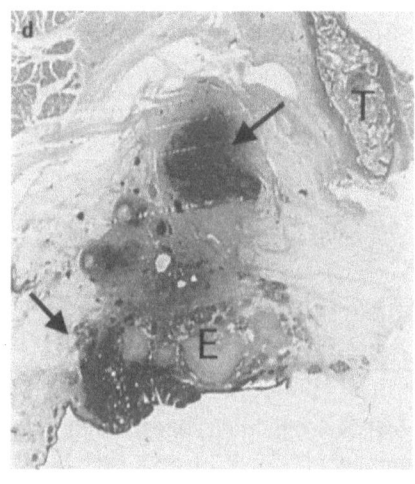

Fig. 1a-d. *Neoplastic invasion of the preepiglottic space due to supraglottic cancer.* **a** Axial contrast- enhanced CT image at the supraglottic level shows an enhancing mass invading the preepiglottic space (*asterisk*). **b** Axial unenhanced T1-weighted image at the supraglottic level shows a tumor mass with an intermediate signal intensity as it extends into the preepiglottic space (*dashed arrows*). Note the high signal intensity of the noninvaded paraglottic space due to the high content of fatty tissue (*thin arrows*). **c** Axial Gd-enhanced T1-weighted image at the same level shows enhancement of the tumor mass invading the preepiglottic space. **d** Whole-organ axial histologic slice from supraglottic horizontal laryngectomy specimen confirms tumor invasion of the preepiglottic space (*arrows*). Epiglottis (*E*), thyroid cartilage (*T*). (Reproduced from [6] with permission)

intensity and when enhancement of the preepiglottic mass is observed (Fig. 1) [3, 6]. Although sagittal images are best suited for delineating the extent of tumor spread within the preepiglottic space (Fig. 2), standard axial images are sufficient to establish the diagnosis. Similarly, on CT, the diagnosis of preepiglottic space invasion is made when an enhancing mass is seen within the preepiglottic fat (Fig. 1). Supraglottic tumors originating from the false cord, laryngeal ventricle, or aryepiglottic fold primarily infiltrate the paraglottic space. The primary sign of tumor spread to the paraglottic space on MRI or CT is replacement of fatty tissue by tumor tissue (Fig. 2) [3, 6, 7]. The sensitivities of MRI and CT for the detection of neoplastic spread to the preepiglottic and paraglottic space are high; however, the corresponding specificities are limited due to the fact that peritumoral inflammatory changes may lead to overestimation of tumor spread with both methods, therefore resulting in false-positive assessments. The primary lymphatic spread of supraglottic carcinomas is directed toward the superior jugular lymph nodes. Lymph node metastases are common and often bilateral.

Glottic carcinoma typically arises from the anterior half of the vocal cord and primarily spreads into the anterior commissure. Invasion of the anterior commissure is seen on CT and MRI as a soft tissue thickening of more than 1-2 mm. Once the tumor has reached the anterior commissure, it may easily spread into the thyroarytenoid muscle, contralateral cord, paraglottic space, supraglottis or subglottis. On axial CT or MR images, neoplastic invasion occurring at the subglottic level below the anterior commissure appears as an irregular thickening of the cricothyroid membrane. Further spread occurs mainly in a cephalad or caudad direction or, via the cricothyroid membrane, into the perilaryngeal tissue. Paraglottic tumor spread in glottic cancer may be entirely occult clinically and detectable only by means of CT or MRI. Subglottic spread is relatively common in glottic cancer and may either occur superficially or deep in the elastic cone. Deep subglottic spread is difficult to detect endoscopically, and underestimation of the tumor may occur

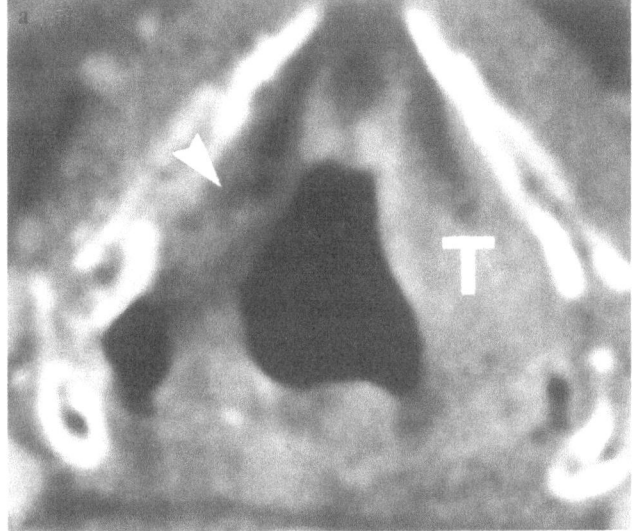
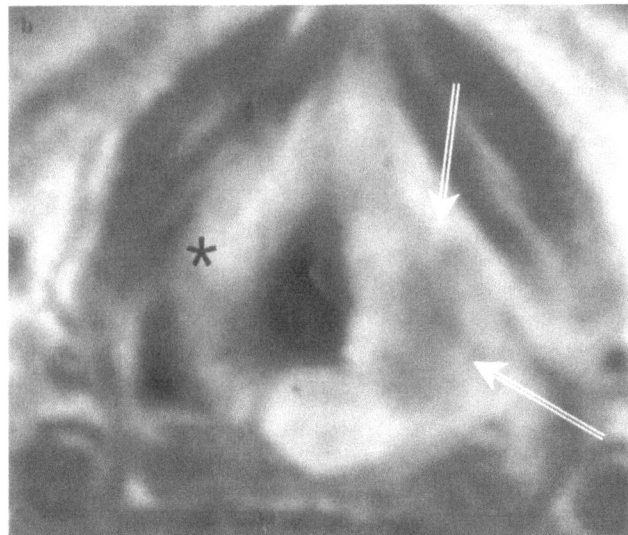
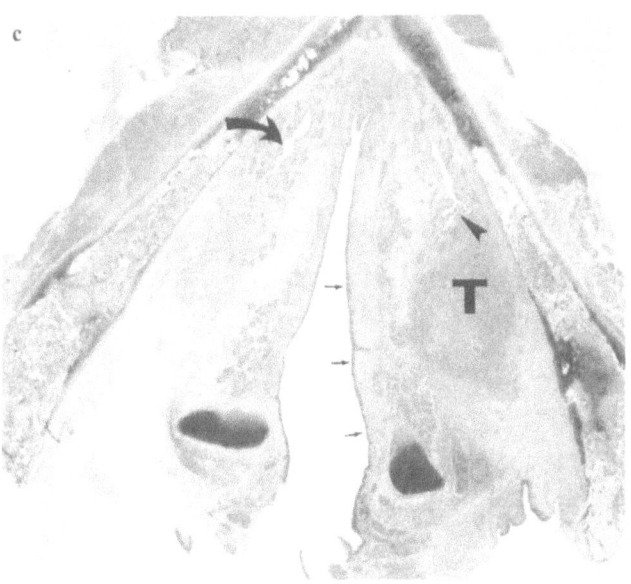

Fig. 2a-c. *Neoplastic invasion of the left paraglottic space due to ventricular cancer.* Endoscopically only a very small mucosal lesion was present within the left laryngeal ventricle. **a** Axial contrast-enhanced CT image at the supraglottic level shows a tumor mass (*T*) invading the left paraglottic space. Note normal appearance of the contralateral paraglottic space (*arrowhead*). **b** Axial contrast-enhanced T1-weighted image shows an enhancing tumor mass (*arrows*) invading the left paraglottic fat. Normal right paraglottic fat space (*asterisk*). **c** Whole-organ axial slice from specimen confirms extensive paraglottic space invasion by a predominantely submucosal tumor mass (*T*). The tumor mass originated from the left laryngeal ventricle (*arrowhead*). *Curved arrow,* right laryngeal ventricle. Note the normal aspect of the laryngeal mucosa overlying the tumor mass (*thin arrows*). (Reproduced from [7] with permission)

unless CT or MRI is performed. The degree of subglottic spread is best displayed on axial images (Fig. 3). Coronal images are of limited help in the assessment of subglottic spread, because they are difficult to interpret except in the midcoronal plane. Lymphatic metastases from glottic carcinoma are uncommon as long as the tumor is confined to the endolarynx. However, once the tumor has spread into the soft tissues of the neck, the frequency of lymph node metastases increases significantly.

Primary *subglottic carcinoma* is uncommon and tends to spread to the trachea or invade the thyroid gland and the cervical esophagus. Lymph node metastases are much more common than in glottic carcinoma and they affect the paratracheal and pretracheal nodes. These nodes drain to the lower jugular or upper mediastinal nodes. Cross-sectional imaging performed in patients with primary subglottic tumors should, therefore, include the upper mediastinum.

Carcinoma of the *hypopharynx* may arise in the piriform sinus (65%), post-cricoid area (20%) and posterior pharyngeal wall (15%) [3, 6]. *Carcinoma of the piriform sinus* is readily detected with endoscopy while very early superficial spreading tumors that are limited to the mucosa may be invisible at cross-sectional imaging. In most cases, however, patients with piriform sinus tumors initially present with advanced lesions and diagnosis with CT or MRI is straightforward. Because the piriform sinus is usually collapsed during quiet respiration, the exact tumor location (medial wall vs. lateral wall) may be difficult to determine radiologically and a close cooperation with the head and neck surgeon is essential. Tumors originating from the lateral wall of the piriform sinus have a tendency to infiltrate early the soft tissues of the neck. Tumors originating from the medial wall or the angle of the piriform sinus may infiltrate the larynx by growing anteriorly into the paraglottic space.

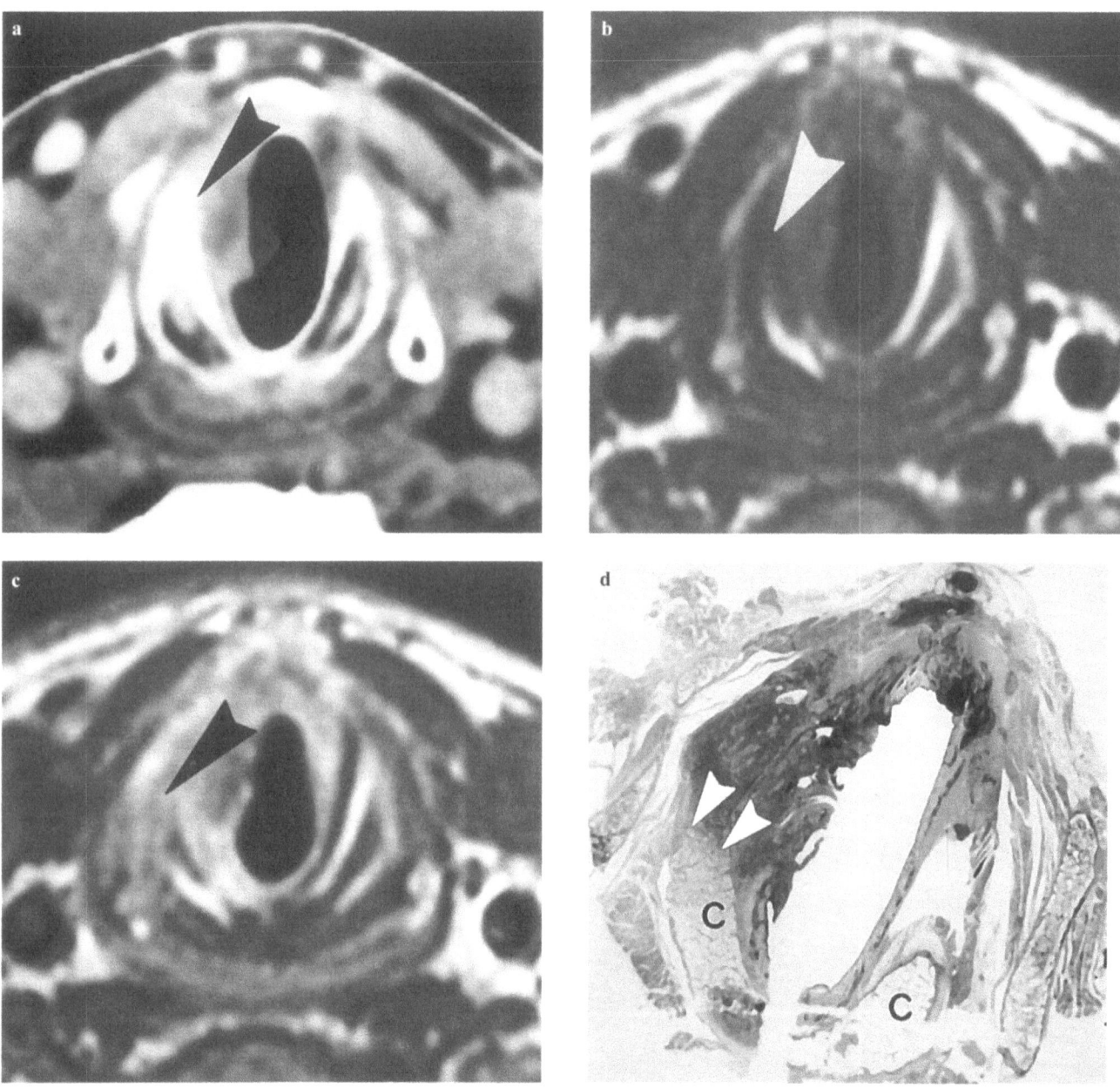

Fig. 3a-d. *Neoplastic invasion of the cricoid cartilage.* Glottosubglottic carcinoma of the larynx in a 46-year-old man. **a** Contrast-enhanced CT at the subglottic level shows a right-sided tumor mass adjacent to a sclerotic cricoid cartilage. Sclerosis suggests invasion of the adjacent cricoid cartilage. **b** Axial T1-weighted image. A mass with intermediate signal intensity infiltrates the right subglottic region. The right cricoid cartilage shows decreased signal intensity (*arrowhead*). **c** Contrast-enhanced axial T1-weighted image shows extensive contrast enhancement of the right subglottic tumor mass, as well as of the adjacent cricoid cartilage. The extensive enhancement of the right cricoid cartilage (*arrowhead*) suggests tumor invasion. **d** Axial slice from specimen at the same level shows a large subglottic tumor mass invading the right cricoid cartilage (*arrowheads*). *C*, cricoid cartilage. (Reproduced from [1] with permission)

Piriform sinus carcinoma frequently invades the paraglottic space and the laryngeal cartilages (discussed later).

Post-cricoid carcinoma is uncommon in general but observed in certain groups at risk (e.g. patients with Plummer-Vinson syndrome). These tumors spread submucosally most often toward the cervical esophagus. Because tumor growth is mainly submucosal, the true extent only becomes apparent with axial or sagittal MR images.

Carcinoma of the posterior pharyngeal wall commonly involves both the oropharynx and hypopharynx. On axial MR images, these tumors appear as asymmetrical thickenings of the posterior pharyngeal wall. Invasion of the prevertebral muscles is unusual at initial presentation.

Squamous cell carcinoma of the hypopharynx has a relatively poor prognosis, with up to 75% of patients having metastases to cervical lymph nodes at initial presentation.

Neoplastic Cartilage Invasion

Invasion of the hyaline laryngeal cartilage by squamous cell carcinoma alters staging, prognosis and, in most centers, the therapeutic approach [1-4, 6-12]. Most authors believe that radiation therapy cannot eradicate tumor within cartilage but may result in perichondritis and chondronecrosis, although some others believe that radiation therapy can sterilize tumor even in invaded cartilage. Invasion of the thyroid, cricoid and both arytenoid cartilages precludes classic voice-sparing partial laryngectomy and necessitates total laryngectomy, an extremely invasive procedure. Recent direct comparison studies with histologic correlation have shown that CT has a high sensitivity and a high negative predictive value for the detection of carti-

lage invasion provided that the following criteria are used: sclerosis, erosion, lysis and extralaryngeal spread [4].

– *Sclerosis* is a sensitive sign for the detection of neoplastic cartilage invasion and enables diagnosis of early or microscopic intracartilaginous tumor spread (Fig. 3). It corresponds to bone remodeling and new bone formation induced by the presence of tumor cells in immediate vicinity. The specificity of this sign varies considerably from one cartilage to another, and is lowest in thyroid cartilage (40%) and higher in cricoid and arytenoid cartilages (76% and 79%, respectively). Therefore, if a tumor mass is seen adjacent to a sclerotic cartilage, this does not automatically imply that tumor cells are found within the remodelled marrow cavity (Fig. 4). Conversely, failing at surgery to re-

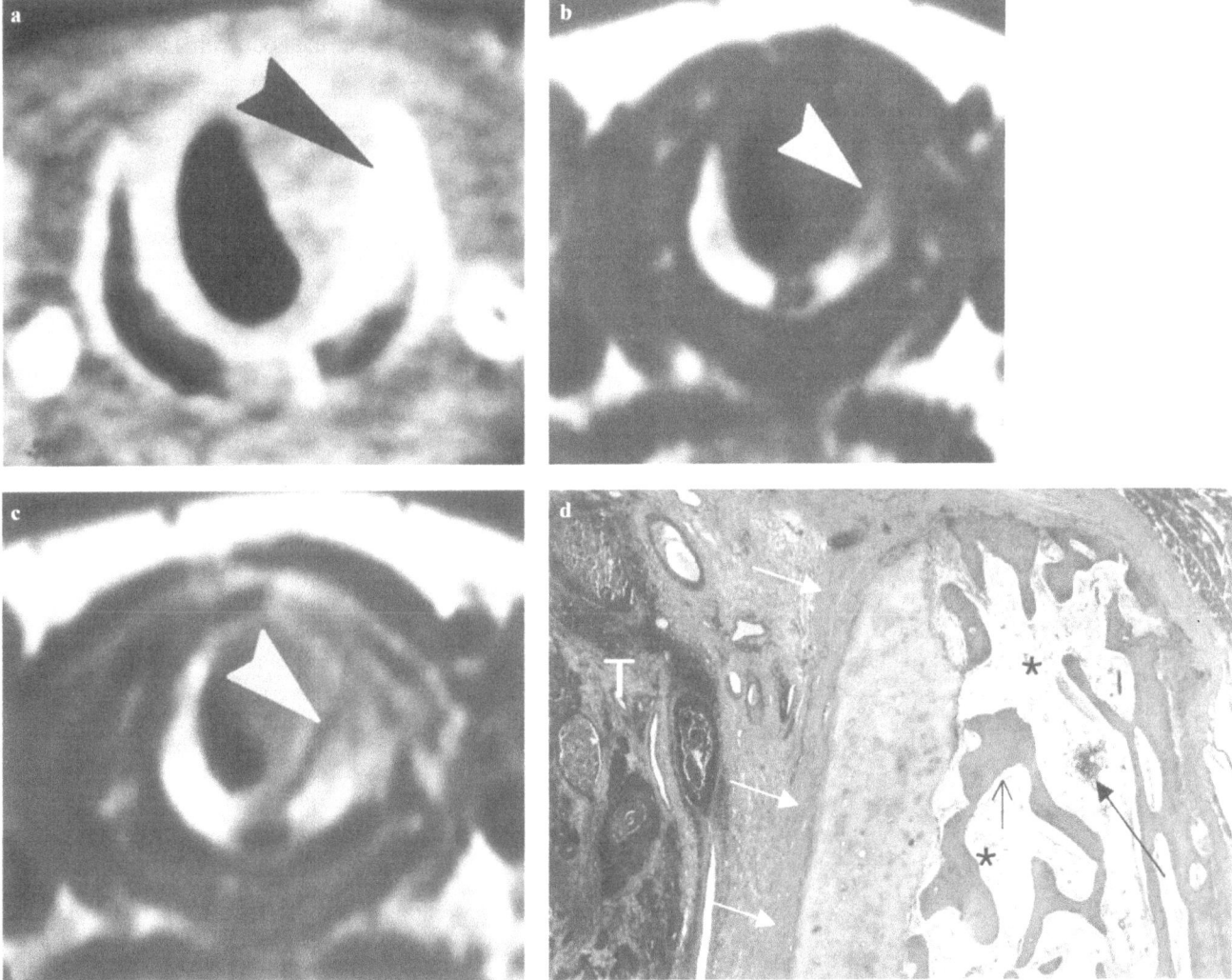

Fig. 4a-d. *Inflammatory changes appearing as false-positive neoplastic cartilage invasion on CT and MRI.* Glottosubglottic carcinoma of the larynx in a 71-year-old woman. **a** Contrast-enhanced CT image shows sclerosis of the left cricoid cartilage suggesting invasion by the adjacent tumor. **b** T1-weighted axial image. A mass with low signal intensity infiltrates the left subglottic region. The adjacent left cricoid cartilage shows decreased signal intensity (*arrowhead*). **c** Contrast-enhanced T1-weighted image. Contrast enhancement is seen within the left cricoid cartilage (*arrowhead*), as well as within the subglottic tumor mass suggesting invasion. **d** Axial slice from specimen shows a large, left-sided subglottic tumor mass (*T*) but no evidence of cartilage invasion. The cricoid cartilage shows extensive inflammatory changes with lymph follicles (*black arrow*), fibrosis (*asterisks*) and bone resorption (*open arrows*), but with an intact perichondrium (*white arrows*). (Reproduced from [1] with permission)

move a cartilage that exhibits sclerosis on CT carries a 50%-60% risk of leaving tumor behind.

- As the process of cartilage invasion progresses, minor and major areas of osteolysis are seen within the areas of new bone formation. Minor areas of osteolysis correspond to the CT criterion of *erosion*, while major areas of osteolysis correspond to the CT criterion of *lysis*. Histologically, erosion and lysis correspond to destruction of bone due to osteoclastic activity. As a consequence, erosion and lysis can be considered specific criteria for the detection of neoplastic invasion in all cartilages. The overall specificity of erosion and lysis is 93%. However, both of these criteria are not very sensitive as they are bound to the presence of more advanced invasion of laryngeal cartilage [4].

- *Extralaryngeal spread* occurs due to tumor invasion through a cartilage into the extralaryngeal soft tissues. This CT criterion is highly specific (overall specificity, 95%), but because it is only seen very late in the disease process its sensitivity is as low as 44%.

By applying the combination of sclerosis, erosion-lysis, and extralaryngeal spread to all cartilages, one may obtain an overall sensitivity as high as 91%. Because the negative predictive value of this combination is 95%, CT may be considered an excellent test to exclude cartilage invasion prior to treatment.

MRI has a high sensitivity for the detection of cartilage invasion. The reported sensitivity of MRI for the detection of neoplastic cartilage invasion is 89%-94%. the specificity is 74%-88%, and the negative predictive value is 94%-96%. Extensive tumor invasion involving both inner and outer aspects of the cartilage can be diagnosed with a high accuracy with MRI. In addition, MRI enables detection of intracartilaginous tumor spread. If tumor is present only adjacent to the inner aspect of a cartilage, the radiologist can differentiate between tumor and nonossified cartilage by comparing the different MR pulse sequences. Cartilage invaded by tumor displays an intermediate or low signal intensity on T1-weighted images, a higher signal intensity on proton-density and T2-weighted images, and areas of enhancement within the cartilage adjacent to the tumor after injection of gadolinium chelates (Fig. 3). If these signs are absent, cartilage infiltration can be ruled out with a high level of confidence, since the negative predictive value of MRI is high (Fig. 5). Unfortunately, the MRI findings suggesting neoplastic cartilage invasion are not as specific as expected ini-

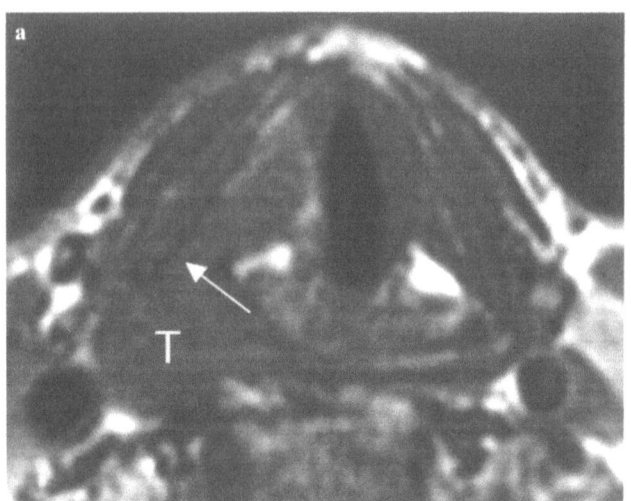

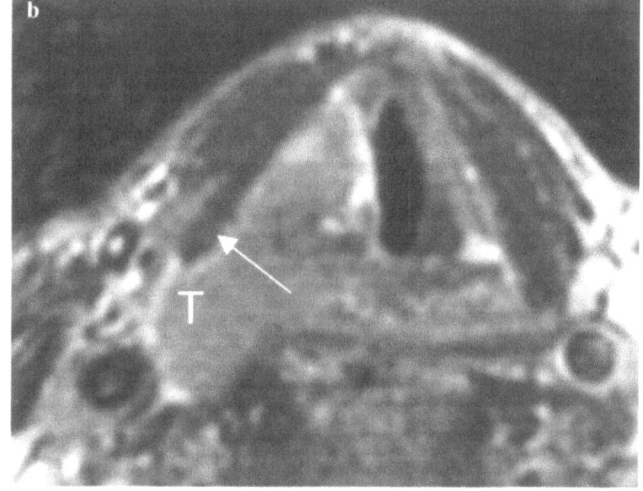

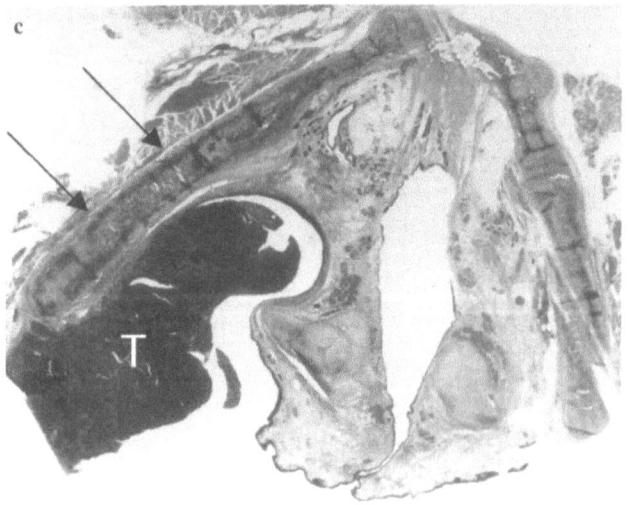

Fig. 5a-c. *True-negative MRI findings for neoplastic invasion of the thyroid cartilage.* **a** T1-weighted image obtained at the supraglottic level shows a right-sided piriform sinus tumor with intermediate to low signal intensity (*T*). The adjacent right thyroid lamina also has intermediate to low signal intensity (*arrow*). **b** T1-weighted SE image obtained after intravenous administration of contrast medium shows contrast enhancement of the tumor mass (*T*), however no enhancement of the adjacent thyroid lamina (*arrow*). This suggests that the thyroid cartilage is composed of nonossified hyaline cartilage and that no intracartilaginous tumor spread is present. **c** Corresponding axial slice from surgical specimen at the same level confirms that the right thyroid lamina is composed of nonossified hyaline cartilage (*arrows*). No cartilage invasion was found at histological analysis. The tumor (*T*) arose from the lateral wall of the right piriform sinus. (Reproduced from [6] with permission)

tially, but may be false positive in a considerable number of instances; the positive predictive value is only 71%. This is because reactive inflammation, edema, fibrosis, and ectopic red bone marrow in the vicinity of the tumor may display diagnostic features similar to those of cartilage infiltrated by tumor (Fig. 4). Since inflammatory changes are most common in the thyroid cartilage, the specificity of MRI in detecting neoplastic invasion of the thyroid cartilage is only 56%, as opposed to 87% and 95% in the cricoid and arytenoid cartilages, respectively [1]. The positive diagnosis of neoplastic invasion of the thyroid cartilage should, therefore, be made with extreme caution at MRI.

TNM Classification of Laryngeal and Hypopharyngeal Carcinomas

Laryngeal and hypopharyngeal carcinomas are staged according to the criteria recommended by the International Union Against Cancer (UICC) or according those of the American Joint Cancer Committee (AJCC) [15]. The guidelines of both UICC and AJCC, which are now almost identical, recommend the use of cross-sectional imaging. Several studies as well as experience at my institution have shown that the use of CT or MRI greatly improves the accuracy of the pretherapeutic T classification of laryngeal and hypopharyngeal tumors. In our experience, the overall pretherapeutic staging accuracy is 80% with CT and 85% with MRI [6, 17].

Non-squamous Cell Laryngeal Neoplasms

Carcinomas with other histological traits different from the squamous cell type occur only occasionally in the laryngohypopharyngeal region [2]. *Adenocarcinoma* and *adenosquamous carcinoma* typically originate and extend beneath the mucosal surface. Therefore, these carcinomas are more difficult to detect with endoscopy than squamous cell carcinoma. Although none of the unusual types of carcinoma has any signal characteristics allowing its distinction from squamous cell carcinoma on CT or MRI, the discrepancy between the presence of a tumoral soft tissue mass on MRI and an intact mucosa at endoscopy should always raise the suspicion of a non-squamous neoplasm [2, 7]. In such cases, both CT and MRI serve not only to assess the degree of tumor spread, but also to direct the endoscopist to the appropriate site where to perform deep, aggressive biopsies necessary to establish the correct histologic diagnosis.

Laryngeal *chondrosarcoma* predominantly affects men in the sixth or seventh decade and more commonly originates from the cricoid than from the thyroid cartilage [2, 3, 16]. As in chondrogenic tumors of other locations, the tumor matrix has high signal intensity on T2-weighted images corresponding to hyaline cartilage with its low cellularity and high water content (Fig. 6). Small areas of low signal intensity correspond to stippled calcifications; these changes are, however, not as well demonstrated as

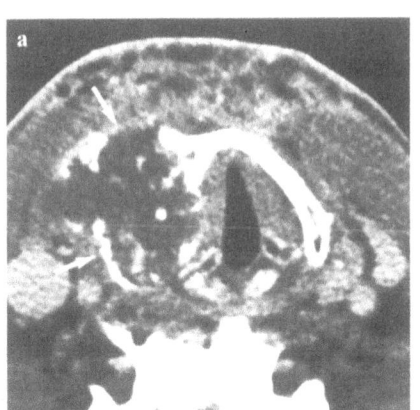
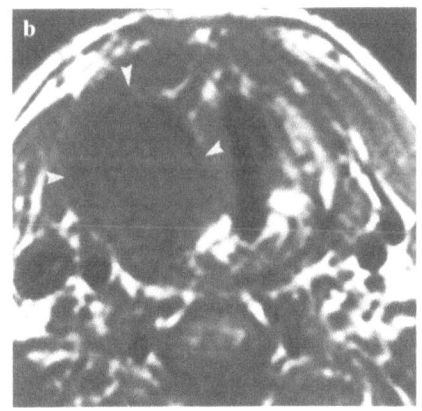
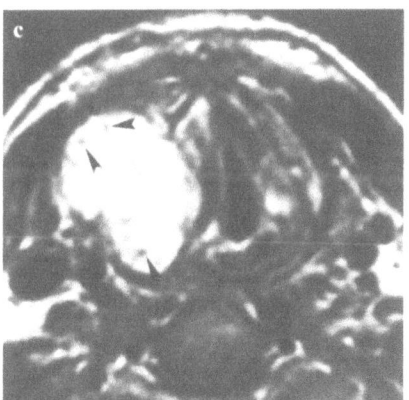
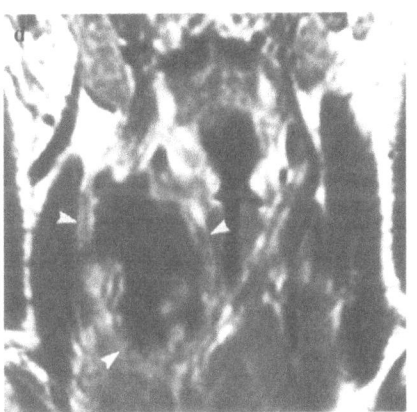

Fig. 6a-d. *CT and MRI appearances of chondrosarcoma of the thyroid cartilages in a 47-year-old man presenting with a hard lump in the neck.* **a** Axial contrast-enhanced CT scan shows a large, lobulated mass with coarse and stippled calcifications characteristic of chondrosarcoma (*arrows*). **b** T1-weighted axial MR image shows a lobulated mass with low signal intensity that arises from the right thyroid lamina (*arrowheads*). Note normal aspect of the left thyroid lamina. **c** T2-weighted FSE image. The tumor mass has high signal intensity due to high water content. The hypointense areas within the tumor correspond to intratumoral calcifications (*arrowheads*). **d** T1-weighted, contrast-enhanced, coronal image. Moderate peripheral enhancement (*arrowheads*). Note extramucosal tumor location. The patient underwent voice-preserving laryngeal resection and he is free of recurrence five years later. (*Panel a*, reproduced from [6] with permission; *panels b-d*, reproduced from [2] with permission)

with CT, where characteristic "popcorn" calcifications may be seen. Although the injection of gadolinium chelates may lead to a diffuse central or peripheral enhancement on T1-weighted images, these findings are non-specific and do not help in differentiating low-grade chondrosarcoma from benign chondroma [16]. Although the diagnosis of laryngeal chondrosarcoma can be strongly suspected on CT or MRI, it must be confirmed with deep biopsy. Surgery is regarded as the treatment of choice and is increasingly done in the form of function-preserving laryngeal resection. Imaging studies are important for follow-up after treatment, since chondrosarcoma has a tendency to recur locally.

Cysts and Laryngoceles

Laryngeal cysts arise from the mucosa and are related to minor salivary glands, whereas laryngoceles (also called saccular cysts) are dilatations of the saccule of the laryngeal ventricle. A laryngocele occurs when there is obstruction of the ventricle, sometimes by a small cancer located near the neck of the saccule. Laryngoceles may contain air or fluid. An internal laryngocele extends superiorly in the paralaryngeal space, and may present as a submucosal supraglottic mass at endoscopic evaluation. If the laryngocele extends through the thyrohyoid membrane into the soft tissues of the neck, it is called an external laryngocele. On CT or MRI, a laryngocele presents as a well-circumscribed, air- or fluid-filled structure extending from the laryngeal ventricle into the paralaryngeal space or through the thyrohyoid membrane into the soft tissues of the neck.

Vocal Cord Paralysis

Paralysis of the recurrent laryngeal nerve is the most common type of vocal cord paralysis. The CT and MRI features of recurrent laryngeal nerve paralysis are explained by atrophy of the thyroarytenoid muscle and include an enlarged ventricle, ipsilateral enlargement of the piriform sinus, and decreased size or fatty infiltration seen at the level of the true vocal cord. A patient with recurrent laryngeal nerve paralysis of unknown origin should undergo imaging of the entire pathway of the vagus and recurrent laryngeal nerves to exclude a tumor mass.

Inflammatory Lesions

Epiglottitis and croup are diagnosed clinically and do not require imaging. In the Western Hemisphere, the larynx is rarely affected by granulomatous diseases. Tuberculosis, numerous mycotic infections, leprosy and syphilis appear to be more common in Asia and Africa and may affect the larynx and pharynx. Relapsing polychondritis affects laryngeal cartilages,

and rheumatoid arthritis affects the cricoarytenoid and the cricothyroid joints.

Necrotizing fasciitis of the head and neck is a severe, acute, and potentially life-threatening bacterial soft tissue infection with a rapid clinical evolution [5]. It affects both immunocompetent and immunocompromised patients and, unless immediate surgical treatment is given, leads invariably to mediastinitis and fatal sepsis. CT and MRI findings include cellulitis, multiple fluid collections with or without gas in various neck compartments, diffuse enhancement of neck fasciae and myositis. The inflammatory, edematous process often involves the larynx, necessitating intubation. Myositis with or without abscess formation or myonecrosis is seen in the pharyngeal constrictor muscles. In the acute and subacute phases, CT and MRI may demonstrate contrast enhancement of the pharyngeal constrictor muscles or frank disruption of the pharyngeal wall.

Trauma

Trauma to the larynx can cause mucosal tears, submucosal hematomas, avulsion of the epiglottis, fractures of the laryngeal cartilages, and joint dislocation [3]. Both fractures and hematomas may lead to severe airway compromise. Fractures of the thyroid cartilage may be vertical or horizontal, or the entire thyroid cartilage may be shattered (Fig. 7). Fractures of the cricoid cartilage tend to occur bilaterally. Cricothyroid dislocations tend to occur with severe trauma, while cricoarytenoid dislocations tend to occur with minor trauma. Most patients with laryngeal trauma undergo CT, which allows excellent delineation of most traumatic lesions. However, MRI may provide significant additional information in young patients, in whom laryngeal cartilages are not ossified and therefore not well visualized on CT.

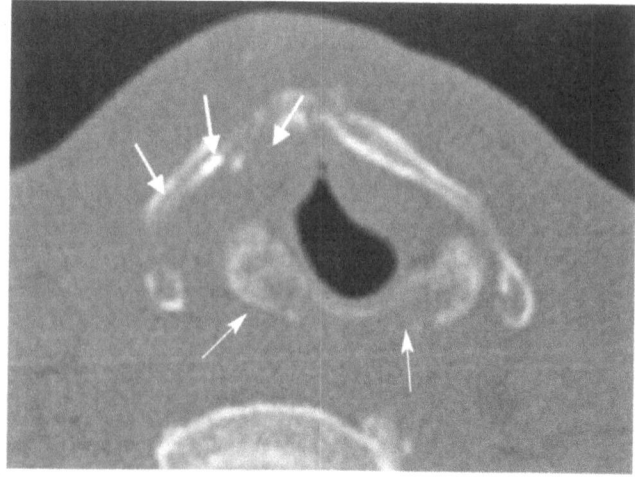

Fig. 7. Laryngeal trauma following motor vehicle accident. Comminutive fracture of the thyroid cartilage (*arrows*) and bilateral fracture of the cricoid cartilage (*thin arrows*)

Stenosis of the larynx or cervical trachea can be a sequela of trauma or prolonged intubation. MRI (axial, coronal and sagittal images) and CT with 2D reconstructions are useful in exactly defining the vertical extent of a stenosis.

References

1. Becker M, Zbären P, Laeng H et al (1995) Neoplastic invasion of the laryngeal cartilage: comparison of MRI and CT with histopathologic correlation. Radiology 194:661-669
2. Becker M, Moulin G, Kurt AM et al (1998) Non-squamous cell neoplasms of the larynx: radiologic-pathologic correlation. Radiographics 18(5):1189-1209
3. Becker M (2004) The larynx. In: Valvassouri G, Mafee M, Becker M (eds) Imaging of the head and neck. Thieme, New York Stuttgart, in press
4. Becker M, Zbären P, Delavelle J et al (1997) Neoplastic invasion of the laryngeal cartilage: reassessment of criteria for diagnosis at CT. Radiology 203:521-532
5. Becker M, Zbären P, Hermans R et al (1997) Necrotizing fasciitis of the head and neck: role of CT in diagnosis and management. Radiology 202:471-476
6. Becker M (1998) Larynx and hypopharynx. Radiol Clin N Am 36:891-920
7. Becker M (2001) Malignant lesions of the larynx and hypopharynx. In: Baert AL, Sartor K, Hermans R (eds) Imaging of the larynx. Springer, Berlin Heidelberg New York, pp 55-84
8. Becker M, Moulin G, Kurt AM et al (1998) Atypical squamous cell carcinoma of the larynx and hypopharynx: radiologic features and pathologic correlation. Eur Radiol 8:1541-1551
9. Castelijns JA, Gerritsen GJ, Kaiser MC et al (1988) Invasion of laryngeal cartilage by cancer: comparison of CT and MRI. Radiology 167:199-206
10. Castelijns JA, Becker M, Hermans R (1996) The impact of cartilage invasion on treatment and prognosis of laryngeal cancer. Eur Radiol 6:156-169
11. Castelijns JA, van den Brekel MWM, Tobi H et al (1996) Laryngeal carcinoma after radiation therapy: correlation of abnormal MRI signal patterns in laryngeal cartilage with the risk of recurrence. Radiology 198:151-155
12. Curtin HD (1996) The larynx. In: Som PM, Curtin HD (eds) Head and neck imaging, 3rd edn. Mosby, St. Louis, pp 612-707
13. Loevner LA, Yousem DM, Montone KT et al (1997) Can radiologists accurately predict preepiglottic space invasion with MRI? AJR Am J Roentgenol 169:1681-1687
14. Mancuso AA (1991) Evaluation and staging of laryngeal and hypopharyngeal cancer by computed tomography and magnetic resonance imaging. In: Silver CE (ed) Laryngeal cancer. Thieme, New York Stuttgart, pp 46-94
15. Sobin LH, Wittekind C (2002) TNM classification of malignant tumors, 6th edn. UICC, Wiley-Liss, New York
16. Stiglbauer R, Steurer M, Schimmerl S et al (1992) MRI of cartilaginous tumors of the larynx. Clin Radiol 46:23-27
17. Zbären P, Becker M, Laeng H (1996) Pretherapeutic staging of laryngeal cancer: clinical findings, computed tomography and magnetic resonance imaging versus histopathology. Cancer 77(7):1263-1273

Paranasal Sinuses and Nose: Normal Anatomy and Pathologic Processes

L.A. Loevner

Neuroradiology Division, Department of Radiology, University of Pennsylvania Medical Center, Philadelphia, PA, USA

Introduction

The development of the paranasal sinuses has been well described [1]. The maxillary sinuses are the first of the paranasal sinuses to develop; development begins in the first trimester of gestation and usually is completed by adolescence. The ethmoid air cells arise from numerous evaginations from the nasal cavity, beginning with the anterior air cells, and progressing to the posterior air cells. The ethmoid air cells begin to develop between the end of the first trimester and the mid-second trimester of gestation, and reach final adult proportions during puberty. The sphenoid sinus is present by the second trimester, and is fully developed in early adolescence. The frontal sinuses are the only sinuses consistently absent at birth. Their development is variable: it begins during the first few years of life and completes in adolescence.

The paranasal sinuses and nasal cavity are lined by ciliated columnar epithelium that also has mucinous and serous glands. The common drainage pathway for the frontal sinuses, maxillary sinuses, and anterior ethmoid air cells is through the paired ostiomeatal complex made up of the maxillary sinus ostium, the infundibulum, the hiatus semilunaris, and the middle meatus [2]. Secretions within the maxillary sinuses circulate towards the maxillary sinus ostium propelled by ciliated epithelium. From the maxillary ostium, mucous circulates through the infundibulum located lateral to the uncinate process (an osseous extension of the lateral nasal wall). From the infundibulum, secretions progress through the hiatus semilunaris, an air-filled channel anterior and inferior to the ethmoidal bulla (the largest ethmoid air cell), and then pass into the middle meatus, the nasal cavity, and the nasopharynx where they are swallowed.

The frontal sinuses drain inferiorly through the frontal ethmoidal recess (the channel between the inferomedial frontal sinus and the anterior part of the middle meatus) into the middle meatus (the common drainage site also for the anterior ethmoid air cells that have ostia in contact with the infundibulum of the ostiomeatal complex)

[2]. The anterior-most ethmoid air cells, the agger nasi cells, are located in front of the middle turbinates, which are in turn located anterior, lateral, and inferior to the frontal ethmoidal recess. Inconstant ethmoid air cells located along the anterosuperior maxillary surface just inferior to the orbital floor are called maxilloethmoidal or Haller cells.

The posterior ethmoid air cells are located behind the middle turbinate; secretions drain through the superior and supreme meatus, and through other tiny ostia under the superior turbinate into the sphenoethmoidal recess, the nasal cavity and finally the nasopharynx. Secretions in the sphenoid sinus are propelled by cilia to the ostia of this sinus that is located above the sinus floor.

The three sets of turbinates in the nasal cavity include the superior, middle, and inferior turbinates. Occasionally there may be a supreme turbinate located above the superior turbinate. When the middle turbinate is aerated, it is termed a concha bullosa, present in up to 30%-50% of patients. Large or opacified conchae bullosa may obstruct the ostiomeatal complex.

The nasal septum separates the right and left nasal turbinates, dividing the nasal cavity in half. The anterior and inferior aspects of the nasal septum are made of cartilage. The posterior portion of the nasal septum is osseous. The superoposterior portion is the perpendicular plate of the ethmoid bone, while the inferoposterior portion is the vomer. The nasal septum is lined by squamous epithelium, while the remainder of the nasal cavity is lined by columnar epithelium. There is normal cyclical passive congestion and decongestion of each side of the nasal cavity and ethmoid air cells that result in temporary mucosal thickening in these structures [2]. The nasolacrimal duct extends from the lacrimal sac at the medial canthus along the anterior and lateral nasal walls, and drains into the inferior meatus.

Blood supply to the sinonasal structures comes from both the internal and external carotid arteries. The arterial supply to the frontal sinuses is from supraorbital and supratrochlear branches of the ophthalmic artery, while venous drainage is through the superior ophthalmic veins. The ethmoid air cells and sphenoid sinus receive blood from branches of the sphenopalatine artery (arising from the external carotid circulation) as well as from the ethmoidal branches of the ophthalmic artery (arising from the internal carotid circulation). Venous drainage is through nasal veins into the nasal cavity, or through ethmoidal veins that drain into ophthalmic veins, which subsequently drain into the cavernous sinus. The maxillary sinuses are supplied predominantly by branches of the maxillary artery from the external carotid circulation, and drain through facial and maxillary veins, the latter communicating with the pterygoid venous plexus. It is the venous drainage of the paranasal sinuses (ultimately communicating with the cavernous sinus and pterygoid venous plexus) that is responsible for the potential intracranial complications of sinusitis including meningitis, subdural empyema, and cavernous sinus thrombosis.

Disease Processes of the Paranasal Sinuses

Congenital Lesions

Many congenital abnormalities of the nasal cavity and skull base are related to aberrant invagination of the neural plate [3]. During neural plate retraction in embryogenesis, the dura contacts the dermis. Normally this dermal connection regresses; when it does not congenital abnormalities that may develop include sinus tracts, dermoid cysts, encephaloceles (Fig. 1), and nasal gliomas [3, 4]. With nasal gliomas (not true neoplasms), there is a fibrous connection with the intracranial compartment.

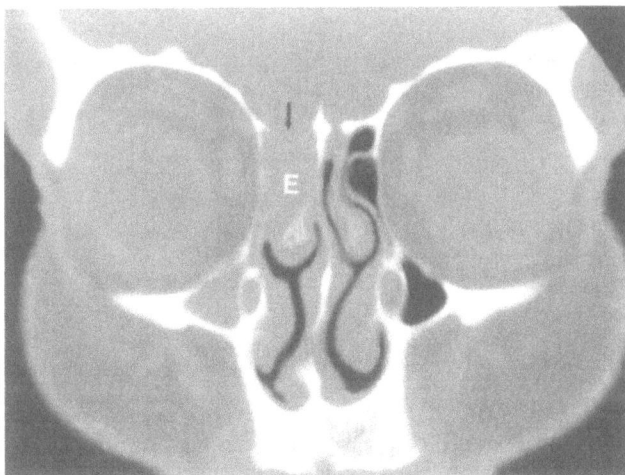

Fig. 1. A 47-year-old patient with recurrent right nasal drainage. Coronal CT image shows a defect in the right cribriform plate (*arrow*). Soft tissue (*E*) in the adjacent right sinonasal cavity represents an encephalocele

Inflammatory Disease and Sinusitis

Most cases of acute sinusitis are related to an antecedent viral upper respiratory tract infection. Swelling of the mucosal surfaces within the paranasal sinuses results in apposition, leading to obstruction of the normal drainage pathways and inadequate drainage that results in bacterial overgrowth.

When evaluating patients for sinusitis and potential fundoscopic sinus surgery (FESS), it is important to evaluate certain anatomical landmarks. Specifically, the medial orbital walls, cribiform plate, and roof and lateral walls of the sphenoid sinus should be evaluated for osseous defects or thinning. A defect in the lamina papyracea may result in orbital penetration and subsequent hematoma formation or optic nerve injury, whereas a dehiscence in the cribiform plate or sphenoid sinus can result in meningitis, encephalocele (Fig. 2), or carotid artery complications (perforation, pseudoaneurysm). It is important to comment on mucosal apposition or inflammatory changes in the region of the ostiomeatal unit and the sphenoethmoidal recess. The presence of air-fluid levels should be noted. Hyperdense secretions on computed tomography (CT) may suggest the presence of inspissated secretions or fungal disease [5].

Sinonasal secretions have variable signal intensity patterns on magnetic resonance imaging (MRI) related to the protein concentration and mobile water protons within the secretions [6]. The changes in signal intensity are likely due to extensive cross-linking of glycoproteins present within hyperproteinaceous secretions. As a result, the amount of mobile water protons decreases. When the protein concentration is less than 10%, secretions are hypointense on T1-weighted images and hyperintense on T2-weighted images (this is the state in which there is a high concentration of free mobile water). When protein concentrations approach 20%-25%, they typically are hyperintense on both unenhanced T1-weighted (Fig. 3b) and T2-weighted sequences. When protein concentrations exceed approximately 25%, they are typically hypointense on T2-weighted images, and when they exceed 28%, they are hypointense on both T1-weighted and T2-weighted sequences.

Complications of sinusitis include periorbital cellulitis, meningitis, thrombophlebitis (including cavernous sinus thrombosis), subdural empyema, brain abscess, and perineural and perivascular spread of infection (in particular in invasive fungal disease). Infectious "mycotic" aneurysms of the intracranial vasculature are uncommon, accounting for less than 5% of intracranial aneurysms. The causative organism is usually bacterial, although these lesions may occur as a complication of invasive sinonasal fungal infection [7]. Mucoceles may be a complication of sinusitis and are most common in the frontal sinuses and ethmoid air cells. Mucoceles show a spectrum of signal characteristics on MRI that are dependent on their pro-

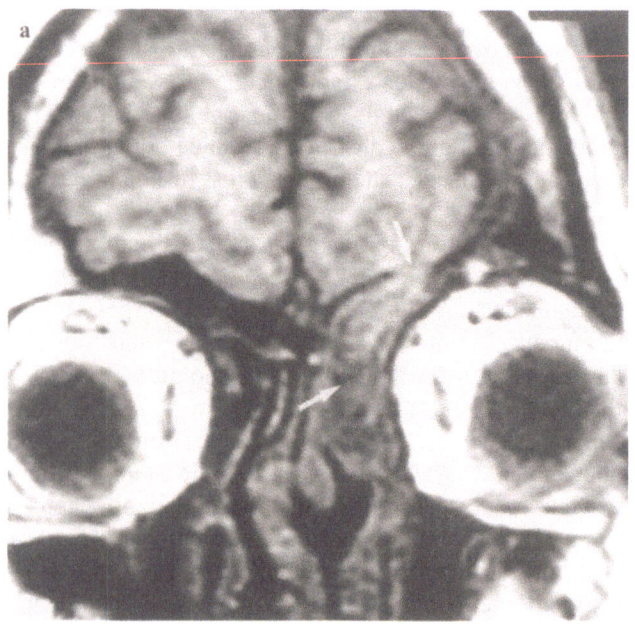

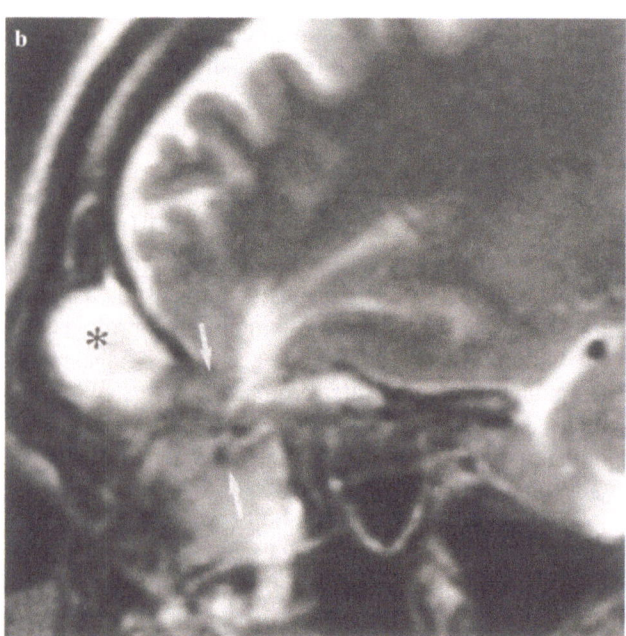

Fig. 2a, b. *A 41-year-old man with encephalocele complicating functional endoscopic sinonasal surgery.* **a** Unenhanced coronal T1-weighted MR image shows an osseous defect in the left frontal sinus and floor of the anterior cranial fossa with an encephalocele (*arrows*) extending into the adjacent sinonasal cavity. **b** Sagittal T2-weighted MR image shows the large defect in the floor of the anterior cranial fossa with the encephalocele (*arrows*). There are secretions and fluid in the frontal sinus (*)

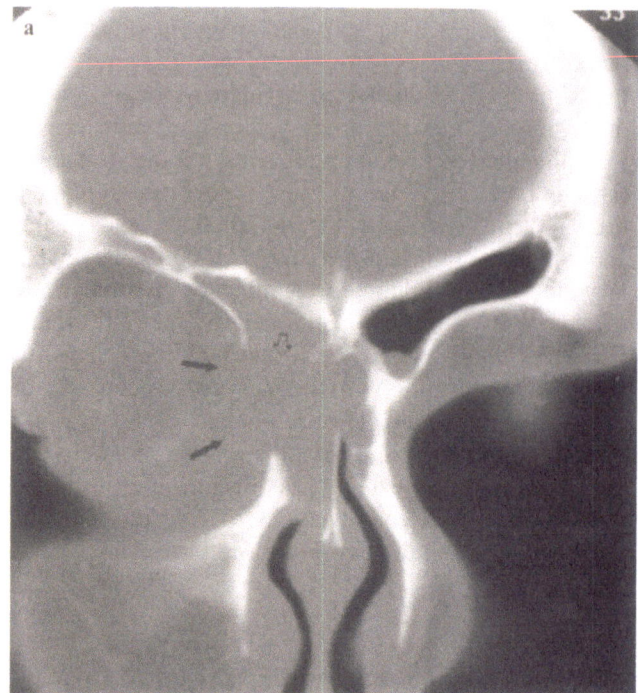

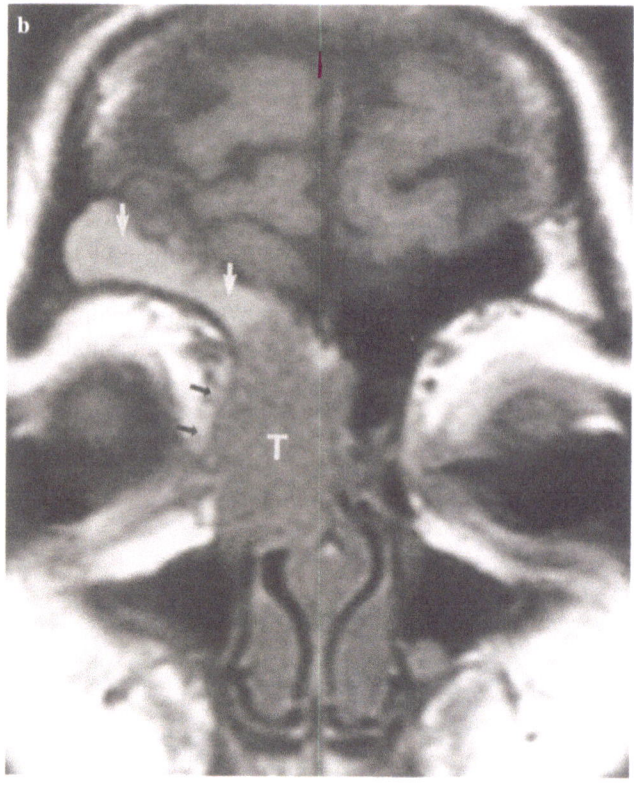

Fig. 3a, b. *A 33-year-old man with squamous cell carcinoma of the sinonasal cavity and orbital extension.* **a** Coronal CT image shows osseous destruction of the superolateral nasal wall and marked thinning and medial bowing of the medial right orbital wall (*arrows*). There is also absence of the bone comprising the floor of the right frontal sinus (*open arrow*). **b** Unenhanced coronal T1-weighted MR image shows tumor (*T*) in the right sinonasal cavity (isointense to brain), hyperintense proteinaceous secretions (*white arrows*) in the right frontal sinus, and soft tissue stranding (*black arrows*) in the extraconal fat in the medial right orbit

tein content, and usually demonstrate rim enhancement compared to tumors that typically show more solid enhancement (Fig. 4) [8-11].

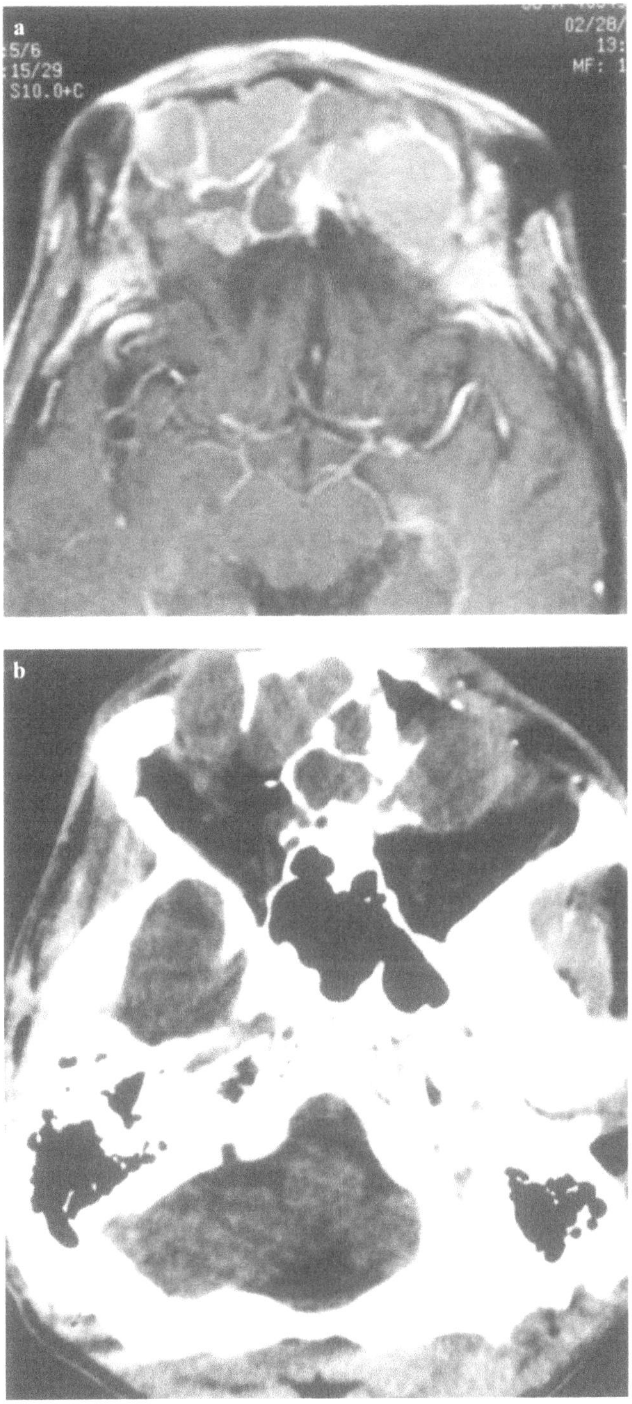

Sinonasal Neoplasms

CT and MRI play complementary roles in evaluating sinonasal tumors. CT provides bone detail, while MRI provides superior soft tissue resolution. MRI is better in evaluating intracranial extension of neoplastic processes. Another advantage of MRI over CT is its ability to help discern complex sinonasal secretions and inflammatory disease from malignancy [8-11].

Typically, benign lesions such as mucoceles and benign neoplasms when large enough expand the paranasal sinus that they are in and remodel the adjacent bone on CT (Fig. 4b). Occasionally, malignant tumors have benign imaging features. The contrary is also true, i.e. benign tumors may appear to be relatively aggressive [12-14]. Caution is always required when evaluating masses within the sinuses. Fibro-osseous lesions that involve the paranasal sinuses include osteomas (Fig. 5), fibrous dysplasia, ossifying or nonossifying fibromas, and chondroid lesions. These can be difficult to diagnose on MRI as the abnormal osseous structures may appear hypointense like "air" (Fig. 6), but fibro-osseous lesions frequently have characteristic sclerotic appearances on CT (Fig. 5) [15].

Fig. 4a, b. *A 38-year-old man with extensive mucoceles complicating prior facial trauma.* **a** Enhanced axial T1-weighted MR image shows multiple, expansile, rim-enhancing mucoceles in the frontal sinuses. The wide spectrum of T1-weighted signal intensities is due to differing protein concentrations. **b** Corresponding unenhanced axial CT image shows multiple expansile lesions in the frontal sinuses with associated long-standing osseous remodeling and expansion

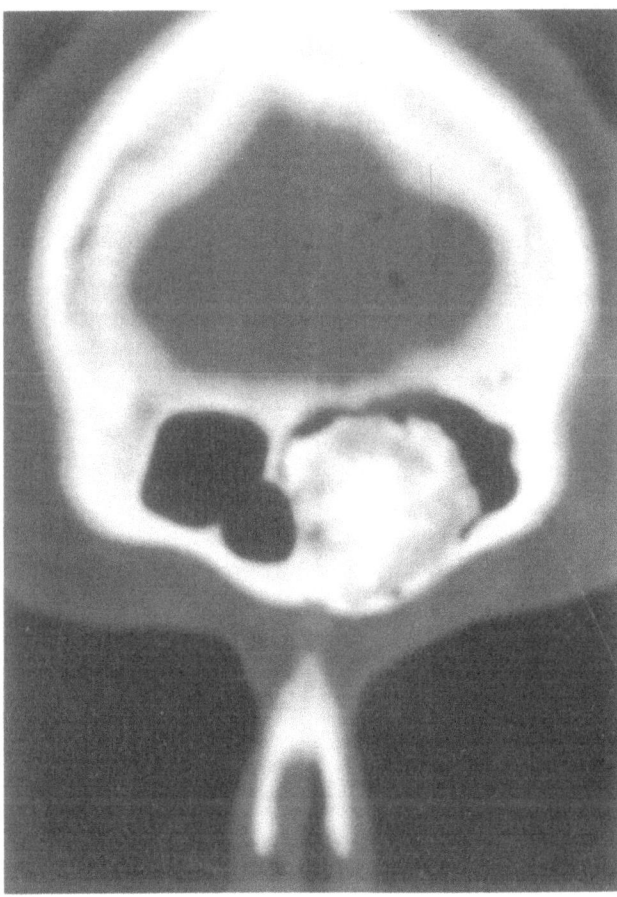

Fig. 5. Coronal CT image of bone detail shows a characteristic osteoma of the left frontal sinus. The benign neoplasm of osseous origin is intrasinus with heterogenous fibrous and sclerotic bone matrix

Most neoplasms may be distinguished from inflammatory conditions due to their imaging characteristics as well as their more solid enhancement pattern (compared to rim enhancement in benign inflammatory disease). In addition, T2-weighted images may be helpful as most malignancies are heterogeneous and intermediate in signal intensity compared to inflammatory secretions that tend to be hyperintense and more homogeneous in character [8].

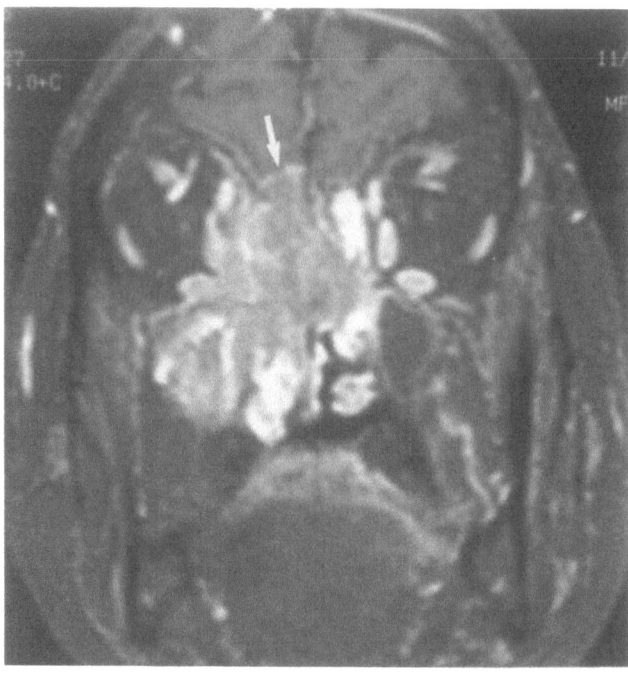

Fig. 7. Squamous cell carcinoma of the paranasal sinuses. Intracranial extension through the floor of the anterior cranial fossa (*arrow*) and right medial intraorbital extension are shown on this fat-suppressed coronal T1-weighted MR image

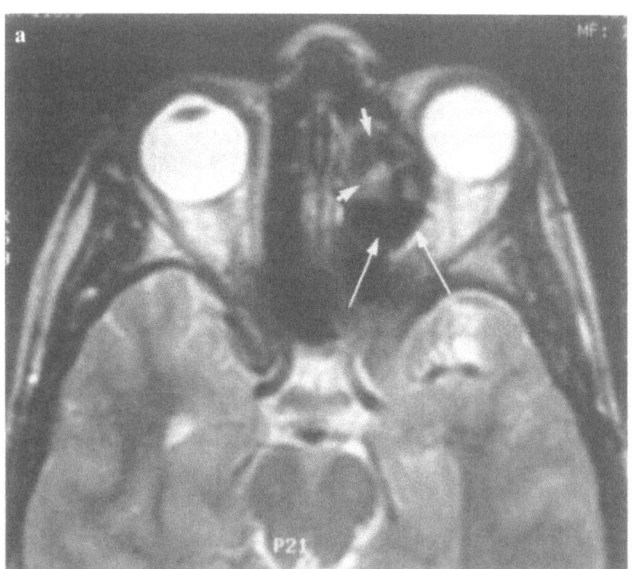

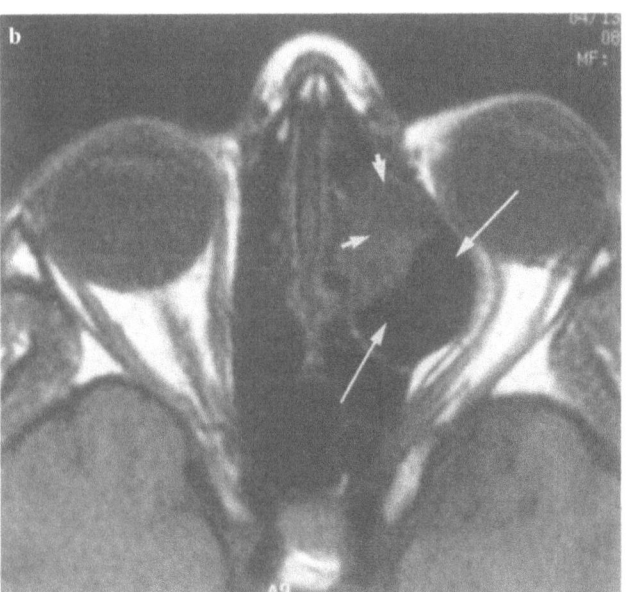

Fig. 6a, b. *Nonossifying fibroma of the left ethmoid air cells.* **a** Axial T2-weighted MR image shows intermediate signal intensity of the ventral portion of the mass (*short arrows*), and hypointensity of the posterior portion of the mass mimicking "air" (*long arrows*). **b** Unenhanced axial T1-weighted image shows expansile mass of the left ethmoid. The ventral portion is isointense to muscle (*short arrows*). The posterior portion is markedly hypointense (isointense to air in the adjacent paranasal sinuses, *long arrows*), consistent with sclerotic bone. There is lateral bowing of the medial orbital wall with lateral displacement of the adjacent medial rectus muscle and optic nerve

In most instances, excellent anatomic resolution may be acquired from an unenhanced and enhanced MRI examination performed with a standard head coil. Imaging of sinonasal malignancies must include high-resolution views not only of the sinonasal cavity, but also of the orbit, skull base, and intracranial compartment (Figs. 3, 7) [11, 16]. Direct extension or perineural spread of tumor may allow for tumor extension outside the sinonasal cavity and into these important adjacent anatomic locations, which significantly impacts upon the patient's staging and operability, the type of resection that will occur, and the necessity for radiation therapy (Tables 1, 2). An especially important anatomic location for detection of tumor spread is the pterygopalatine fossa. When tumor spreads to the pterygopalatine fossa, extension to the adjacent orbit, infratemporal fossa (masticator space), skull base, and intracranial compartment may subsequently occur. Specifically, tumor may spread from the pterygopalatine fossa to the pterygomaxillary fissure, allowing subsequent growth into the infratemporal compartment. From the pterygopalatine fossa, tumor may extend to

Table 1. Criteria for nonresectability of sinonasal malignancies. Depending upon the institution, cavernous sinus and optic chiasm invasion are relative contraindications for surgery

Distance metastases
Invasion of the optic chiasm
Extensive cerebral involvement
Bilateral cavernous sinus or carotid infiltration
Poor general medical conditions

Table 2. T system for staging sinonasal malignancies, according to the American Joint Committee on Cancer (Adapted from [22])

T1	Neoplasm confined to anthral mucosa without associated osseous erosion or destruction
T2	Neoplasm with erosion or destruction of the osseous infrastructure, including the hard palate or middle nasal mediatus
T3	Tumor extension to the anterior ethmoid air cells or posterior wall of the maxillary sinus, or tumor invasion outside of the sinonasal cavity to involve the skin of the cheek or floor or medial wall of the orbit
T4	Tumor extension to the posterior ethmoid air cells, sphenoid sinus, pterygoid plates, nasopharynx, base of skull or cribiform plate, or tumor involving the contents within the orbit

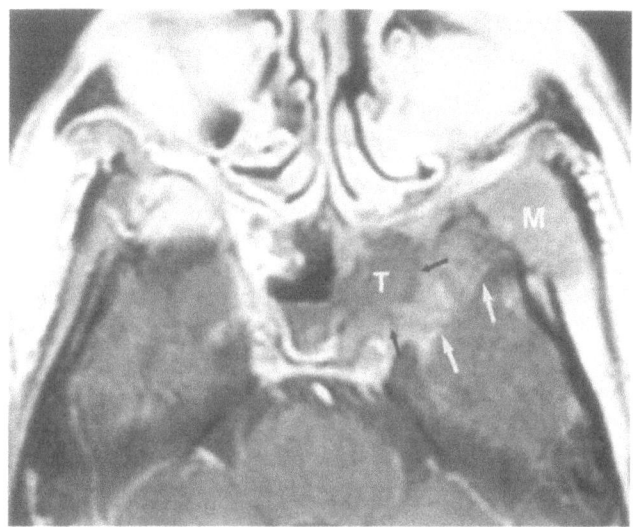

Fig. 8. A 53-year-old man with post-transplantation lymphoproliferative disorder (non-Hodgkin's lymphoma) complicating lung transplantation 8 years previously. The patient presented with multiple acute cranial nerve palsies. Enhanced axial T1-weighted MR image shows fluid in the right sphenoid sinus, tumor (*T*) in the left sphenoid sinus with disruption of the left lateral sphenoid sinus wall (*black arrows*), and abnormal enhancing tissue (lymphoma) in the left middle cranial fossa (*white arrows*) and in the infratemporal fossa and masticator spaces (*M*)

the vidian canal, and from here to foramen lacerum, and then into the intracranial compartment. In addition, tumor may spread from the pterygopalatine fossa to the foramen rotundum, and in such cases patients may present with a fifth cranial nerve neuropathy. From the foramen rotundum, tumor may spread in a perineural fashion to the inferior orbital fissure, and into the orbit or ventral cavernous sinus.

Papillomas arise from columnar epithelium and include three common subtypes: inverted, cylindric, and fungiform [12]. Papillomas tend to occur unilaterally in the sinonasal cavity. The most common papilloma is the inverted papilloma. These are more common in men in the fourth through sixth decades of life. This is a benign neoplasm; however, squamous carcinoma may be present within these in up to 20% of cases. Inverted papillomas may have an aggressive appearance with bone destruction, and occasionally they may erode the skull base (as may benign polyps), simulating an aggressive cancer [13, 14]. This neoplasm typically arises from the lateral nasal wall at the level of the middle turbinate, or less commonly, within the maxillary sinus [12, 13].

Squamous cell carcinoma is the most common malignancy of the paranasal sinuses and nasal cavity, representing two-thirds of all cancers here [11, 12, 17]. Occupational exposures to radium, Thorotrast, and nickel are causative factors. The majority arise in the maxillary sinus anthrum [17], while the next most common site is the septum in the nasal cavity. Adenocarcinomas, lymphoma, undifferentiated carcinomas, esthesioneuroblastomas [18], and sarcomas may also occur in the sinonasal cavity. Following squamous cell carcinoma, minor salivary gland tumors [19] and melanomas [20] (arising from melanocyte rests in the mucosa) are the next most common malignancies to affect the nasal cavity. Minor salivary gland tumors represent a wide spectrum of histologic subtypes including adenoid cystic carcinoma (most common), mucoepidermoid carcinoma, and acinic cell carcinomas [11, 19]. Uncommon, but likely to be recognized more frequently as patients live longer, is post-transplantation lymphoproliferative disorder of the paranasal sinuses, seen in the setting of chronic immunosuppression following organ transplantantation [21]. This is usually aggressive (lymphoma), and may mimic invasive fungal sinusitis (Fig. 8). Treatment is usually a combination of irradiation and chemotherapy. Metastatic disease to the sinuses is unusual, with renal cell carcinoma the most commonly reported.

References

1. Schaeffer JP (1920) The embryology, development and anatomy of the nose, paranasal sinuses, nasolacrimal passageways and olfactory organs in man. Blakiston's Son, Philadelphia
2. Zinreich SJ, Kennedy DW, Kuman AJ et al (1988) MR imaging of normal nasal cycle: comparison with sinus pathology. J Comput Assist Tomogr 12:1014-1019
3. Barkovich AJ, Vandermarch P, Edwards MSB et al (1991) Congenital nasal masses: CT and MR imaging features in 16 cases. AJNR Am J Neuradiol 12:105-116
4. Kallman JE, Loevner LA, Yousem DM, Chalian AA, Lanza DC, Jin L, Hayden RE (1996) Heterotopic brain in the pterygopalatine fossa. AJNR Am J Neuroradiol 18:176-179
5. Babbel RW, Harnsberger HR, Sonkens J et al (1992) Recurring patterns of inflammatory sinonasal disease demonstrated on screening sinus CT. AJNR Am J Neuroradiol 13:903-912
6. Dillon KB, Som PM, Fullerton GD (1990) Hypointense MR signal in chronically inspissated sinonasal secretions. Radiology 174:73-78
7. Hurst RW, Judkins A, Bolger W, Chu A, Loevner LA (2001) Mycotic aneurysm and cerebral infarction resulting from fungal sinusitis: imaging and pathologic correlation. AJNR Am J Neuroradiol 22:858-863
8. Som PM, Shapiro MD, Biller HF et al (1988) Sinonasal tumors and inflammatory tissues: differentiation with MR. Radiology 167:803-808
9. Lanzieri CF, Shah M, Krauss D et al (1991) Use of gadolinium-enhanced MR imaging for differentiating mucoceles from neoplasms in the paranasal sinuses. Radiology 178:425-428

10. Loevner LA, Yousem DM, Lanza DC, Kennedy DW, Goldberg A (1995) MR evaluation of frontal osteoplastic flaps using autogenous fat grafts to obliterate the sinus. AJNR Am J Neuroradiol 16:1721-1726
11. Loevner LA, Sonners AI (2002) Imaging of neoplasms of the paranasal sinuses. Magn Reson Imaging Clin N Am 10:467-493
12. Lasser A, Rothfeld PR, Shapiro RS (1976) Epithelial papilloma and squamous cell carcinoma of the nasal cavity and paranasal sinuses: a clinicopathologic study. Cancer 38:2503-2510
13. Woodruff WW, Vrabec DP (1994) Inverted papilloma of the nasal vault and paranasal sinuses: spectrum of CT findings. AJR Am J Roentgenol 162:419-423
14. Som PM, Lawson W, Lidov MW (1991) Simulated aggressive skull base erosion in response to benign sinonasal disease. Radiology 180:755-759
15. Tobey JD, Loevner LA, Yousem DM, Lanza DC (1996) Tension pneumocephalus: a complication of invasive ossifying fibroma of the paranasal sinuses. AJR Am J Roentgenol 166:711-713
16. Eisen MD, Yousem DM, Loevner LA, Thaler ER, Bilkner WB,

Goldberg AN (2000) Preoperative imaging to predict orbital invasion by tumor. Head Neck Surg 22:456-462
17. St. Pierre S, Baker SR (1983) Squamous cell carcinoma of the maxillary sinus: analysis of 66 cases. Head Neck Surg 5:508-513
18. Som PM, Lidov M, Brandwein M et al (1994) Sinonasal esthesioneuroblastoma with intracranial extension: marginal tumor cysts as a diagnostic MR finding. AJNR Am J Neuroradiol 15:1259-1262
19. Sigal R, Monnet O, de Baere T et al (1992) Adenoid cystic carcinoma of the head and neck: evaluation with MR imaging and clinical-pathologic correlation in 27 patients. Radiology 184:95-101
20. Yousem DM, Li C, Montone KT, Montgomery L, Loevner LA, Rao V et al (1996) Primary malignant melanoma of the sinonasal cavity: MR evaluation. Radiographics 16:1101-1110
21. Gordon AR, Loevner LA, Sonners AI, Bolger WE, Wasik MA (2002) Posttransplantation lymphoproliferative disorder of the paranasal sinuses mimicking invasive fungal sinusitis. AJNR Am J Neuroradiol 23:855-857
22. American Joint Committee on Cancer (1997) Manual for staging of cancer, 4th edn. Lippincott, Philadelphia

Nose, Paranasal Sinuses and Adjacent Spaces

R. Maroldi[1], D. Farina[1], P. Nicolai[2]

[1] Department of Radiology, University of Brescia, Brescia, Italy
[2] Department of Otorhinolaryngology, University of Brescia, Brescia, Italy

Introduction

Cross-sectional imaging has achieved an essential role in the diagnosis and treatment planning of both inflammatory and neoplastic diseases of the sinonasal tract. Particularly, the development of endonasal surgery techniques during the last two decades has been possible as a result of the detailed preoperative assessment of the extent of lesions and of the individual anatomy of the nose and paranasal sinuses, usually by computed tomography (CT). With multislice CT, reliable information in the sagittal plane is obtained, making the assessment of key structures, such as the frontal recess, more feasible.

External surgical approaches still have a role in the management of selected cases of inflammatory diseases and benign tumors, and are considered the gold standard for malignant tumors. In this setting, magnetic resonance imaging (MRI) maintains a primary role, as its superior contrast resolution enables clinicians to more clearly differentiate normal tissues and structures from adjacent lesions. Improvements in both time and spatial resolutions of the new MRI equipment help minimize the rate of non-diagnostic examinations, and enable an accurate demonstration even of the thin and complex anatomic structures of the sinonasal area. Therefore, MRI is generally used to obtain a precise pretreatment assessment of intraorbital or intracranial invasion.

Nowadays, a multidisciplinary approach to the complex variety of sinonasal lesions is considered the best strategy to a successful management of these diseases. Consequently, thorough knowledge of the essential information for planning endonasal and external approaches is necessary.

Essential Anatomy of the Sinonasal Area

Three anatomic areas, corresponding to the narrowest tracts of drainage pathways, are crucial for endoscopic surgery planning: the ostiomeatal complex, the frontal recess, and the spheno-ethmoid recess.

The *ostiomeatal complex* is the crossroads of anterior ethmoid, frontal sinus and maxillary sinus mucus drainage. It includes the maxillary sinus ostium, the ethmoid infundibulum, the ethmoid bulla and the uncinate process. The ethmoid infundibulum is the air passage connecting the maxillary sinus ostium to the middle meatus. It is bordered superiorly by the ethmoid bulla, the most posterior cell within the anterior ethmoid, protruding in the middle meatus. The vertical portion of the uncinate process is a key structure of the ostiomeatal complex (Figs. 1-4).

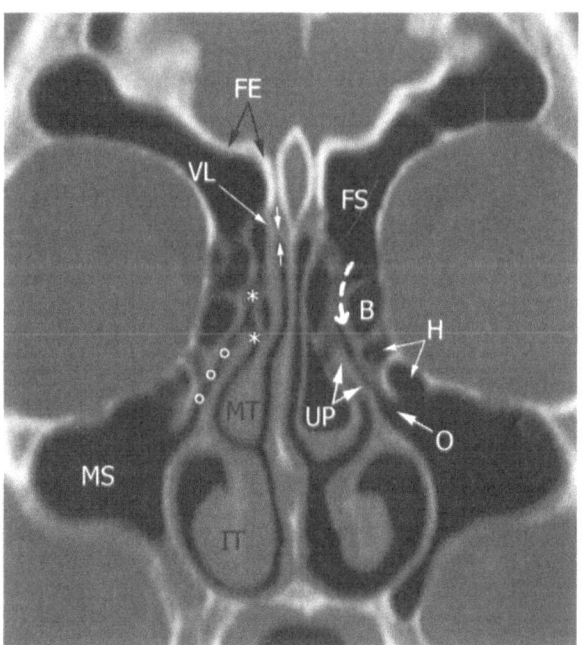

Fig. 1. Multislice CT with coronal multiplanar reconstruction shows key structures of the ostiomeatal complex. The ethmoid bulla (*B*) faces the uncinate process (*UP*), and borders the ethmoidal infundibulum (*small circles*). Both the ethmoidal infundibulum and the frontal recess (*interrupted arrows*) empty into the middle meatus (*asterisks*). The thin horizontal (*small opposite arrows*) and vertical (*VL*) cribriform plates appear less dense than the thicker orbital plate of the frontal bone. *FE*, fovea ethmoidalis; *MS*, maxillary sinus; *FS*, frontal sinus; *O*, maxillary sinus ostium; *MT*, middle turbinate; *IT*, inferior turbinate; *H*, inferior orbital "Haller" cells

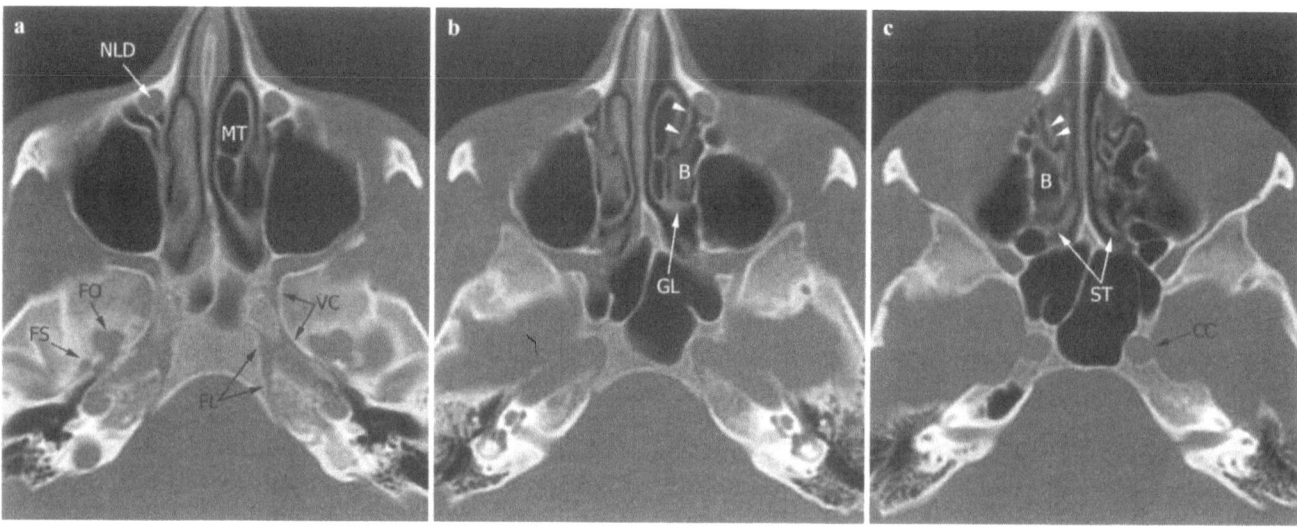

Fig. 2a-c. *Multislice CT in axial plane.* **a** The plane crosses the skull base at the level of the body of the sphenoid bone. The vidian canal (*VC*), foramen ovale (*FO*), spinosum (*FS*), lacerum (*FL*), and nasolacrimal duct (*NLD*) are shown. Large pneumatized middle turbinate (*MT*) on left side. **b** Anterior attachment of the uncinate process onto the nasolacrimal duct wall is demonstrated. The ethmoidal infundibulum empties between the uncinate process (*arrowheads*) and the ethmoid bulla (*B*). Lateral attachment of the middle turbinate (ground lamella, *GL*) marks the limit between anterior and posterior ethmoidal sinuses. **c** A few millimeters above, the bulla appears larger. Part of the superior turbinate (*ST*) is shown. *CC*, carotid canal

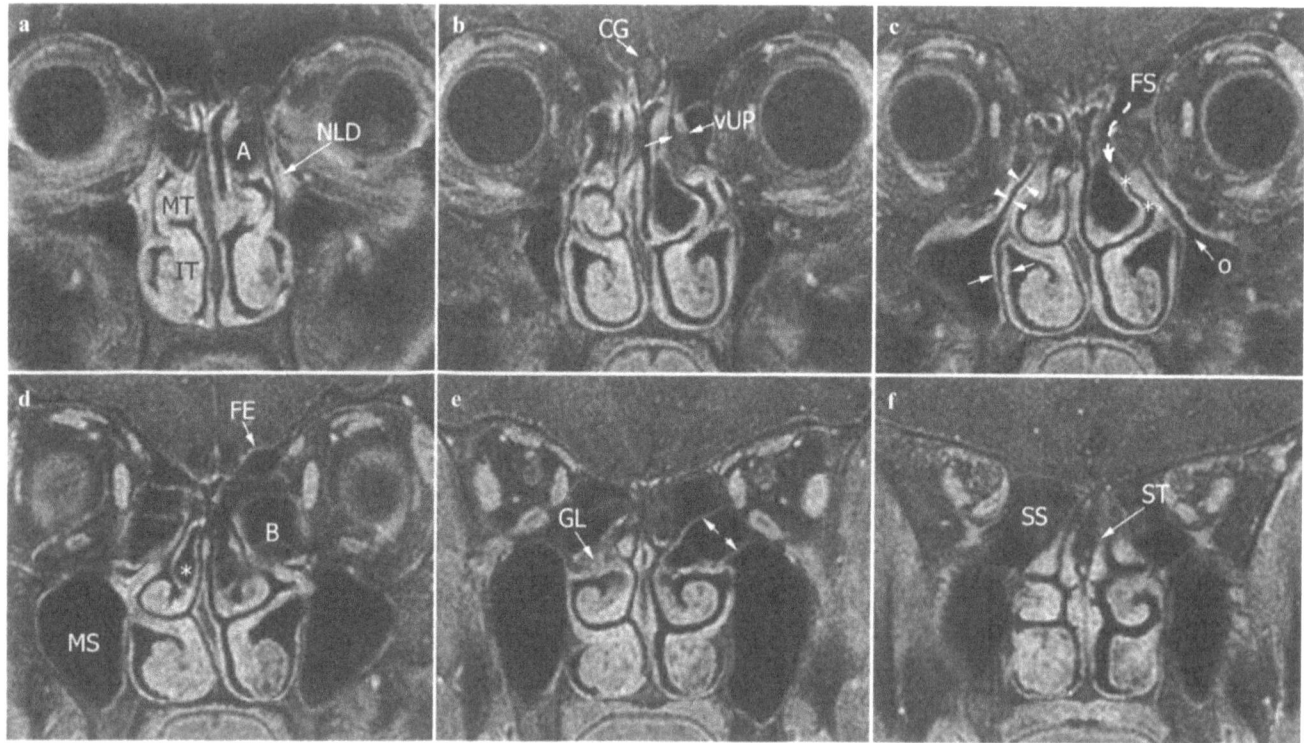

Fig. 3a-f. *Three-dimensional gradient echo enhanced (VIBE) sequence in the coronal plane, 0.5-mm sections.* **a** The most anterior ethmoidal cell is the agger nasi cell (*A*), medially bordered by the pneumatized vertical lamella of the middle turbinate. **b** The vertical portion of the uncinate process (*vUP*) attaches superiorly at the fovea ethmoidalis. **c** Ethmoidal infundibulum (*opposite arrowheads*) and frontal recess (*interrupted arrow*) empty into the middle meatus (*asterisks*). *Opposite arrows* point to the sandwich-like appearance of the "nasal mucosa-medial maxillary wall-maxillary sinus mucosa" complex. **d** A large ethmoid bulla (*B*) on left side, a pneumatized vertical lamella of the middle turbinate on right side; lamellar concha (*asterisk*). **e** Posterior to the ethmoid bulla, the retrobullar space is seen on the left (*arrows*); attachment of the ground lamella (*GL*) on the right. **f** Right sphenoid sinus (*SS*) and superior turbinates (*ST*) are detected. *IT*, inferior turbinate; *MT*, middle turbinate; *NLD*, nasolacrimal duct; *CG*, crista galli; *FS*, frontal sinus; *o*, maxillary sinus ostium; *MS*, maxillary sinus; *FE*, fovea ethmoidalis

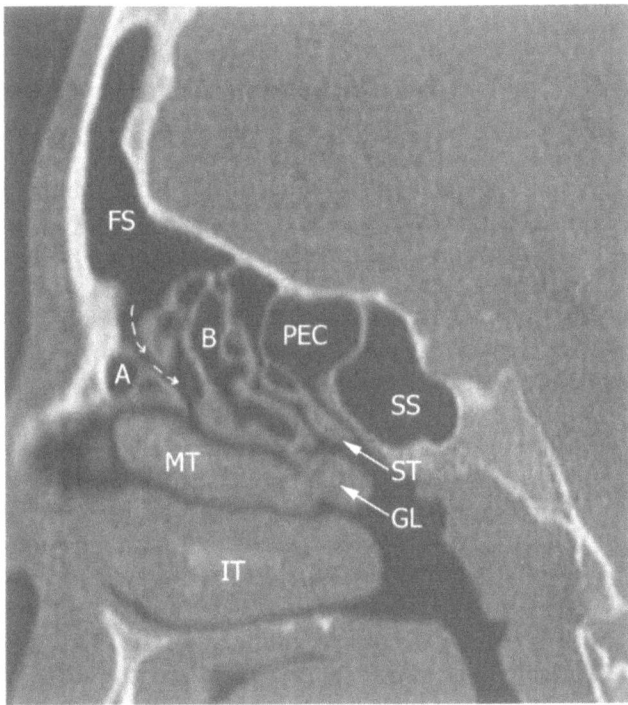

Fig. 4. Multislice CT in sagittal plane through the frontal recess (*interrupted arrow*) passing posteriorly to the agger nasi (*A*) and anteriorly to the anterior ethmoidal cells, the ethmoid bulla (*B*) being the largest. Posterior ethmoidal cells (*PEC*) are located behind the ground lamella (*GL*) of the middle turbinate (*MT*). *IT*, inferior turbinate; *ST*, superior turbinate; *FS*, frontal sinus; *SS*, sphenoid sinus

Depending on the type of its superior attachment, the *frontal recess* (i.e. the mucus drainage path of the frontal sinus) may open into the middle meatus medially or into the uncinate process laterally [1]. Correct assessment of the frontal recess opening is essential in planning the proper endonasal approach to the frontal recess and the adequate exposure of the frontal sinus. Medially, the middle turbinate borders the ostiomeatal complex; its vertical lamina is anchored on the cribriform plate while its ground lamella inserts laterally onto the posterior part of lamina papyracea.

The *spheno-ethmoid recess* is outlined by the anterior sphenoid sinus wall and by the posterior wall of posterior ethmoid cells. It conveys sphenoid sinus secretions in the superior meatus; it is more clearly shown on axial CT images.

Several variants of sinonasal anatomic structures may be observed. Most of them are due to the variable extent of ethmoid sinus pneumatization into adjacent sinuses – infra-orbital ethmoidal cells, frontal cells and Onodi cells derive, respectively, from pneumatization of maxillary, sphenoid and frontal sinuses. Other anatomic variants are created by pneumatization of bones adjacent to the ethmoid as the agger nasi cells from lacrimal bone and the supraorbital ethmoid cells from frontal bone. Finally, pneumatization of laminae belonging to the ethmoid bone itself give rise to concha bullosa. Extensive pneumatization of the sphenoid sinus may result in de-

hiscence of its bony boundary with the internal carotid artery or the optic nerve. Similarly, dehiscences of the lamina papyracea increase the risk of complications due to damage of intraorbital structures.

The pterygopalatine fossa is a narrow space between the pterygoid process and the vertical process of the palatine bone (merged with the posterior maxillary sinus wall). Both CT and MRI demonstrate the foramina and canals, through which the pterygopalatine fossa directly communicates with: the middle cranial fossa (vidian canal and foramen rotundum); the orbit (inferior orbital fissure); the masticatory space (pterygomaxillary fissure); the choana (sphenopalatine foramen); and the oral cavity (greater and lesser palatine canals). Within the pterygopalatine fossa are the pterygopalatine ganglion, part of the maxillary nerve, terminal branches of the internal maxillary artery (the sphenopalatine artery), and fat.

Imaging Patients with Acute and Chronic Rhinosinusitis

Acute rhinosinusitis does not require radiological studies of the paranasal sinuses because documenting the patient's symptoms and performing an endoscopic examination are sufficient for a correct diagnosis [2]. Contrast-enhanced CT is indicated in the suspicion of an orbital complication (generally secondary to acute ethmoiditis) or an intracranial complication. CT may help discriminate among preseptal cellulitis, subperiosteal inflammation and intraorbital (extra- or intraconal) spread [3]. Overall, CT permits a correct diagnosis of orbital complications in up to 91% of cases, and is significantly more accurate than clinical examination alone (81%) [4].

Intracranial complications are generally secondary to frontal sinusitis. They are observed even in the absence of sinus wall defects because they may be secondary to thrombophlebitis of valveless diploic veins [5]. Imaging is mandatory for correctly assessing the degree of involvement of intracranial structures. In this setting, MRI is considered the technique of choice because its accuracy is superior to that of CT, in particular in differentiating dural reaction from epidural, subdural or intracerebral abscess and in demonstrating thrombosis of sagittal or cavernous sinus [4, 6].

CT evaluation of patients complaining of chronic rhinosinusitis and nasal polyposis is essentially focused on accurate delineation of the extent of the lesion and of those elements (e.g. inflammatory mucosal changes and predisposing anatomic factors) that may impair mucociliary drainage (Fig. 5).

Patients affected by chronic rhinosinusitis should receive adequate medical treatment before CT examination of the paranasal sinuses, in order to treat acute infection and resolve mucosal edema. Oral antibiotics, nasal steroids and antihistamines, prescribed at least three weeks before CT, decrease the risk of overestimating chronic inflammation and polypoid reaction of the mucosa.

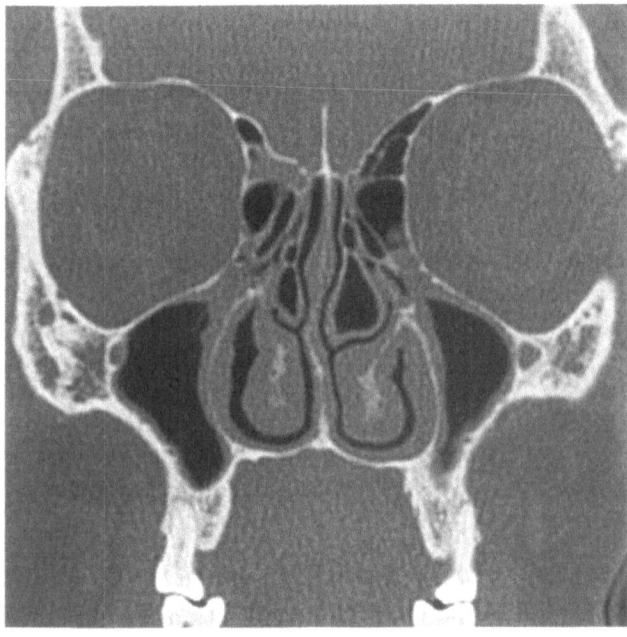

Fig. 5. Single-slice coronal CT image of a patient with chronic rhinosinusitis reveals infundibular pattern, mucosal thickening along maxillary walls. and both ethmoidal infundibula without blockage of mucus drainage

one of these patterns is based on the obstruction of different mucus-drainage pathways:

1. *Infundibular pattern* is mainly due to the presence of mucosal thickenings or isolated polyps along the ethmoid infundibulum with blockage of maxillary sinus drainage alone.
2. *Ostiomeatal unit pattern* reflects the obstruction of all drainage systems in the middle meatus, leading to maxillary, frontal, and anterior ethmoid sinusitis. Most frequent causes are non-specific mucosal thickenings and nasal polyps. This pattern may also be observed in the presence of benign or malignant neoplasms arising from the lateral nasal wall.
3. *Spheno-ethmoid recess pattern* is rather rare and consists of sphenoid sinusitis or posterior ethmoiditis, secondary to spheno-ethmoid recess obstruction.
4. The pattern of *nasal polyposis* is usually characterized by bilateral involvement of middle meatus, ethmoidal infundibulum and paranasal cavities by inflammatory polyps. At CT, they appear as solid lobulated lesions filling the ethmoidal sinus, the nasal fossae and sinusal cavities. Bone remodelling is associated, triggered by mechanical pressure exerted by the polyps but also by the local release of inflammatory mediators and by bacterial invasion of bone and periosteum [10] (Fig. 6).

Because of the high contrast between air, mucosa and bone, low-dose protocols may be adopted using single-slice CT (SSCT) equipment and decreasing the tube current to 30-50 mA [7]. This results in a considerable decrease of the eye-lens dose [8] without a significant loss of diagnostic information. With multislice CT (MSCT), patient exposure is a primary issue, as recent data demonstrate eye-lens doses higher than with single-slice scanners, even when low-dose protocols are used.

With SSCT, images are primarily acquired on the coronal plane, as perpendicular as possible to the hard palate by tilting the gantry and encouraging the patient to cooperate. This plane permits demonstrating patency, width, and morphology of the middle and superior meatus and the ethmoidal infundibulum, which are hidden by turbinates and therefore difficult to access at clinical examination. Moreover, coronal imaging clearly shows both the superior and lateral insertions of the middle turbinate, and the cribriform plate. In our experience, optimal demonstration of the ostiomeatal unit and of natural drainage pathways is achieved with:

- Thin slice collimation (1-2 mm), to minimize partial volume artifacts that may mimic mucosal thickening along small-caliber drainage pathways, and
- Scanning with 3- or 4-mm increments and 1.5 pitch (sequential or single-slice spiral equipment, respectively) as a trade-off between dose reduction and the necessity of not missing anatomical structures such as the uncinate process.

According to Sonkens et al. [9], five different patterns of chronic rhinosinusitis may be described at CT. All but

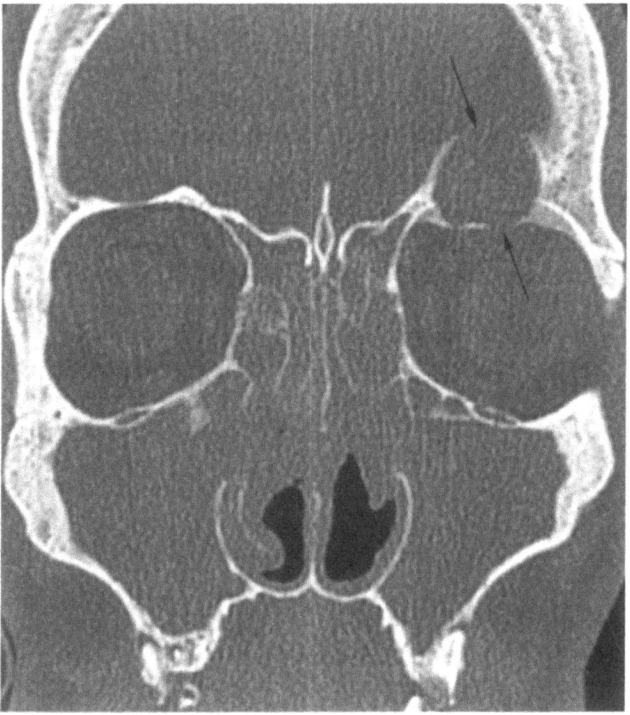

Fig. 6. Single-slice coronal CT image of a patient with chronic rhinosinusitis and nasal polyposis reveals air within the maxillary sinuses. The normal signal of the ethmoidal sinuses and nasal cavities has been replaced by soft tissue density. Outward bowing and thickening of both laminae papyraceae are due to the pressure exerted by polyps. A mucocele developing within the left frontal sinus is secondary to drainage blockage. Resorption of the orbital roof and superior frontal sinus wall is present (*arrows*)

Widening of the ethmoidal infundibulum and truncation of the middle turbinates (observed bilaterally in up to 80% of cases) are signs indicating nasal polyposis. A peculiar variant of sinonasal polyp is the *antrochoanal polyp*, which arises from the maxillary sinus and bulges into the middle meatus, where it extends between the middle turbinate and the lateral nasal wall to reach the choana. CT density of an antrochoanal polyp is low (fluid-like), while MRI appearance resembles that of inflammatory polyps. Because the waist of the polyp may be strangled as it passes through constrictive ostia, dilation and stasis of feeding vessels combined with edema lead the lesion to show non-homogeneous enhancement, a sign of an angiomatous polyp [11].

5. *Sporadic pattern* includes a wide list of different conditions (such as isolated sinusitis, retention cyst, mucocele, post-surgical changes) unrelated to impairment of any of mucociliary drainage patterns. CT findings consist of partial or complete obliteration of a sinusal cavity by means of thickened mucosa with smooth, occasionally lobulated surface and homogeneously low density [12].

Imaging Patients with Fungal Rhinosinusitis and Aggressive Inflammatory Lesions

Fungal infections may manifest in different forms that are grouped as noninvasive or invasive, according to the absence or presence of fungal invasion of mucosa, submucosa, vessels and bone.

- *Noninvasive forms*, generally occurring in immunocompetent patients, consist of fungus ball (mycetoma) and allergic fungal sinusitis (AFS). The CT and MRI appearances of fungus ball are conditioned by the high content of heavy metals and calcium within fungal hyphae. Therefore, fungus ball is spontaneously hyperdense at CT [13, 14], while both T2- and T1-weighted sequences demonstrate a hypointense lesion bordered by hyperintense (T2) and enhancing (T1, after contrast administration) mucosa [6]. In some cases, T1 and T2 shortening may be so relevant to result in signal void, making discrimination between fungus ball and intrasinusal air nearly impossible. AFS is currently considered an immune disorder rather than an infectious disease. The combination of immunologic predisposing factors and drainage pathways obstruction (due to chronic rhinosinusitis, nasal polyposis) leads to accumulation of allergic eosinophilic mucin within sinusal cavities. Intrasinusal fungal material as well as progressive dehydration of eosinophilic mucin produces CT and MRI patterns similar to fungus ball [14, 15].
- Acute fulminant and chronic courses are the two most frequent forms of *invasive mycoses*. A third rarer invasive form has been referred to as "indolent" fungal rhinosinusitis. Imaging findings of acute fulminant my-

cosis consist of aggressive destruction of bony sinusal walls and invasion of adjacent soft tissues [16] characterized by ischemic necrosis. CT and MRI appearances of chronic and indolent forms are not yet clearly defined. In these varieties, the diagnosis is primarily based on the less aggressive clinical course, as compared to acute fulminant form.

Imaging Patients with Sinonasal Masses: CT and MRI Techniques

The first step in the diagnostic work-up of both benign and malignant sinus neoplasms consists of fiberoptic examination. Endoscopy allows adequate demonstration of the superficial spread of the lesion and may guide biopsy. The discrimination between benign and malignant tumors and the precise characterization of the lesion are, in most cases, far beyond the capabilities of CT [17]. Main goals of imaging are, therefore, to provide a precise map of deep tumor extension in all areas blinded at fiberoptic examination, especially the anterior cranial fossa, orbit and pterygopalatine fossa.

In this setting, MRI is the technique of choice because it clearly differentiates tumor from retained secretions, it allows early detection of perivascular and perineural spread, and provides higher contrast resolution. On the other hand, the strengths of CT consist of a superior definition of bone structures even in the case of subtle erosions, faster and easier performance, superior accessibility and inferior costs.

Despite the relevant improvements provided by multislice technology (e.g. fast coverage of the volume of interest, thin collimation, and acquisition of nearly isotropic voxels), CT is nowadays restricted to patients not preliminarily examined by the otolaryngologist (to rule out non-neoplastic lesions) and to those with contraindications to MRI.

A key point of the MRI protocol is represented by spatial resolution: nasal cavity and paranasal sinuses are a complex framework of airspaces bordered by thin bony boundaries. Moreover, a thin osteoperiosteal layer separates the sinonasal region from the anterior cranial fossa (cribriform plate and dura) and the orbit (lamina papyracea and periorbita). An adequate depiction of these structures mandates high-field equipment and a dedicated circular coil (head coil). In addition, a high-resolution matrix (512×512) should be applied along with the smallest field of view (FOV) achievable. It is also recommended to acquire images not exceeding 3.0-3.5 mm in thickness, with an interslice gap ranging from 1.5 to 2.4 mm (50%-70%). These parameters, applied to both turbo spin echo (TSE) T2-weighted and SE T1-weighted sequences, represent an acceptable compromise between the need to attain small pixel size and the risk of significantly decreasing signal-to-noise ratio.

Inverted Papilloma and Juvenile Angiofibroma: CT and MRI Findings

Inverted papilloma (IP) is a benign epithelial neoplasm characterized by the infolding of the mucosa in the underlying stroma without crossing the basement membrane. It is one of the most common benign neoplasms of the sinonasal tract [18, 19]. Its association with sinonasal malignancies, in particular squamous cell carcinoma, is well established (incidence, 1.5%-56%). IP may be suspected whenever an isolated, unilateral polypoid lesion is detected by imaging studies. At CT, IP appears as a mass with soft-tissue density, non-homogeneous contrast enhancement and calcifications that represent residues of involved bone [20]. TSE T2-weighted and enhanced T1-weighted images may reveal a pattern described as "septate striated appearance" [21], "convoluted cerebriform pattern" [22] or "columnar pattern" that corresponds to the peculiar macroarchitecture of the lesion. The juxtaposition of several epithelial and stromal layers results in a quite regular columnar pattern on MRI: the first layer is hypointense on TSE T2-weighted images (because it is highly cellular) and mildly enhancing on post-contrast SE T1-weighted images; the second layer is hyperintense on TSE T2-weighted images (because it is edematous) and highly enhancing on post-contrast SE T1-weighted images. Thin SE T1-weighted sections and acquisition of slices in the three planes of space improve the detection of this pattern.

Juvenile angiofibroma (JA), a lesion composed of vascular and fibrous elements, typically occurs in adolescent males. It has been recently suggested that the lesion must be considered a vascular malformation [23] (or hamartoma) rather than a tumor. Peculiar findings of JA are its tendency to grow in the submucosal plane and early invasion of cancellous bone of the pterygoid root, from which the lesion may grow laterally into the greater wing of the sphenoid bone. From its site of origin in the pterygopalatine fossa, the JA extends: (a) medially into the nasal cavity (and nasopharynx) via enlargement and erosion of the sphenopalatine foramen; (b) anteriorly with bowing of the maxillary sinus wall [24]; (c) laterally via the pterygomaxillary fissure; and (d) superiorly into the apex of the orbit through the inferior orbital fissure, and into the middle cranial fossa via the superior orbital fissure (Fig. 7). Enhanced CT and MRI provide a precise map of the extent into these spaces by detecting the enhancing "finger-like projections" of JA, characterized also by sharp and lobulated margins.

At CT, intradiploic spread may be demonstrated by differentiating the normal medullary content from the strongly enhancing JA. On MRI, this discrimination may be achieved by combining a plain T1-weighted image with a post-contrast T1-weighted image without or with fat saturation. The latter permits easy distinction of the hyperintense enhanced JA from the suppressed signal of the surrounding bone marrow. Intracranial extent is mainly due to finger-like projections running along canals or through foramina. Rarely does it occur through the de-

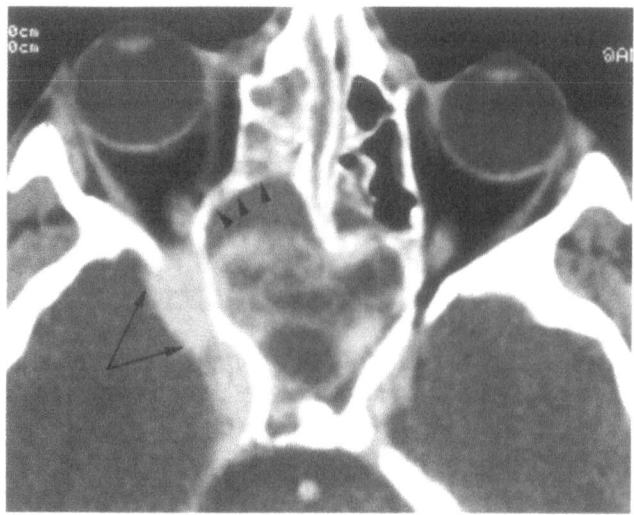

Fig. 7. Single-slice axial CT image of a juvenile angiofibroma with non-homogeneous enhancement occupying the sphenoid sinuses. Displacement and thinning of the anterior wall (*arrowheads*) are due to a secondary mucocele. Intracranial extradural extent of the enhancing lesion runs through the right superior orbital fissure (*arrows*)

struction of the inner table of the greater wing or the lateral sphenoid sinus walls.

Essential Information in Managing Nasosinusal Neoplasms

Although infrequent, sinonasal neoplasms are characterized by numerous, different histotypes, a distinctive feature which reflects the peculiar density of diverse anatomic structures present in this area. About 80% arise from the maxillary sinus (up to 73% are squamous cell carcinoma [25]), and most of the remaining tumors arise from the ethmoid sinus [26]; among these malignancies, adenocarcinoma, squamous cell carcinoma and olfactory neuroblastoma are prevalent. As a result, patterns of tumor spread may be generalized into two different models, according to their site of origin (e.g. maxillary area vs. naso-ethmoidal area).

Mapping Maxillary Sinus Malignancies

The critical areas of neoplasms arising from the maxillary area include the posterior wall of the maxillary sinus, the infratemporal and pterygopalatine fossae, and the orbital floor. The main goal of imaging is to assess the integrity of the bone-periosteal barrier. MRI is less accurate than CT in the assessment of focal bony erosions, since its calcium content cannot be adequately detected [27, 28]. Nevertheless, the most effective barrier to spread of aggressive lesions beyond sinusal walls is the periosteum rather than the mineralized bony walls [29]. Therefore, neoplastic spread beyond the periosteum of the sinusal walls is,

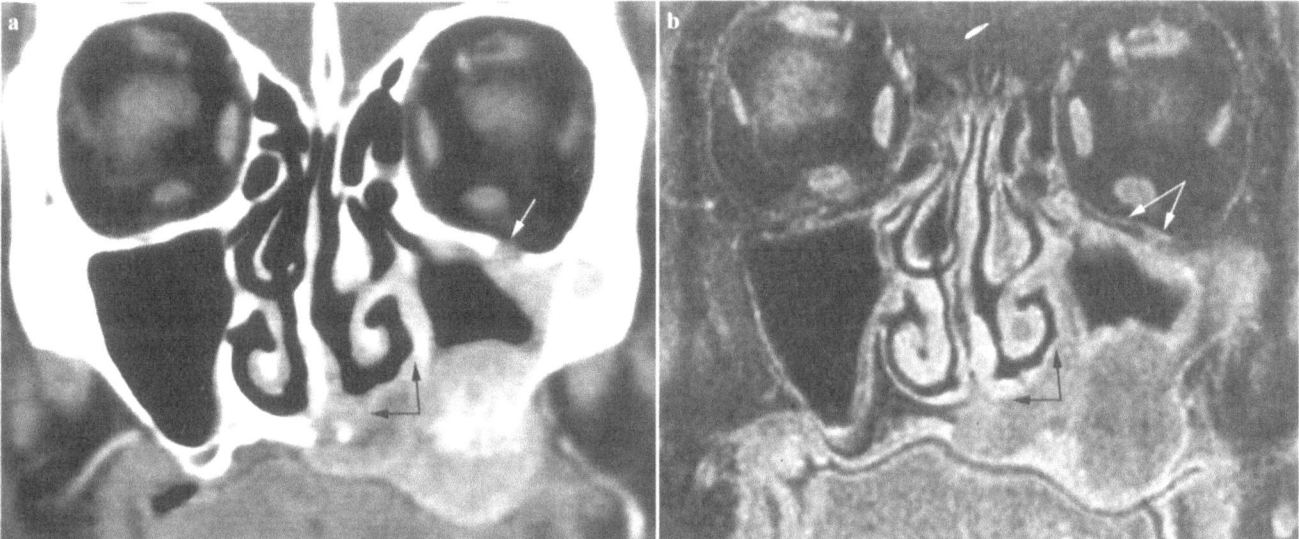

Fig. 8a,b. *Maxillary sinus squamous cell carcinoma.* **a** Enhanced multislice CT image in coronal plane. **b** VIBE sequence in coronal plane. Both imaging techniques show the subperiosteal extent of tumor, covered by residual mucosa (*black arrows*). Invasion of the hard palate, nasal septum, right nasal floor, medial wall of the left maxillary sinus, and left zygomatic bone is demonstrated. Periosteal thickening at the orbital floor is shown on MRI (a). Residual bone at the left alveolar process is appreciated on CT (b)

in effect, the critical information for therapeutic planning because it is related to extrasinusal infiltration (Fig. 8).

The thin sinusal walls appear hypointense in every MR sequence because of the reduced water contents of cortical bone and periosteum. The entire thickness of the wall can be appreciated when invested by thickened mucosa or when the air on one or both sides has been replaced by mucous secretions or neoplastic tissue [30]. Of course, the proper frequency-encoding direction has to be selected in order to avoid asymmetric appearance of cortical bone due to chemical shift artifact [31].

Pterygopalatine Fossa Invasion: CT and MRI Findings

Posterior spread into the pterygopalatine fossa is a relevant element in treatment planning. On MRI, neoplastic invasion of the pterygopalatine fossa is suspected whenever its fat content has been replaced or effaced by soft tissue intensity [32]. Pterygoid canal and nerve, foramen rotundum and maxillary nerve are well demonstrated on axial and coronal MR sequences. Segmental thickening or asymmetric enhancement of the nerves may raise the suspicion of perineural spread [33]. Perineural spread has a significant impact on therapeutic planning: it is associated with poor prognosis, and a reduction of more than 30% of the local control rate has been reported [34]. In fact, progression of tumor along trigeminal nerve branches may lead to cavernous sinus invasion. In this case, MRI shows enlargement, lateral bulging, and replacement of the hyperintense venous signal by the tumor on coronal and axial T2-weighted and on enhanced T1-weighted sequences. Encasement of the internal

carotid artery may also be detected on both T1- and T2-weighted sequences.

Mapping Naso-ethmoidal Malignancies

In managing naso-ethmoidal neoplasm, the most critical areas include the orbit (particularly the roof and the posterior lamina papyracea where most postoperative recurrences occur), the floor of the anterior cranial fossa), and the sphenoid sinus. Nowadays, even though its bony walls have been completely eroded, the orbit is preserved at surgery, on condition that the periorbita is not (or is minimally) invaded. In fact, it has been recently demonstrated that a more aggressive approach does not improve survival [35].

Displacement and distortion of orbital walls by ethmoidal neoplasms occur frequently. The mineral content of the wall may be partially or completely resorbed, leading to a questionable CT evaluation. On MRI, when a thin and regular hypointense area is still detectable - between neoplasm and orbital fat - the periorbita should be considered intact. The assessment of the integrity of the periorbita, however, it is not crucial since in most cases the lamina itself is partly or completely resected at surgery for intra-operative pathologic examination. Nevertheless, if imaging suggests orbital infiltration, the patient should be informed that orbital exenteration may be required. Assessment of invasion of the anterior cranial fossa floor has a great impact on surgical planning.

Similarly to orbital wall invasion, bone destruction of the skull base is better demonstrated by CT. However, at the skull base level, imaging findings differ from those observed at other bone interfaces of the paranasal sinuses.

This is because when the skull base is invaded, the dura mater usually shows abnormal thickening and enhancement that can be due either to neoplastic invasion or to an inflammatory, non-neoplastic reaction. Since dural invasion implies both a worse prognosis and a surgical resection not limited to the eroded bone, the goals of imaging focus on determining the depth of skull base invasion [36, 37].

MRI has been reported to be more precise than CT. At the anterior cranial fossa level, a key aspect regards the analysis of the MRI signal intensity of the structures located at the interface between the ethmoid roof (below) and brain (above): the cribriform plate and its double periosteal covering (lower layer); the dura mater (middle layer), and the subarachnoid space (superior layer). On enhanced sagittal and coronal SE T1-weighted sequences or 3D gradient echo (GE) fat-saturated T1-weighted (VIBE) sequences, the three layers compose a "sandwich" of different signals (bone-periosteum complex, dura mater, cerebrospinal fluid) [38]. When a sinonasal neoplasm abuts against the cribrifom plate interface, without interrupting its hypointense signal, the lesion should be considered limited to the ethmoid and nasal fossae. Replacement of this lower layer hypointense signal by tumor implies bone-periosteum penetration. In this case, a thickened enhancing dura mater (middle layer) usually borders the neoplasm. If uninterrupted, the neoplasm may be graded as intracranial-extradural. Conversely, focal or more extensive replacement of enhanced, thickened dura mater by tumor indicates intracranial-intradural invasion. Brain invasion is suspected in the presence of edema [17] (Fig. 9).

Determination of the resectability of tumors invading the brain does not stand only upon the assessment by imaging of the depth of tumor extent into the brain or on the detection of bilateral brain invasion. It requires a thorough evaluation of several other issues, the most important being the histotype and patient's status. Patients with limited brain invasion treated by craniofacial resection have a nonsignificantly shorter mean survival compared to those with dural invasion only.

References

1. Landsberg R, Friedman M (2001) A computer-assisted anatomical study of the nasofrontal region. Laryngoscope 111(12):2125-2130
2. Phillips CD (1997) Current status and new developments in techniques for imaging the nose and sinuses. Otolaryngol Clin North Am 30(3):371-387
3. Hahnel S, Ertl-Wagner B, Tasman AJ, Forsting M, Jansen O (1999) Relative value of MR imaging as compared with CT in the diagnosis of inflammatory paranasal sinus disease. Radiology 210(1):171-176
4. Younis RT, Lazar RH, Bustillo A, Anand VK (2002) Orbital infection as a complication of sinusitis: are diagnostic and treatment trends changing? Ear Nose Throat J 81(11):771-775
5. Lerner DN, Choi SS, Zalzal GH, Johnson DL (1995) Intracranial complications of sinusitis in childhood. Ann Otol Rhinol Laryngol 104(4 Pt 1):288-293
6. Rao VM, Sharma D, Madan A (2001) Imaging of frontal sinus disease: concepts, interpretation, and technology. Otolaryngol Clin North Am 34(1):23-39
7. Hagtvedt T, Aalokken TM, Notthellen J, Kolbenstvedt A (2003) A new low-dose CT examination compared with standard-dose CT in the diagnosis of acute sinusitis. Eur Radiol 13(5):976-980
8. Sohaib SA, Peppercorn PD, Horrocks JA, Keene MH, Kenyon GS, Reznek RH (2001) The effect of decreasing mAs on image quality and patient dose in sinus CT. Br J Radiol 74(878):157-161
9. Sonkens JW, Harnsberger HR, Blanch GM, Babbel RW, Hunt S (1991) The impact of screening sinus CT on the planning of functional endoscopic sinus surgery. Otolaryngol Head Neck Surg 105(6):802-813
10. Giacchi RJ, Lebowitz RA, Yee HT, Light JP, Jacobs JB (2001) Histopathologic evaluation of the ethmoid bone in chronic sinusitis. Am J Rhinol 15(3):193-197
11. De Vuysere S, Hermans R, Marchal G (2001) Sinochoanal polyp and its variant, the angiomatous polyp: MRI findings. Eur Radiol 11(1):55-58
12. Scuderi AJ, Babbel RW, Harnsberger HR, Sonkens JW (1991) The sporadic pattern of inflammatory sinonasal disease including postsurgical changes. Semin Ultrasound CT MR 12(6):575-591
13. Eloy P, Bertrand B, Rombeaux P, Delos M, Trigaux JP (1997) Mycotic sinusitis. Acta Otorhinolaryngol Belg 51(4):339-352
14. Dhong HJ, Jung JY, Park JH (2000) Diagnostic accuracy in sinus fungus balls: CT scan and operative findings. Am J Rhinol 14(4):227-231
15. Mukherji SK, Figueroa RE, Ginsberg LE et al (1998) Allergic fungal sinusitis: CT findings. Radiology 207(2):417-422
16. Saleh HA, Bridger MW (1997) Invasive aspergillosis of the paranasal sinuses: a medical emergency. J Laryngol Otol 111(12):1168-1170
17. Maroldi R, Farina D, Battaglia G, Maculotti P, Nicolai P, Chiesa A (1997) MR of malignant nasosinusal neoplasms. Frequently asked questions. Eur J Radiol 24(3):181-190

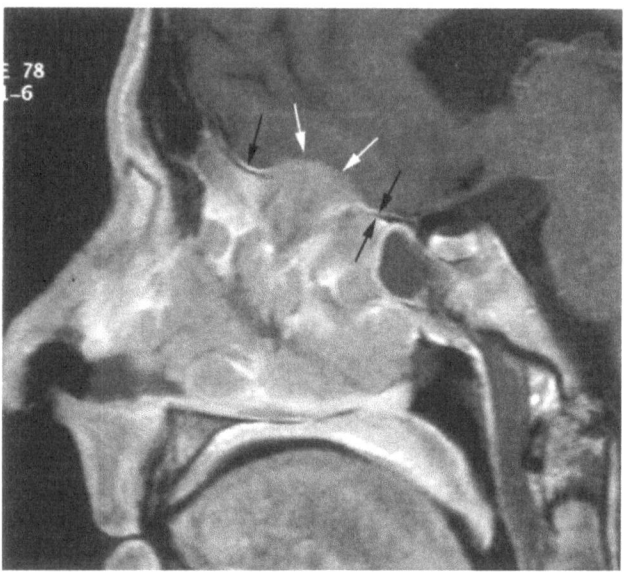

Fig. 9. Adenocarcinoma of the ethmoid sinus revealed by sagittal T1-weighted spin echo image after gadolinium administration. Ethmoid and nasal fossae are occupied by a non-homogeneous enhancing mass. At the level of the planum sphenoidalis, the tumor (*white arrows*) replaces the hypointense signal of bone (*opposite black arrows*) and the hyperintense signal of the thickened dura (*single black arrow*), suggesting intracranial intradural extent

18. Outzen KE, Grontveld A, Jorgensen K, Clausen PP, Ladefoged C (1996) Inverted papilloma: incidence and late results of surgical treatment. Rhinology 34(2):114-118
19. Hyams VJ (1971) Papillomas of the nasal cavity and paranasal sinuses. A clinicopathological study of 315 cases. Ann Otol Rhinol Laryngol 80(2):192-206
20. Som PM, Lidov M (1994) The significance of sinonasal radiodensities: ossification, calcification, or residual bone? AJNR Am J Neuroradiol 15(5):917-922
21. Yousem DM, Fellows DW, Kennedy DW, Bolger WE, Kashima H, Zinreich SJ (1992) Inverted papilloma: evaluation with MR imaging. Radiology 185(2):501-505
22. Ojiri H, Ujita M, Tada S, Fukuda K (2000) Potentially distinctive features of sinonasal inverted papilloma on MR imaging. AJR Am J Roentgenol 175(2):465-468
23. Schick B, Plinkert PK, Prescher A (2002) Die vaskulare Komponente: Gedanken zur Entstehung des Angiofibroms. Laryngorhinootologie 81(4):280-284
24. Lloyd GA, Phelps PD (1986) Juvenile angiofibroma: imaging by magnetic resonance, CT and conventional techniques. Clin Otolaryngol 11(4):247-259
25. Tiwari R, Hardillo JA, Mehta D et al (2000) Squamous cell carcinoma of maxillary sinus. Head Neck 22(2):164-169
26. Cantù G, Solero CL, Mariani L et al (1999) Anterior craniofacial resection for malignant ethmoid tumors – a series of 91 patients. Head Neck 21(3):185-191
27. Lund VJ, Howard DJ, Lloyd GA, Cheesman AD (1989) Magnetic resonance imaging of paranasal sinus tumors for craniofacial resection. Head Neck 11(3):279-283
28. Som PM, Shapiro MD, Biller HF, Sasaki C, Lawson W (1988) Sinonasal tumors and inflammatory tissues: differentiation with MR imaging. Radiology 167(3):803-808
29. Kimmelman CP, Korovin GS (1988) Management of paranasal sinus neoplasms invading the orbit. Otolaryngol Clin North Am 21(1):77-92
30. Som PM, Braun IF, Shapiro MD, Reede DL, Curtin HD, Zimmerman RA (1987) Tumors of the parapharyngeal space and upper neck: MR imaging characteristics. Radiology 164(3):823-829
31. Dick BW, Mitchell DG, Burk DL, Levy DW, Vinitski S, Rifkin M (1988) The effect of chemical shift misrepresentation on cortical bone thickness on MR imaging. AJR Am J Roentgenol 151(3):537-538
32. Woodruff WW Jr, Yeates AE, McLendon RE (1986) Perineural tumor extension to the cavernous sinus from superficial facial carcinoma: CT manifestations. Radiology 161(2):395-399
33. Laccourreye O, Bely N, Halimi P, Guimaraes R, Brasnu D (1994) Cavernous sinus involvement from recurrent adenoid cystic carcinoma. Ann Otol Rhinol Laryngol 103(10):822-825
34. Jiang GL, Ang KK, Peters LJ, Wendt CD, Oswald MJ, Goepfert H (1991) Maxillary sinus carcinomas: natural history and results of postoperative radiotherapy. Radiother Oncol 21(3):193-200
35. Perry C, Levine PA, Williamson BR, Cantrell RW (1988) Preservation of the eye in paranasal sinus cancer surgery. Arch Otolaryngol Head Neck Surg 114(6):632-634
36. Kraus DH, Lanzieri CF, Wanamaker JR, Little JR, Lavertu P (1992) Complementary use of computed tomography and magnetic resonance imaging in assessing skull base lesions. Laryngoscope 102(6):623-629
37. Shah JP, Kraus DH, Bilsky MH, Gutin PH, Harrison LH, Strong EW (1997) Craniofacial resection for malignant tumors involving the anterior skull base. Arch Otolaryngol Head Neck Surg 123(12):1312-1317
38. Ishida H, Mohri M, Amatsu M (2002) Invasion of the skull base by carcinomas: histopathologically evidenced findings with CT and MRI. Eur Arch Otorhinolaryngol 259(10):535-539

Degenerative Diseases of the Spine

B.C. Bowen

Neuroradiology Section, MRI Center, Department of Radiology, University of Miami School of Medicine, Miami, FL, USA

Degenerative Disk Disease

The intervertebral disk consists of three components: cartilaginous endplate (hyaline cartilage), nucleus pulposus (fibrocartilage with ground substance containing hyaluronic acid and glycosaminoglycans), and anulus fibrosus (inner part contains fibrocartilage, while the outer part has dense fibrous lamellae with fibers, called Sharpey fibers, that insert on the vertebral ring apophysis). The inner part of the anulus and the nucleus pulposis are indistinguishable on magnetic resonance imaging (MRI). In the normal adult disk, a hypointense band or cleft is observed at the center of the nucleus pulposus and inner anulus on T2-weighted sagittal images and has been attributed to a higher concentration of collagen in this region of the disk. The adult disk normally lacks innervation and vascularity.

With aging, the composition of the disk changes. Increases in collagen and decreases in glycosaminoglycans are believed responsible for a decrease in hydrophilicity and hence a decrease in water content, which results in a small (few percent) decrease in the signal intensity of the disk on T2-weighted images. Considerable loss of signal and loss of normal intervetebral disk height are not considered typical of normal aging, but rather indicate disk degeneration. The outer anulus manifests small concentric and transverse tears as part of normal aging; however, radial tears are considered a marker of disk degeneration. Concentric tears are characterized as delamination of the lamellae of the anulus fibrosus, and transverse tears represent disruptions of the anulus near the insertion of Sharpey fibers into the ring apophysis. The radial tear involves all layers of the anulus and appears on MRI as a band of hyperintensity penetrating the normally hypointense outer anulus on T2-weighted images and as a strip of enhancement on post-contrast T1-weighted images. Contrast enhancement on MRI has been attributed to the ingrowth of granulation tissue into the tear as a consequence of healing. The clinical significance of anular tears is not known. Some investigators attribute back pain in patients without nerve root compression to scar tissue within an annular tear or to a disk herniation that irritates nerve endings in the peripheral anulus ("diskogenic pain"). Many patients, though, have asymptomatic annular tears, suggesting that additional factors play a role in back pain. Nerves, which may be nociceptors, have been identified in the vertebral endplates, facet joints, posterior longitudinal ligament (PLL), and anterior longitudinal ligament (ALL), thus enabling these structures to be potential sources of pain.

Disk Degeneration

Although the pathogenesis of intervertebral disk degeneration is not well understood, the results of this process are characterized by loss of height, loss of signal intensity, bulging or herniation of the disk [1]. These morphological changes are consistently accompanied by the anular tears described previously, and occasionally gas or calcification develops within a degenerating disk. A classification system for lumbar disk degeneration based on routine T2-weighted MRI has been developed and shown to be reliable in distinguishing among grades of degeneration based on intra- and interobserver kappa statistics [2]. Grades ranging from I (normal) to V (collapsed disk space) are assigned based on disk signal intensity, disk structure, distinction between nucleus and annulus, and disk height. Recent studies [3] have attempted to relate such grading schemes for disk degeneration to the biomechanical characteristics of individual lumbar motion segments subjected to loading forces in the direction of flexion-extension, axial rotation, or lateral bending.

In addition to the degenerative changes involving the disk structure, biochemical and structural changes also occur within the bone marrow near the endplates of the vertebral bodies adjacent to the degenerating disk [4]. These so-called endplate changes have been classified into three types, and some authors have proposed adding this classification to the disk degeneration grading scheme in order to further specify degenerative disease. On MRI, the signal intensity within the marrow bordering the endplate may be increased or decreased compared to normal marrow. The combination of signal intensity changes on T1-weighted and T2-weighted images reflects the underlying histopathological changes and has been categorized by Modic, Ross, and others as type I, II, or III endplate changes. For type I changes (low signal intensity on T1-weighted and high intensity on T2-weighted images), fibrovascular tissue replaces the hematopoietic and lipid elements of normal marrow. Type I changes may mimic the MRI findings for vertebral osteomyelitis; however, osteomyelitis is usually accompanied by diskitis, resulting in an abnormal configuration and high signal intensity of the intervertebral disk space. These disk space abnormalities differ from the usual observation of low signal intensity for the degenerated disk; however, some degenerated disks contain cystic areas that are bright on T2-weighted images and thus may be indistinguishable from early infection.

For type II changes (high signal intensity on T1-weighted images and intermediate-high intensity on T2-weighted images), there is an increase in the lipid content of the marrow space (i.e. more "yellow marrow") compared to normal. Type II changes are slightly more common than type I. The signal intensity on T2-weighted images depends in part on the pulse sequence used – the fast spin echo sequence typically yields higher signal than the standard spin echo sequence. Type I changes have been observed to convert to type II changes with time, while type II changes are relatively stable. Type III changes most likely represent areas of marrow replacement by dense woven bone, since type III changes correspond to areas of bony sclerosis on radiographic studies. On post-contrast T1-weighted images, the regions of type I or type II change may enhance with gadolinium, mimicking infection.

Although there is no universally accepted classification system for describing degenerative disk disease, a standardized nomenclature for classifying morphological changes in lumbar disk degeneration, focused on the posterior aspect of the disk, has been accepted and endorsed by a number of North American medical societies [5]. In this nomenclature, disks are either bulging or herniated. A bulging disk is one in which disk tissue extends diffusely (50%-100% of the total circumference of the disk) beyond the margins of the vertebral endplates. The anulus remains grossly intact. Herniated disks are subclassified into protrusions and extrusions, which may be focal (<25% of disk circumference) or broad-based (25%-50% of disk circumference). At least one study has shown that the frequency of protrusions (27%) is much greater than the frequency of extrusions (1%) in asymptomatic patients.

A protrusion has a roughly conical shape, so that the distance between edges of the disk material extending beyond the vertebral endplates is *narrower* than the distance between the edges at the base of the protrusion. Anatomically, some of the outer anular fibers remain intact; however, identification of these fibers on MRI or computed tomography (CT) is difficult or impossible. In an extrusion, the distance between the edges of the disk material extending beyond the vertebral endplates is *wider* than the distance at the base in at least one plane of view. In other words, extrusion is identifiable when the portion ("cap") of the herniated disk beyond the end-

plates is wider than the "neck" connecting the cap to the bulk of the disk in the interspace. An extrusion is a larger herniation than a protrusion and extends through the entire anulus. MRI is not accurate in determining whether the extruded disk also disrupts the PLL. A sequestration is a specific form of extrusion in which the displaced disk material has completely lost continuity with the parent disk. Sequestration may reside anterior or posterior to the PLL, or rarely may be intradural. Extruded disks, including sequestrations, can migrate either superiorly or inferiorly from the level of the parent disk space.

In a herniation, any combination of disk constituents – nucleus pulposus, cartilage, fragmented apophyseal bone, anulus – may be displaced. To describe the location of a herniated disk in the axial (horizontal) plane, several terms, which refer to "anatomic zones", have been proposed as part of the standardized nomenclature (Fig. 1).

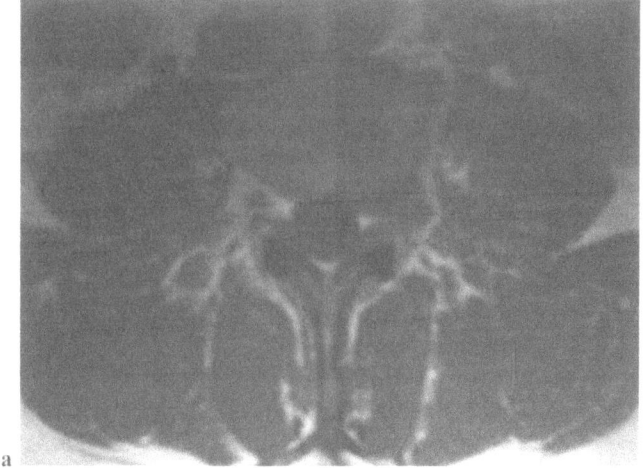

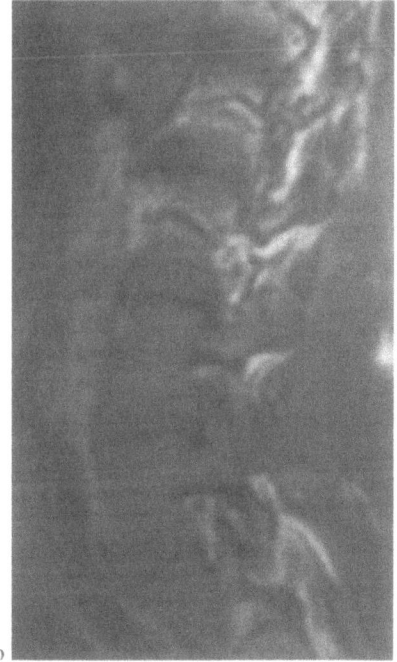

Fig. 1a, b. *Left foraminal (or lateral) disk herniation.* Axial (a) and parasagittal (b) T1-weighted images of the lumbar spine demonstrate loss of the normal epidural fat signal in the left neural foramen at L4-5. The herniated disk appears to be an extrusion in the parasagittal image and is encroaching on the exiting left L4 nerve root, which is located in superior portion of the neural foramen. Loss of disk space height at L4-5 is not evident on the parasagittal image

Moving from central to lateral for a left-sided herniated disk, the location would be identified as "central", "left central", "left subarticular", "left foraminal", or "left extraforaminal" (synonymous with "far lateral"). Of course, a large herniated disk may span more than one zone. In the sagittal (craniocaudal) plane, anatomic zones, which can be used to describe the extent of migration, are loosely defined as the "disk level", the "infrapedicular level", the "pedicular level", or the "suprapedicular level".

When lumbar herniated disks migrate either superiorly or inferiorly, the migrated component is found predominantly in either the left or right half of the anterior epidural space in 94% of cases. This lateralization is due to the presence of a collagenous, sagittal midline septum (adherent to the PLL and the vertebral body periosteum, yet potentially detachable) which divides the anterior epidural space opposite the vertebral body into a left and a right compartment [6]. There is no consensus in the literature regarding the relative frequency of superior versus inferior migration of lumbar herniated disks.

The portion of an extruded disk extending beyond the vertebral endplates may or may not have high signal intensity on T2-weighted images compared with the intervertebral (parent) portion. For sequestered disk fragments (free fragments), some investigators have noted that initial high signal intensity may decrease with time, perhaps as a result of water loss. It is important to remember that disk herniation may occur in the absence of significant degeneration. This is uncommon and tends to occur in young persons participating in strenuous activities, or as a result of trauma.

In unoperated patients, enhancement of the margin of a herniated disk due to peridiskal scar may occasionally be observed on post-contrast T1-weighted images, especially when there is a sequestered fragment. A separate, but perhaps related, finding that has been reported is the abnormal enhancement of lumbosacral nerve roots in approximately 5% of unoperated patients with low back pain or radiculopathy. In one study, the nerve root enhancement was associated with disk herniation in the majority of cases. There is no consensus, though, as to whether a correlation exists between the observed root enhancement and clinical radiculopathy, and investigators caution that nerve root enhancement may be mimicked by the normal enhancement of intramedullary veins in the lumbosacral region [7].

A herniation through a break in the vertebral body endplate is referred to as an intravertebral herniation and gives rise to a Schmorl's node (SN). Chronic SNs are asymptomatic and most frequently found in the thoracolumbar region. The thin invaginated rim of the chronic SN has decreased signal intensity on all MR imaging sequences. The surrounding vertebral body marrow may have variable signal but lacks the diffuse hyperintensity on T2-weighted images associated with edema. Acute SNs can be symptomatic, and they exhibit MRI evidence of diffuse marrow edema [8]. Indentation of the endplate may be focal or diffuse. Loss of height of the parent disk space is atypical for acute SNs.

Spinal Stenosis, Spondylosis Deformans and Degenerative Facet Disease

In addition to the changes in disk morphology described previously, disk degeneration is also implicated in the development of other structural and biomechanical abnormalities: spinal stenosis, facet arthrosis, and malalignment-instability (e.g. spondylolisthesis).

The presence of osteophytes arising from the vertebral body margins at the site of attachment of the anulus fibrosus is generally referred to as spondylosis deformans. It has been considered the most common degenerative process of the spine, probably occurring secondary to degenerative disk disease with disruption of Sharpey's fibers and increased stress on the vertebral body margins. Some investigators, though, suggest that spondylosis deformans should be defined narrowly as anterior and lateral changes in vertebral body apophyses that may accompany normal aging and occur in vertebra that are normal or slightly decreased in height. This definition distinguishes spondylosis from osteophyte formation occurring as part of *intervertebral osteochondrosis*, a degenerative process involving the vertebral endplates, the nucleus pulposus, and the anulus fibrosus. In intervertebral osteochondrosis, disk space narrowing, vacuum phenomenon, and vertebral endplate changes are observed.

Degenerative disease (osteoarthritis) of the facet joints typically occurs in combination with degenerative disk disease. Synovial joints like the facet joints (and the cervical uncovertebral joints) are susceptible to the development of joint space narrowing, osteophyte formation, subchondral sclerosis, cyst formation, and subluxation. These degenerative changes affecting the nociceptors in the synovium and joint capsule, as well as nerve root impingement (in the neural foramen or lateral recess) from hypertrophied facets, may produce symptoms of pain and radiculopathy. Enlargement, buckling or redundancy of the ligamentum flavum may be seen in association with degenerated, hypertrophied, and sclerotic facets. Juxta-articular (synovial, or rarely ganglion) cysts occur secondarily and may compress the thecal sac or nerve roots, also resulting in pain, with or without radiculopathy.

The findings that help to characterize intraspinal, juxta-articular cyst are its location (epidural, posterolateral), its apparent continuity with a hypointense, degenerated facet joint, and its hypointense rim on T2-weighted images. These cysts may have variable signal intensity depending on whether they contain synovial or other watery fluid, hemorrhage, proteinaceous material or air. The hypointensity of the rim on T2-weighted images has been attributed to the presence of a fibrous capsule with hemosiderin deposits or fine calcification. Post-contrast enhancement of the rim probably reflects the presence of inflammation, and may be useful to better define the lesion in suspected cases. Hemorrhage into a cyst has been proposed as a mechanism to explain acute exacerbation of chronic low back pain. Conversely, spontaneous resolution of symptoms has been attributed to decompression of the cyst into the adjacent facet joint as inflammation resolves.

Lumbar Spinal Stenosis

The bone proliferation and enlargement that accompany vertebral body marginal osteophyte formation and facet degeneration frequently coexist and contribute, along with soft tissue changes, to degenerative spinal stenosis. In lumbar spinal stenosis, narrowing of the central spinal canal (central stenosis), lateral recesses, and neural formina may coexist or occur independently. Measurements of the dimensions of the bony canal for central stenosis are no longer recommended, because frequently they are not accurate predictors of clinical symptoms and because MRI provides better depiction of thecal sac narrowing due to degenerative osseous and soft tissue (e.g. ligamentous) changes. Obliteration of the epidural fat that accompanies spinal stenosis is usually well shown on T1-weighted MR images. In symptomatic patients with only mild degenerative disease, CT or MRI is useful to detect developmentally shortened pedicles that are associated with a narrowed canal, predisposing to symptoms ("congenital stenosis").

The lateral recess is bordered posteriorly by the superior articular facet, laterally by the pedicle, and anteriorly by the vertebral body and disk. Lumbar lateral recess stenosis results when a hypertrophic superior facet encroaches on the the recess, often in combination with narrowing due to a bulging disk and osteophyte. Compression of the nerve root sleeve in the stenosed lateral recess can mimic a herniated disk clinically. MRI is useful to differentiate lateral recess stenosis from central stenosis and to determine whether or not disk herniation is present.

Foraminal stenosis occurs when a hypertrophic facet, vertebral body osteophyte, or bulging disk narrows the neural foramen and encroaches on the lumbar nerve roots, which are located in the superior portion of the foramen. Fortunately, degenerated disks first narrow the inferior portion of the foramen. When obliteration of the fat normally surrounding the ventral nerve root and the dorsal root ganglia in the foramen is detected on sagittal T1-weighted images, marked encroachment has occurred (Fig. 1).

Cervical Spinal Stenosis

In the cervical spine, central canal stenosis is usually secondary to osteophytosis (spondylosis deformans) and ligamentous thickening or redundancy (PLL and ligamentum flavum). Vertebral endplate changes, as described earlier, are often present. Osteophytic ridging and disk bulge or herniation may be inseparable on MRI and CT and thus are sometimes referred to as disk-osteophyte complex or chon-

dro-osseous spur. Disk degeneration with loss of disk space height contributes to overriding and degeneration of the uncoverterbral joints. Hypertrophy of the uncinate processes and the facets as a result of uncovertebral joint and facet joint osteoarthritis produces foraminal stenosis, and the hypertrophied facets also contribute to the multifactorial central canal stenosis. Symptoms of myelopathy, called cervical spondylotic myelopathy, develop as the central stenosis worsens; radiographic or CT measurements that are predictive for the diagnosis include: (i) decrease in the anteroposterior (AP) diameter of the canal (between C3 and C7) from the normal value of approximately 17 mm to a value in the range from 10 to 14 mm (11 mm is frequently quoted), (ii) decrease in the ratio of the AP diameter of the canal to the AP vertebral body diameter from a value of 1.0 or greater for a normal canal to a value of 0.8 or less, and (iii) a cross-sectional area of the canal less than 60 mm^2. In the diagnosis of foraminal stenosis, CT has been favored, although two- or three-dimensional gradient recalled echo (GRE) MR images are increasingly being used to confirm clinical evidence of radiculopathy due to foraminal stenosis. MRI is the procedure of choice in assessing myelopathy because of the ability to detect abnormalities in size, shape, and signal intensity of the cord. Patients who have abnormal signal intensity within the cervical cord tend to have more severe myelopathic symptoms and signs than patients with normal cord signal. Abnormal signal typically appears as hyperintensity on T2-weighted images and has been attributed to cord compression from the hypertrophic bony and ligamentous changes responsible for central canal stenosis. The intramedullary hyperintensity results from any or all of the following pathological processes: edema, demyelination, gliosis and myelomalacia. Edema is almost certainly a contributor to the hyperintensity in cases where the abnormal signal intensity disappears or diminishes following surgery, as has been observed by several investigators.

Ossification of the posterior longitudinal ligament (OPLL) generally produces severe central canal stenosis and significant myelopathy (Fig. 2). Patients typically present in the sixth decade with upper and lower extremity weakness, dysesthesias, and neck pain. OPLL begins with calcification and progresses to frank ossification, first in the upper cervical spine and then later in the lower cervical and upper thoracic spine. Four types of OPLL have been proposed on the basis of the CT appearance: (i) continuous, with OPLL extending confluently over multiple levels (27% of cases); (ii) segmental, with OPLL limited to the posterior margins of the vertebral bodies (39%); (iii) mixed continuous and segmental OPLL (29%); and (iv) OPLL crossing the disk space only (5%).

CT and plain radiography are probably preferable to MRI in identifying subtle calcification and ossification, yet MRI is valuable for identifying cord compression. The ossified ligament may have fatty marrow and thus increased signal on T1-weighted images. OPLL can be associated with ligamentum flavum calcification and ossification, and when combined, these processes may result

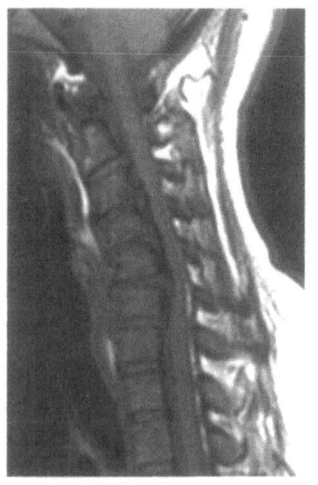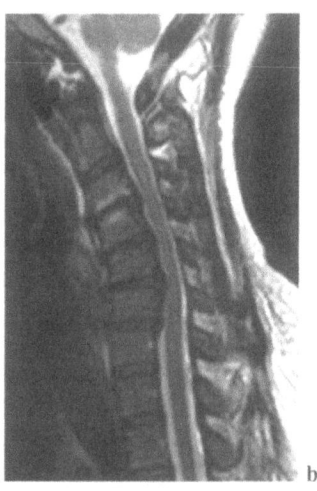

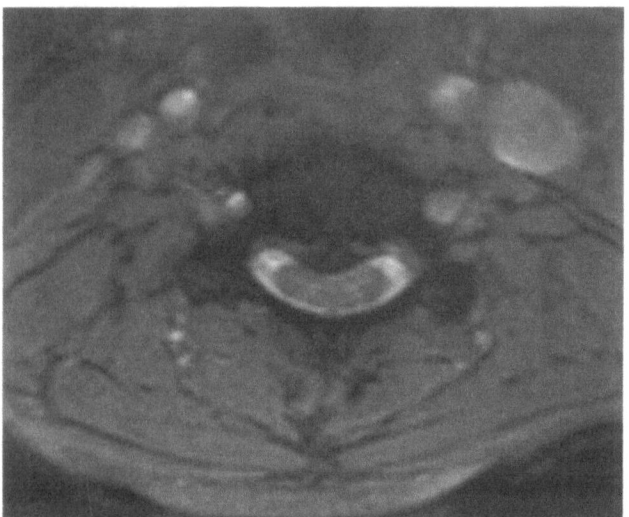

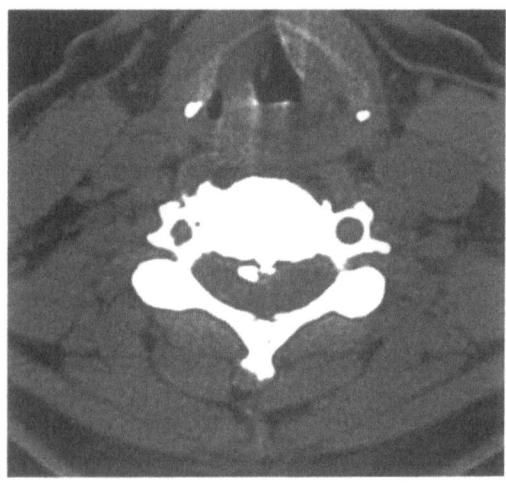

in circumferential compression of the cord. An association of OPLL with diffuse idiopathic skeletal hyperostosis (DISH) has also been reported.

An important finding on CT or MRI is the detection of calcification and ossification at the level of the vertebral body either segmentally or continuously over several levels. This helps to differentiate OPLL (95% of cases) from osteophytes and calcified herniated disks, which should be present at the level of the disk space only. For patients with myelopathy, surgical treatment is aimed at decompressing the cord. Both anterior and posterior approaches are used. In the last decade, numerous studies have shown clinical benefits when multilevel disease is treated with a canal-expansive laminoplasty procedure [9]. This procedure is usually done at each level from C3 to C7, and then bone grafts are placed across the opening at alternate levels (usually C3, C5, and C7) in order to keep the "door" open and the cord uncompressed. The same procedure has been used for many years to successfully treat multilevel cervical spondylotic myelopathy.

Spondylolisthesis

Spondylolisthesis, which is the most frequently observed example of malalignment, is defined as anterior slippage of a vertebra relative to the subjacent vertebra. The slippage is graded on a scale of 1 to 4: one-fourth or less of the vertebral body width is grade 1, one-fourth to one-half is grade 2, one-half to three-fourths is grade 3, and three-fourths to the entire width is grade 4. Grade 1 accounts for more than 90% of cases. The two most common causes are bilateral isthmic (pars interarticularis) defects, referred to as isthmic or spondylolytic spondylolisthesis, and degenerative facet disease resulting in degenerative spondylolisthesis. The pars abnormalities in isthmic spondylolisthesis probably result from a combination of hereditary dysplasia of the pars and repeated stress fractures that result in persistent defects or healing with sclerosis and elongation of the isthmus.

Spondylolisthesis is readily detected with MRI, using direct sagittal imaging, or with CT, using sagittal reformatted images. The pars defects in spondylolysis, though, are more reliably demonstrated with CT and plain radiography. On MRI, evaluation of the pars is optimally done using T1-weighted sagittal images. When the hyperintense signal from marrow extends continuously from the superior articular process through the pars to the inferior articular process, then the pars is intact. Unfortunately, if signal abnormality or discontinuity is present in the pars region, the MRI findings are not specific for a pars defect since they may be due to other etiologies such as partial volume averaging with a degenerated facet, osteoblastic metastasis, or benign sclerosis. Spondylolisthesis is usually accompanied by bulging or "pseudobulging" of the disk. Elongation of the foramina due to vertebral slippage and foraminal encroachment by the bulging disk typically leads to compromise of the

Fig. 2a-d. *Cervical spondylosis with ossification of the posterior longitudinal ligament (OPLL).* Sagittal T1-weighted image (**a**) and fast spin echo T2-weighted image (**b**) reveal osteophytes or disk osteophytes at each intervertebral disk space from C2-3 to C6-7, with cord compression at C4-5 and C5-6. The posterior longitudinal ligament appears to be thickened at several vertebral levels, including C5 where the axial gradient-echo MR image (**c**) and the axial CT image (**d**) demonstrate evidence of OPLL. Note the type 1 endplate changes at C3-4, and the loss of normal cervical lordotic curvature

nerve roots in the foramina. Disk herniation is less common at the level of spondylolisthesis and more common at the level immediately above.

Several congenital clefts of the neural arch have been described. From anterior to posterior along the neural arch, these include persistent neurocentral synchondrosis, retrosomatic cleft, retroisthmic cleft, and spina bifida. Retrosomatic and retroisthmic clefts are usually detected incidentally and should be distinguished from the pars (isthmic) defect in spondylolysis. The frequency of contralateral spondylolysis involving a vertebra with a retroisthmic cleft is many times greater than the prevalence of spondylolysis in the general population.

Postoperative Lumbar Spine

Recurrent or residual low back pain in a patient after lumbar disk surgery has a reported incidence of 5%-40%, and the syndrome has been called the "failed back" or "failed back surgery" syndrome (FBSS). Potential causes include epidural fibrosis ("scar"), recurrent or persistent disk herniation, arachnoiditis, spondylolisthesis, and residual bony stenosis. Ross [10] demonstrated a significant association between the presence of extensive peridural scar and the occurrence of recurrent radicular pain.

Typically, a physician who is caring for a patient with symptoms of FBSS wants to know if the clinical symptoms (recurrent back pain, radiculopathy, and functional incapacitation) are primarily due to scar or disk. The reported accuracy of post-contrast MRI in distinguishing between scar and disk in patients at least 6 weeks after surgery is 96%-100%. Whether the time elapsed since surgery is months or years, scar consistently enhances on images acquired immediately following injection of contrast material. Because it is avascular, the disk does not enhance on these early images (Fig. 3). On delayed images (≥30 min following injection), disk material may enhance because of diffusion of the low molecular weight contrast material (gadolinium chelate) into the disk from adjacent scar, especially when there is a relatively large volume of scar compared to the volume of herniation. A secondary sign that favors scar over recurrent or persistent disk is retraction of the thecal sac toward the region of aberrant epidural soft tissue. The presence of mass effect is not helpful since both epidural scar and disk can produce this finding. The addition of a frequency-selective fat-saturated pulse sequence to the routine post-contrast T1-weighted images has been found to improve visualization of enhancing scar, help distinguish scar from recurrent herniated disk, and more clearly show the relationship of scar to nerve roots and thecal sac.

Lumbar arachnoiditis, which has been cited as a cause of FBSS in up to 16% of cases, can have a variable appearance and has been categorized into three groups or patterns. These patterns, which may overlap, can be observed with myelography, CT myelography, or MRI, and

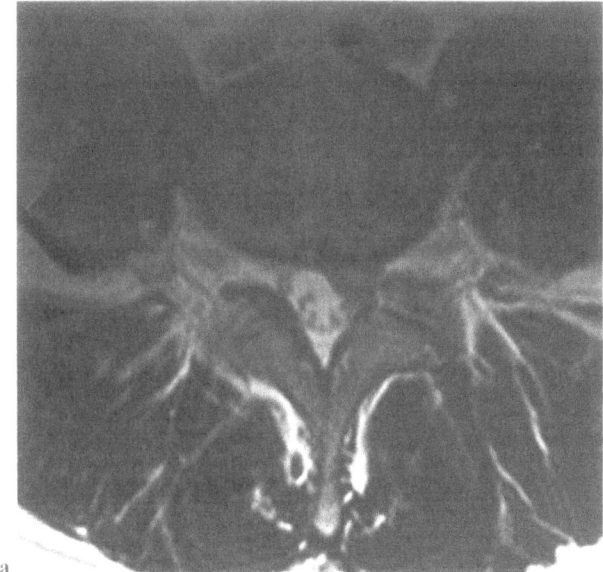

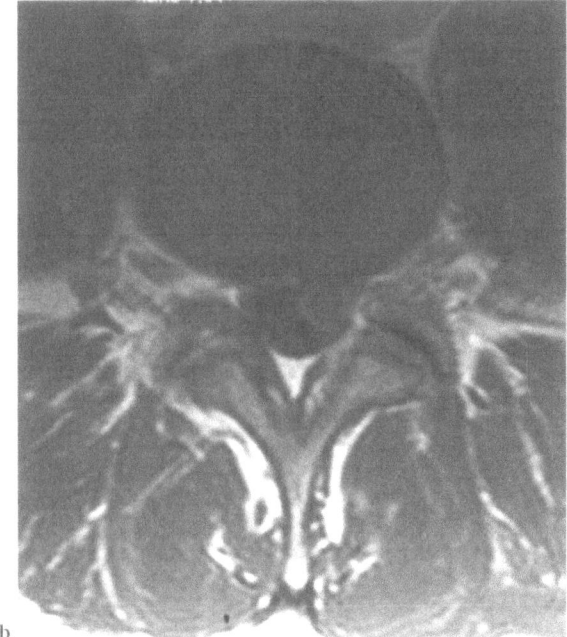

Fig. 3a, b. *Postoperative, recurrent lumbar disk herniation.* Axial T2-weighted (**a**) and post-contrast T1-weighted (**b**) images at the L4-5 level show thinning and disruption of the left ligamentum flavum, consistent with a previous left partial laminectomy. On the T2-weighted image, the soft tissue mass in the left side of the canal could be scar or recurrent disk herniation. On the post-contrast T1-weighted image, the bulk of the mass does not enhance, which is consistent with recurrent disk herniation. The thin rim of enhancement bordering the mass represents mild adjacent scarring

differ from the normal feathery appearance of the nerve roots surrounded by fluid. Pattern 1 is clumping of nerve roots into cords and represents central adhesion of the roots within the thecal sac. Pattern 2 is referred to as the "empty thecal sac" sign and represents adhesion of the nerve roots to the meninges. In pattern 3, the thecal sac is filled by a mass, representing the end-stage of the inflammatory response. On myelography, this appears as a block with an irregular "candle-dripping" appearance, whereas CT myelography and MRI show only a non-specific soft tissue mass. Arachnoiditis may or may not show enhancement on post-contrast T1-weighted images, and the diagnosis is best made on the basis of the morphology of the roots and sac.

References

1. Bowen BC (2001) Spine imaging: case review. Mosby, Philadelphia
2. Pfirrmann CW, Metzdorf A, Zanetti M, Hodler J, Boos N (2001) Magnetic resonance classification of lumbar intervertebral disc degeneration. Spine 26:1873-1878
3. Tanaka N, An HS, Lim TH, Fujiwara A, Jeon CH, Haughton VM (2001) The relationship between disc degeneration and flexibility of the lumbar spine. Spine J 1:47-56
4. Czervionke LF, Haughton VM (2002) Degenerative disease of the spine. In: Atlas SW (ed) Magnetic resonance imaging of the brain and spine, 3rd edn. Lippincott Williams Wilkins, Philadelphia, pp 1633-1713
5. Fardon DE, Milette PC (2001) Nomenclature and classification of lumbar disc pathology: recommendations of the combined task forces of the North American Spine Society, American Society of Spine Radiology, and American Society of Neuroradiology. Spine 26:E93-E113
6. Schellinger D, Manz HJ, Vidic B, Patronas NJ, Deveikis JP, Muraki AS, Abdullah DC (1990) Disk fragment migration. Radiology 175:831-836
7. Lane JI, Koeller KK, Atkinson LD (1994) Enhanced lumbar nerve roots in the spine without prior surgery: radiculitis or radicular veins? AJNR Am J Neuroradiol 15:1317-1325
8. Wagner AL, Murtagh FR, Arrington JA, Stallworth D (2000) Relationship of Schmorl's nodes to vertebral body endplate fractures and acute endplate disk extrusions. AJNR Am J Neuroradiol 21:276-281
9. Lee TT, Manzano GR, Green BA (1997) Modified open-door cervical expansive laminoplasty for spondylotic myelopathy: operative technique, outcome, and predictors for gait improvement. J Neurosurg 86:64-68
10. Ross JS (1999) MR imaging of the postoperative lumbar spine. Magn Reson Imaging Clin N Am 7:513-524

Degenerative Diseases and Pain Syndromes

J.L. Drapé

CHU Cochin, Radiology Service B, Paris, France

Introduction

Degenerative disease of the lumbar spine is very common, affecting two-thirds of adults during their lifetimes. It represents a real public health challenge due to costs resulting in lost days of work and a high rate of invalidity.

Imaging modalities may demonstrate physiological mechanisms of low back pain as well as radiculalgia and allow adequate therapy to be administered. Radioclinical correlation is mandatory due to the high rate of abnormal findings demonstrated even in asymptomatic patients. This presentation is not exhaustive but discusses particular points concerning diskopathies (erosive or calcifying), annular tears, Schmorl's nodes, C1-C2 osteoarthritis and lumbar spine stenosis.

Erosive Disk Disease

Common degenerative disk disease (DDD) is usually easily diagnosed. Nevertheless, DDD may be erosive in some cases, resulting in inflammatory type pain, and may be confused with infectious diskitis. These erosive disk diseases (EDDs) may cause disk lysis (loss of 50% of disk height in less than two years) or vertebral instability [1]. Erosions of vertebral endplates, with disk space narrowing on plain films or abnormal signal intensity of disk or vertebral endplates on magnetic resonance imaging (MRI), are suggestive of spondylodiskitis [2].

Lumbar spine involvement and higher frequency in males are common in both DDD and EDD. In case of multiple EDD, calcium pyrophosphate deposition disease (CPPD) must be suspected.

On plain radiography and computed tomography (CT), four signs suggest EDD [3]:
- Small erosions with peripheral sclerosis and well-defined margins,
- Osteosclerosis of adjacent vertebral endplates, anterior in location, with large, well-defined dome-shaped limits,
- "Excentered" osteophytes suggestive of instability [4],

- Intradiskal gas [5] phenomenon that may be better demonstrated on stress view in hyperextension.

On MRI examination, disk and vertebral endplates demonstrate low signal intensity on T2-weighted images, although areas of high signal intensity may be present in case of intradiskal gas bubbles secondarily filled with fluid in decubitus [6]. Linear or focal contrast enhancement of vertebral endplates suggests lesions of annulus or vertebra [7]. Displacement of the common vertebral ligament by osteophytes must not be confused with abscess. Edematous signal intensity (Modic 1) of the vertebral endplates is poorly suggestive. These modifications occur in 4% of DDD but in 100% of EDD [8]. An area of fatty infiltration (Modic 2) commonly surrounds these areas of low signal intensity on T1-weighted images. Evolution of Modic 1 into Modic 2 is possible.

In rare cases, imaging does not allow diagnosis and percutaneous bone, and disk biopsies are mandatory.

Idiopathic Calcifying Disk Disease

Disk calcification, a common and incidental finding, is idiopathic in origin [9]. In children, calcification is commonly seen in cervical spine. In adults, it is more common in thoracic and lumbar spines. Cadaveric correlations in elderly people demonstrated calcifications of the annulus fibrosus in 71% of cases [10].

Symptomatic calcifications are usually central in location and suggestive of apatite depositions. Thinner and peripheral calcifications are more suggestive of CPPD.

Clinical findings are variable and include asymptomatic manifestations and central cord compression due to large thoracic calcified disk herniation. Inflammatory type pain may simulate diskitis. Linear calcifications may suggest calcified disk herniation with associated fissure of the annulus. As in calcified tendinitis, calcification may disappear following pain manifestation.

During the inflammatory phase, uptake on bone scans is common in disk as well as in vertebral bodies. Signal hyperintensity on T1-weighted images, close to the calcification, may be seen [11].

Painful Disk without Herniation

The diskoradicular impingement by herniated disk is the commonest etiology of lumboradiculalgia. The acute compression of a normal peripheral nerve is usually painless but accompanied by dysesthesiae. The radicular suffering may be mechanical but also secondary to inflammatory, chemical or scarring reactions or disturbed microvascularization. Some pains of the lower limbs associated with low back pain may be not situated along a dermatoma; therefore the term "radiculopathy" is used [12]. These atypical pains are often associated with disk abnormalities without diskoradicular impingement. Imaging may reveal intradiskal tears.

Three types of CT abnormalities may be evocative of disk tear:
- Disk hypodensity. Normally the disk is homogeneous with a density (80 HU) greater than that of muscle. Posterior peripheral hypodensity may be observed at a median or paramedian location. This hypodensity may be more or less extensive. It is usually associated with a small disk irregularity, without a true herniation.
- Irregularities or notch of the inferior or superior vertebral plates. The defect of the listel of the vertebral plate is more or less regular, concave, and median or paramedian. It is evocative of an avulsion of the peripheral fibers of the annulus and may favor the development of a true herniation.
- Soft tissue abnormalities in front of the defect of the vertebral plate. The association of a small convex area of intermediate or disk density surrounding the defect is in favor of an annular abnormality. Some small iso- or hyperdense areas at the periphery of the disk may be due to inflammatory reaction or disk microfragments.

On MRI, diffuse low signal intensity of the disk is suggestive of DDD. Peripheral areas of the disk as well as the posterior common vertebral ligament must be carefully studied. Focal signal abnormalities (high T2 focus or contrast enhancement) may be noted. Fast T1-weighted spin echo sequences are sensitive. Clinical significance of these abnormalities is debated since they may be present in asymptomatic patients [13]. In contrast, obvious signal abnormalities on T2-weighted images may correspond to annular tear demonstrated by diskography or diskoCT [14].

Spreading, linear or oval-shaped, peripheral signal abnormalities are suggestive of causal disk , particularly in association with abnormalities of the bone-annulus junction.

Schmorl's Nodes

Schmorl's nodes (SN) are commonly found in cadaveric studies and are frequently seen on MRI in asymptomatic patients [15]. Less than one-third of SN are demonstrated by plain films. Plain film sensitivity depends on node size and surrounding adjacent bony osteosclerosis. Large nodes are commonly symptomatic. They must not be confused with a tumoral or infectious process. They are idiopathic in origin or secondary to axial stress. Repair mechanisms are possible with secondary ossification; incidence declines with age [16].

The nature of Schmorl's nodes is variable and includes cartilage matrix, fibrous scary tissue and peripheral vascular proliferation. MRI demonstrates vascularized nodes following gadolinium infusion. Enhancement is more suggestive of repair phenomenon than symptomatic node. Associated edematous manifestations of vertebral endplates (similar to Modic 1 in DDD) are noted in one-third of enhancing nodes and are more common when symptomatic [15].

C1-C2 Osteoarthritis

C1-C2 osteoarthritis (C1-C2 OA) may cause obstinate cervical or occipital pain. It is responsible for unilateral cervical or occipital pain, head ache and retroauricular pain [17], and usually occurs in aged women with multiple osteoarthritic locations. Limitation of rotation is frequent. Only 4% of patients with peripheral OA present C1-C2 OA.

Diagnosis is made on the open mouth view. Lateral or rotating instabilities of C1-C2 result from severe asymmetric cartilage narrowing. Most often, lesions are unilateral in location, at the right side, better demonstrated by volumic CT with multiplanar reconstructions.

MRI may be confusing, demonstrating bone edema or synovial proliferation. Medical treatment includes C1-C2 block with steroid administration by a posterior or lateral approach.

Atlanto-odontoid osteoarthritis is more frequent than lateral C1-C2 OA. Symptoms include occipital pain [18]. Lateral view is more informative than the open mouth view due to multiple superimpositions (e.g. styloids, mandible).

On the anteroposterior view, osteophytes of the superior and lateral aspects of C1 result in a horseshoe calcification mimicking CPPD. Lateral view may emphasize lesions [19]. Volumic CT remains the best modality to demonstrate C1-C2 OA. Joint space narrowing, articular gas bubbles, ostephytes and periarticular ossifications are common, as are transverse ligament calcifications. Direct intra-articular steroid administration is uncommon and rather difficult due to the dangerous anatomic relationship. Lateral C1-C2 steroid administration remains possible but communication with atlanto-odontoid joint occurs only in 20% of cases [20].

Lumbar Spine Stenosis and MR Myelography

Degenerative lumbar spine stenosis (DLSS) is common in elderly people. Stenosis may be central or lateral in location due to osseous or ligamental hypertrophy. Usually, stenosis involves multiple levels and is symmetrical. Plain films, CT and myelography are commonly used techniques but may emphasize lesions.

The value of routine MR myelography remains poor (6%) except for evaluation of DLSS [21]. Three-dimensional (3D) myelographic sequences with maximum intensity projection (MIP) reformations or ultrafast thick single slices are informative about the degree of stenosis as well as effusions in facet joints [22]. Facet joint effusion is common in OA. It results from active OA but not always at the most severely involved level. Synovial cyst may occur, causing nerve root impingement.

Communication between facet joints at the same level may be present through the interspinous bursa. This communication is seen by facet joint arthrography [23]. Interspinous bursitis may be symptomatic (Baastrup's disease or kissing spine).

Plain films demonstrate facet joint OA, DDD causing disk space narrowing and bony remodeling of large spinous processes particularly at the L4-L5 level [24]. Only MRI directly demonstrates interspinous bursitis that may be inflammatory or calcified. Steroid administration is possible during bursography, which may also demonstrate communication with facet joints or intracanalar diverticulae.

References

1. Revel M, Beaudreuil P, Dieude S, Poiraudeau S (1998) La discopathie destructrice rapide. In: Morvan G, Deburge A, Bard H, Laredo JD (eds) Le rachis lombaire dégénératif. Sauramps Médical, Montpellier, pp 279-283
2. Stoller DW, Steinkirchner TM, Porter BA (1997) The spine. In: Stoller DW (ed) Magnetic resonance imaging in orthopaedics and sports medicine, 2nd end. Lippincott Williams Wilkins, Philadelphia, pp 1059-1162
3. Modic MT, Masaryk TJ, Ross JS (1988) Imaging of degenerative disk disease. Radiology 168:177
4. McNab I (1971) The traction spur. An indicator of segmental instability. J Bone Joint Surg Am 53:663-670
5. Lardé D, Mathieu D, Frija J (1982) Spinal vacuum phenomenon: CT diagnosis and significance. J Comput Assist Tomogr 6:671
6. Malghem J, Maldague B, Labaisse MA (1993) Intervertebral vacuum cleft: changes in content after supine positioning. Radiology 187:483
7. Stabler A, Weiss M, Scheidler J (1996) Degenerative disk vascularisation on MRI: correlation with clinical and histopathologic findings. Skeletal Radiol 25:119-126
8. Modic MT, Steinberg PM, Ross JS (1988) Degenerative disk disease: asssessment of changes in vertebral body marrow with MR imaging. Radiology 166:193
9. Ballou SP, Khan MA, Kushner I (1977) Diffuse intervertebral disc calcification in primary amyloidosis. Ann Intern Med 85:616-617
10. Weinberger A, Myers AR (1978) Intervertebral disc calcification in adults: a review. Semin Arthritis Rheum 1:69-75
11. Bangert BA, Modic MT, Ross JS, Obuchowski NA, Perl PJ, Ruggieri PM, Masaryk TJ (1995) Hyperintense disks on T1-weighted MR images: correlation with calcification. Radiology 195:437-443
12. Millette PC (1994) Radiculopathy, radicuar pain, radiating pain, referred pain: what are we really talking about? Radiology 192:281-282
13. Stadnik TW, Lee RR, Coen HL, Neirynck EC, Buisseret TS, Osteaux MJL (1998) Annular tears and disk herniation: prevalence and contrast enhancement on MR images in the absence of low back pain or sciatica. Radiology 206:49-55
14. Schellhas KP, Pollei SR, Gundry CR, Heithoff KB (1996) Lumbar disc high intensity zone: correlation of magnetic resonance imaging and discography. Spine 21:79-80
15. Stäbler A, Bellan M, Weiss M, Gärtner C, Brossmann J, Reiser MF (1997) MR imaging of enhancing intraosseous disk herniation (Schmorl's nodes). AJR Am J Roentgenol 168:933-938
16. Hamanishi C, Kawabata T, Yosii T, Tanaka S (1994) Schmorl's nodes on magnetic resonance imaging: their incidence and clinical relevance. Spine 19:450-453
17. Ehni G, Benner B (1984) Occipital neuralgia and the C1-C2 arthrosis syndrome. J Neurosurg 61:961-965
18. Zapletal J, Hekster RE, Straver JS, Wilmink JT, Hermans J (1996) Relationship between atlanto-odontoid osteoarthritis and idiopathic suboccipital neck pain. Neuroradiology 38:62-65
19. Zapletal J, Hekster RE, Wilmink JT, Hermans J, Mallens WM (1995) Atlanto-odontoid osteoarthritis: comparison of lateral cervical projection and CT. Eur Spine 4: 238-241
20. Chevrot A, Cermakova E, Vallée C, Chancelier MD, Chemla N, Rousselin B, Langer-Cherbit A (1995) C1-C2 arthrography. Skeletal Radiol 24:425-429
21. O'Connell MJ, Ryan M, Powell, T, Eustace S (2003) The value of routine MR myelography at MRI of the lumbar spine. Acta Radiol 44:665-672
22. Nagayama M, Watanabe Y, Okumura A, Amoh Y, Nakashita S, Dodo Y (2002) High-resolution single-slice MR myelography. AJR Am J Roentgenol 179:515-521
23. Sarazin L, Chevrot A, Pessis E, Minoui A, Drapé JL, Chemla N, Godefroy D (1999) Lumbar facet joint arthrography with the posterior approach. Radiographics 19:93-104
24. Bywaters EG, Evans S (1982) The lumbar interspinous bursae and Baastrup's syndrome. An autopsy study. Rheumatol Int 2:87-96

Neoplastic Spinal Cord Disease

D.L. Balériaux

Neuroradiology Clinic, Department of Radiology, Erasme University Hospital, Free University of Brussels, Brussels, Belgium

Introduction

Spinal cord tumors are rare. Every radiologist should be able to recognize and readily identify those lesions often found in younger patients or children. Early diagnosis plays an important role in the management of the lesions and will interfere with the prognosis and final outcome of the patient. Clinical symptoms of cord tumors are usually of insidious onset: pain may be for long the only complaint while motor deficits often appear later. Before the advent of magnetic resonance imaging (MRI), the diagnosis of a spinal cord tumor was often delayed. It is important, however, to diagnose those tumors at an early stage as new, efficient, surgical techniques including the use of Cavitron ultrasound aspiration (CUSA) may heal the patient or at least stop tumor evolution. Adequate management by using the proper diagnostic tools and careful analysis of the MR images help describe important features such as solid nodule, cystic components, associated hydrosyringomyelia and guide the surgeon. On the other hand, intramedullary lesions with mass effect may mimic spinal cord neoplasm: differential diagnosis is essential to avoid unnecessary surgery and to plan and guide adequate biopsy if required.

Examination Techniques

Plain Radiography

Standard X-ray films provide poor if no information at all concerning the intraspinal content. Still, mainly in young children and infants, a slow-growing intramedullary tumor may enlarge the spinal canal. The lower thoracic canal is often expanded in cases of a myxopapillary ependymoma of the conus. In the literature, scoliosis is classically mentioned as being present in cases of intracanalar intramedullary tumors: any evolving scoliosis should at least raise the question of a possible underlying tumor. Spinal deformity is reported to occur in 46% of pediatric spinal cord neoplasms. Torticolis or even a permanent "stiff neck" should also alert the radiologist and prompt a neurological examination with, if necessary, an immediate MRI examination. Loss of the normal cervical lordosis detected on a sagittal plain film should prompt further investigate into the origin of the major pain presented by the patient.

Computed Tomography

The intracanalar content is increasingly visible with the recently developed computed tomography (CT) protocols. Still, subtle cord enlargement, small cystic components and spinal root anomalies are not easily detected with CT. Calcifications are rare in intramedullary tumors. For those reasons, I recommend not wasting time with plain spinal CT and suggest performing MRI immediately. If MRI is not readily available, CT combined with intrathecal contrast medium injection (myelo-CT) is a good alternative examination. Still, one should be aware that neurological worsening of the patient's status may occur following lumbar puncture in cases of large intramedullary tumors.

Myelography

This has been the standard imaging procedure used for the diagnosis of intraspinal pathology. Still, it provides only an "indirect" approach, showing the contours and shape of the cord without the inner structure. Moreover, in case of myelographic "block", only the inferior (when the injection is made by lumbar route) or superior (with suboccipital injection) limits of the tumor infiltration can be assessed. Myelo-CT is a useful complementary examination, as CT is more sensitive and usually allows determining both limits of the tumor. Myelo-CT also allows progressive or delayed enhancement of intramedullary cavities. Today, both myelography and myelo-CT should still be used by radiologists for the rare cases of patients excluded from MRI, but the techniques should definitely be abandoned in favor of MRI whenever possible.

Magnetic Resonance Imaging

MRI examination of the spine must systematically include the use of at least two different imaging planes (usually sagittal and axial), two different imaging techniques (T1- and T2-weighted imaging) and gadolinium-enhanced T1-weighted images. MRI shows not only the shape of the cord (external contours) but also the internal changes within the cord. I recommend that every signal behavior anomaly as well as every change in shape and morphology of the cord be systematically described to answer some fundamental questions:

- Is the lesion a neoplasm or an inflammatory or infectious mass?
- Is the lesion intra- or extramedullary?
- If the lesion is a neoplasm, where is the solid neoplastic infiltration? Can the tumor limits be described with confidence? Are the borders well defined?
- If there are cystic components, are they intratumoral or extratumoral, the so-called associated cysts due to enlargement of the ependymal canal?
- How do these components change after gadolinium injection? Indeed, the borders of a "satellite" or associated cyst do not enhance, contrary to those of a tumoral cyst.

Secondary dilatation of the ependymal canal (hydromyelia) is often associated with spinal cord tumors: at the C0-C1 level we sometimes observe a focal, more important enlargement of the ependymal canal that we call a "bulbar cyst" (Fig. 1). In fact, a syrinx is more likely to be found above (49%) than below (11%) the tumor level. In 40% of cases, a syrinx can be identified above and below a tumor. Ependymoma and hemangioblastoma are the most common tumors to be associated with syringes.

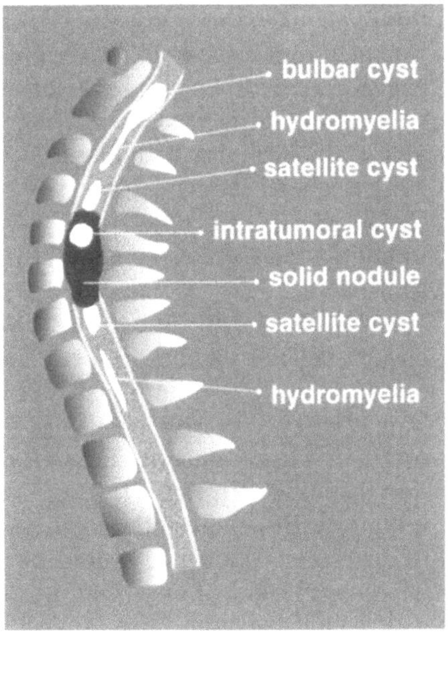

Fig. 1. Various components and anomalies identified on an MR image in cases of intramedullary tumoral lesions. (Reproduced with permission from *MRI of Spinal Cord Lesions*, an educational CD-ROM. Lasion, Aartselaar, Belgium)

MR Myelography

This technique provides heavily T2-weighted images simulating typical myelographic images. This noninvasive and elegant technique shows nicely not only the spinal roots but also the vascular structures on the surface of the cord. It helps to define the intramedullary cyst-like cavities.

Spinal Angiography and MR Angiography

"Conventional" digital angiography is rarely performed for intramedullary tumors. Nevertheless, it should be performed whenever a true arteriovenous malformation is suspected on the basis of standard MR images or in the rare cases in which it is mandatory to know exactly where the artery of Adamkiewicz originates. Nowadays, MR angiography is available but spatial resolution is usually not sufficient to be able to study spinal vessels of small caliber.

Spinal Cord Neoplasms

Tumors of the spinal cord are rare. In a general hospital, only 5% of spinal tumors are intramedullary, while 40% are intradural extramedullary and 55% are extradural. Astrocytoma, ependymoma and hemangioblastoma are the most frequent tumors: they should be recognized preoperatively because surgical management as well as prognosis vary according to tumor histology.

In adults, ependymomas represent 60% of all intramedullary tumors. Astrocytomas account for about 30% of spinal cord gliomas. Hemangioblastomas are less frequent and represent 5%. Clinical presentation is poorly specific; pain is the most common finding and usually the first symptom to be reported. Sensory and motor deficits are variable and occur in function of tumor localization. Urinary disturbances and impotence are rare and appear late in the clinical course of the disease: they occur usually coincident with motor paralysis of the legs.

In children, astrocytoma is far the most frequent intramedullary neoplasm. In fact, my colleagues and I have never observed a case of ependymoma in a child, and the cases reported in the literature are few. In children, pain is equally the most frequent symptom, reported in 42% of cases. Motor regression is present in 36%, gait abnormality in 27%, torticolis in 27% and progressive kyphoscoliosis in 24% of cases; 89% are low-grade lesions.

Astrocytoma, even in adults, is mostly encountered in younger patients (mean age in our series, 29 years) with a predominance of males (63%). Astrocytomas involve mostly large portions of the cord and frequently harbor cystic components. Satellite cysts and secondary hydromyelia can also be observed. Associated edema is often moderate and contrast enhancement is relatively mild and heterogeneous.

Astrocytomas are found more often in the thoracic spine but may occupy any part of the cord. Seventy-five percent of astrocytomas are of low grade and progress slowly, while 25% are aggressive and high grade. An astrocytoma is usually eccentrically located and exhibits heterogeneous, moderate, and partial contrast enhancement after gadolinium injection. Astrocytoma borders are frequently ill defined.

Ependymomas are usually smaller and are preferentially located in the cervical or cervicothoracic spine. They originate from ependymal cells lining the ependymal canal and therefore are typically centered in the middle of the cord. Most are benign although malignant types may occur. They often show associated satellite or bulbar cysts. The enhancement after gadolinium administration is usually more homogeneous and intense compared to that of astrocytoma. Tumor borders are usually well defined. Moreover, a rather specific "cap sign" is often found in ependymomas: it corresponds to the presence of hypointense areas, capping both ends of the tumor. This sign is best seen on gradient echo images as it is in fact due to deposits of hemosiderin, the result of frequent chronic bleeding in ependymoma. Still, intratumoral hemorrhage may also occur in astrocytomas, explaining the sudden worsening of the neurological deficits. Recent bleeding is shown as hyperintense areas on T1-weighted images. In my experience, gross total removal is possible in 70% of cases of ependymoma, in comparison to 33% of astrocytomas.

Hemangioblastomas are richly vascularized tumors, usually located sub-pially. They have two typical presentations: either as a small tumoral nodule associated with extensive edema, or as a small nodular tumor associated with an extensive cystic, often polylobulated cavity. The nodule always enhances strongly after gadolinium injection. These tumors can be either solitary or multiple (if associated with von Hippel-Lindau disease).

An *intramedullary lymphoma* may occur as part of a multifocal lymphoma, with cerebral, cerebellar or brain stem lesions associated with the intramedullary lesion. Primary intramedullary lymphoma is rare.

Spinal cord *metastases* are reported to be rare: in my experience, however, they are easier to diagnose and occur probably more frequently than reported in the literature. Still, it is difficult to ascertain the true incidence of spinal cord metastases, as the clinical picture often is atypical and the lesions are seen in terminally ill patients. Autopsy is also biased, as the cord is often not systematically examined. On the other hand, 2.4% of metastases removed surgically from the central nervous system (CNS) are located in the cord. Clinical symptoms are often non-specific, but usually involve root pain. Today, the exquisite sensitivity of MRI enables intramedullary metastases to be easily detected. No specific MRI characteristics are seen. Usually they are small, nodular, well-defined lesions that are hypointense on T2-weighted images. The enhancement pattern may be either ring-like or homogeneous and intense. It is rare that a primary cancer is discovered by the identification of a solitary intramedullary metastasis.

Gangliogliomas are rare tumors, representing 3.8% of all CNS tumors. They involve the upper cervical cord in the great majority of cases. One-third of gangliogliomas are seen in children, where spinal cord involvement (1.7%) is greater than cerebral (1.4%) or cerebellar (0.7%) involvement.

Oligodendrogliomas are rare in the spinal cord. They exhibit no specific MRI characteristics. However, the few cases in my experience were relatively small tumors (involving two vertebral segments), with ill-defined borders and slight hyperintensity on T1-weighted images. No peritumoral edema or contrast enhancement was seen.

Lipomas are relatively rare spinal cord tumors, representing 6% of intramedullary tumors in our series. True intramedullary lipoma must be differentiated from cauda equina lipomas or lipomas associated with dysraphism, since the clinical, radiological, and surgical issues raised by these lesions are totally different. Although these tumors appear well-defined on MRI, often no cleavage plane from the surrounding spinal cord is found at surgery. Therefore, the tumor usually cannot be completely resected without causing severe neurological damage. The typical hyperintensity of lipomas on T1-weighted images makes these lesions easy to diagnose with MRI.

Cavernomas are vascular malformations that may remain clinically silent for a long period of time. Often they are responsible for an acute or rapidly progressive medullary neurological deficit. Cavernomas represent 2.4% of all intramedullary tumors. All cases present with hemorrhage. Before the advent of MRI, these lesions were extremely difficult to diagnose, especially in the spinal cord, as they usually are small and do not enlarge the spinal cord. On the other hand, on MRI, intramedullary cavernomas (or cavernous hemangiomas) are usually easily recognized. A reticulated appearance with areas of mixed signal intensity on both T1- and T2- or T2*-weighted images is the most common finding. A prominent rim of decreased signal intensity is less commonly seen than in the brain. Contrast enhancement may occur. As cavernomas may be multiple, I recommend cerebral MRI whenever the diagnosis of cavernoma is suspected. If multiple, similar lesions are found in the brain, this should support a final diagnosis of cavernoma of the spinal cord.

Schwannomas originate from Schwann cells and are always located on the posterior nerve root. This explains why schwannomas classically are extramedullary and are responsible for spinal cord compression. Less frequently they may be both extra- and intramedullary. In rare instances, they may be strictly intramedullary. Pure intramedullary schwannomas are well-defined, isointense lesions on T1- and T2-weighted images with homogeneous enhancement after gadolinium injection.

Differential Diagnosis

Numerous non-neoplastic intramedullary lesions may simulate tumor infiltration and should be diagnosed properly in order to avoid unnecessary biopsy. Typically, those lesions include multiple sclerosis (MS) plaques, inflammatory lesions, granulomas, and abscesses. Sarcoidosis is rare in the spinal cord. Diagnosis of an intramedullary lesion is facilitated when the patient has known systemic sarcoidosis. We observed two cases in which the patients had solitary spinal cord lesions presenting as intramedullary tumors. MRI demonstrated non-specific findings of a nodular lesion that strongly enhanced on gadolinium-enhanced T1-weighted images. Sarcoidosis should thus be included in the differential diagnosis of a nodular lesion. Biopsy may be required and should be performed to establish the diagnosis when no systemic signs of sarcoidosis are known.

Important concepts have to be kept in mind: every tumor does not necessarily enhance and conversely every enhancing mass is not a tumor. Extensive mass lesions, on the contrary, are most likely to be neoplasms.

Conclusions

MRI is the optimal imaging modality for the diagnosis of intramedullary neoplasms. The radiologist has an important role to play in carefully identifying and describing the lesion as well as suggesting the proper histological analysis for appropriate management and surgical treatment.

Suggested Reading

Balériaux D, Parizel P, Bank WO (1992) Intraspinal and intramedullary pathology. In: Manelfe C (ed) Imaging of the spine and spinal cord. Raven, New York, pp 513-564

Balériaux D (1999) MRI of spinal cord diseases, 2nd edn. Lasion, (educational CD-ROM) Aartselaar, Belgium

Brotchi J, Dewitte O, Levivier M, Balériaux D, Vandesteene A, Raftopoulos C, Flament Durand J, Noterman J (1991) A survey of 65 tumors within the spinal cord: surgical results and the importance of preoperative magnetic resonance imaging. Neurosurgery 29:651-657

Bourgouin PM, Lesage J, Fontaine S, Konan A, Roy D, Bard C, Del Carpio O'Donovan R (1998) A pattern approach to the differential diagnosis of intramedullary spinal cord lesions on MR imaging. AJR Am J Roentgenol 170(6):1645-1649

Brotchi J (2002) Intrinsic spinal cord tumor resection. Neurosurgery 50(5):1059-1063

Bydder GM, Brown J, Niendorf HP, Young IR (1985) Enhancement of cervical intraspinal tumors in MR imaging with intravenous gadolinium-DTPA. J Comput Assist Tomogr 9:847-851

Colombo N, Kucharczyk W, Brant-Zawadzki M, Norman D, Scotti G, Newton TH (1986) Magnetic resonance imaging of spinal cord hemangioblastoma. Acta Radiol (Diagn) 769:S734-S737

Constantini S, Houten J, Miller DC, Freed D, Ozek MM, Rorke LB, Allen JC, Epstein FJ (1996) Intramedullary spinal cord tumors in children under the age of 3 years. J Neurosurg 85(6):1036-1043

Edal E, Balériaux D, Metens T, David P, Yang P, Roger T, Moreau J (1997) Three-dimensional turbo spin echo cervical magnetic resonance myelography. Int J Neuroradiol 3:130-135

Epstein FJ, Farmer JP, Freed D (1992) Adult intramedullary astrocytomas of the spinal cord. J Neurosurg 77:355-359

Epstein FJ, Farmer JP, Freed D (1993) Adult intramedullary spinal cord ependymomas: the result of surgery in 38 patients. J Neurosurg 79(2):204-209

Fine MJ, Kricheff II, Freed D, Epstein FJ (1995) Spinal cord ependymomas: MR imaging features. Radiology 197(3):655-658

Fischer G, Brotchi J (1996) Intramedullar spinal cord tumors. Thieme, Stuttgart New York

Friedman DP, Hollander MD (1998) Neuroradiology case of the day. Myxopapillary ependymoma of the conus medullaris or filum terminale resulting in superficial siderosis and dissemination of tumor along CSF pathways. Radiographics 18(3):794-798

Hamburger C, Buttner A, Weis S (1997) Ganglioglioma of the spinal cord: report of two rare cases and review of the literature. Neurosurgery 41(6):1410-1415

Innocenzi G, Cervoni L, Caruso R (1997) Intramedullary cervical neurinoma. A case report and review of the literature. Minerva Chir 52(5):679-682

Innocenzi G, Raco A, Cantore G, Raimondi AJ (1996) Intramedullary astrocytomas and ependymomas in the pediatric age group: a retrospective study. Childs Nerv Syst 12(12):776-780

Ijaz T, Jones K (1997) Images in clinical medicine. Intramedullary spinal cord metastases. N Engl J Med 336(11):768

Kahan H, Sklar EML, Donovan Post MJ, Bruce JH (1996) MR characteristics of histopathologic subtypes of spinal ependymoma. AJNR Am J Neuroradiol 17:143-150

Koeller KK, Rosenblum RS, Morrison AL (2000) Neoplasms of the spinal cord and filum terminale: radiologic-pathologic correlation. Radiographics 20:1721-1749

Lahanis S, Vlahos L, Gouliamos A, Papavasiliou C (1993) Arteriovenous malformation of the spinal cord mimicking a tumor. Neuroradiology 35(8):598-599

Levivier M, Brotchi J, Balériaux D, Pirotte B, Flament-Durand J (1991) Sarcoidosis presenting as an isolated intramedullary tumor. Neurosurgery 25:271-276

Li MH, Holtas S (1991) MR imaging of spinal intramedullary tumors. Acta Radiol 32(6):505-513

Lonjon M, Goh KY, Epstein FJ (1998) Intramedullary spinal cord ependymomas in children: treatment, results and follow-up. Pediatr Neurosurg 29(4):178-183

Lunardi P, Licastro G, Missori P, Ferrante L, Fortuna A (1993) Management of intramedullary tumors in children. Acta Neurochir (Wien) 120(1-2):59-65

McCormick PC, Torres R, Post KD, Stein BM (1990) Intramedullary ependymoma of the spinal cord. J Neurosurg 72(4):523-532

Minami M, Hanakita J, Suwa H, Suzui H, Fujita K, Nakamura T (1998) Cervical hemangioblastoma with a past history of subarachnoid hemorrhage. Surg Neurol 49(3):278-281

Nadkarni TD, Rekate KL (1999) Pediatric intramedullary spinal cord tumors. Critical review of the literature. Childs Nerv Syst 15(1):17-28

Ng TH et al (1991) Ganglioneuroma of the spinal cord. Surg Neurol 35(2):147-151

Osborn AG (1994) Tumors, cysts and tumorlike lesions of the spine and spinal cord. In: Osborn AG (ed) Diagnostic neuroradiology. Mosby, St. Louis, pp 876-918

Papadatos D, Albrecht S, Mohr G, Del Carpio O'Donovan R (1998) Exophytic primitive neuroectodermal tumor of the spinal cord. AJNR Am J Neuroradiol 19(4):787-789

Patel U, Pinto R.S, Miller DC, Handler MS, Rorke LB, Epstein FJ, Kricheff II (1998) MR of spinal cord ganglioglioma. AJNR Am J Neuroradiol 19(5):879-887

Przybylski GJ, Albright AL, Martinez AJ (1997) Spinal cord astrocytomas: long-term results comparing treatments in children. Childs Nerv Syst 13(7):375-382

Russo CP, Katz DS, Corona RJ Jr, Winfield JA (1995) Gangliocytoma of the cervicothoracic spinal cord. AJNR Am J Neuroradiol 16:889-891

Samii M, Klekamp J (1994) Surgical results of 100 intramedullary tumors in relation to accompanying syringomyelia. Neurosurgery 35(5):865-873

Scotti G, Scialfa G, Colombo N, Landoni L (1987) Magnetic resonance diagnosis of intramedullary tumors of the spinal cord. Neuroradiology 29:130-135

Sibilla L, Martelli A, Farina L, Uggetti C, Zappoli F, Sessa F, Rodriguez y Baena R, Gaeltani P (1995) Ganglioneuroblastoma of the spinal cord. AJNR Am J Neuroradiol 16:875-877

Sun B, Wang J, Liu A (2003) MRI features of intramedullary spinal cord ependymomas. J Neuroimaging 13(4):346-351

Sze G (1996) Neoplastic disease of the spine and spinal cord. In: Atlas SW (ed) Magnetic resonance imaging of the brain and spine, 2nd edn. Lippincott-Raven, Philadelphia, pp 1339-1385

Timmer FA, van Rooij WJ, Beute GN, Teepen JL (1993) Intramedullary lipoma. Neuroradiology 38(2):159-160

Weiner HL, Freed D, Woo HH, Rezai AR, Kim R, Epstein FJ (1997) Intra-axial tumors of the cervicomedullary junction: surgical results and long-term outcome. Pediatr Neurosurg 27(1):12-18

Spinal Trauma and Spinal Cord Injury

A.E. Flanders

Department of Radiology, Thomas Jefferson University Hospital, Philadelphia, PA, USA

Introduction

Spinal trauma is one of the most common maladies encountered in the emergency room setting. This is especially true in major trauma centers. While the majority of these patients requires minimal supportive care for ligamentous or muscular sprain, a significant proportion of these patients will endure vertebral fractures, spinal instability, neurologic deficits and associated visceral injury depending upon the severity of the initial trauma and mechanism of injury. In the most severe cases, the patient develops a concomitant spinal cord injury.

Spinal cord injury (SCI) is the most devastating consequence of spinal injury. Approximately 11 000 new cases of SCI occur each year in the United States; there are about 250 000 living survivors of SCI [1]. SCI primarily affects young males during their most productive years. The most common etiology of SCI includes motor vehicular collisions and falls, however, the proportion of SCI resulting from violence continues to rise in the United States. The cumulative medical expenses to care for the most severely injured patients (with high cervical injuries) can exceed one million US dollars per patient. Unfortunately, despite the incorporation of better passenger safety devices in automobiles and the increased public awareness of SCI, the overall incidence of SCI has not decreased appreciably. The average age of the typical SCI patient has increased in the past decade.[1]

Imaging of Spinal Trauma

The clinical management and diagnostic assessment of spinal trauma and spinal cord injury have changed drastically in the past decade. Clinicians primarily rely on imaging modalities to diagnose and classify spinal-injured patients. While pluridirectional tomography and myelography have given way to more modern techniques such as computed tomography (CT) and magnetic resonance imaging (MRI), plain radiography is the primary method for assessing bony injury in spinal trauma. The recommended minimum radiographic evaluation of the injured spine includes good quality anteroposterior (AP) and lateral views. In the cervical region, special attention must be given to the C1-2 articulation and to the cervicothoracic (C7-T1) junction. CT evaluation is mandatory for instances in which a portion of the spine is obscured on radiography or when the findings are equivocal.

The advent of multidetector computed tomography (MDCT) has changed the clinical landscape for evaluation of spinal injury. The limitation or trade-off for single-detector CT study of the spine was in-plane resolution for coverage; that is, in order to obtain high resolution isotropic voxels of the spine (suitable for generation of reformatted images), only a limited area of coverage was possible. Alternatively, if a large section of the spine needed to be interrogated, it could only be accomplished at lower resolution. Multidetector CT permits both greater slice resolution and increased coverage. The isotropic voxels that are created from the volumetric dataset are suitable for reconstructions at an infinite number of projections.

The much larger imaging datasets of MDCT have created an even greater need for digital manipulation, review and storage of the resulting imagesets. Formerly, a 3-mm single-slice CT study of the entire cervical spine would result in the creation of 35-45 images. A volumetric dataset created on an MDCT unit at sub-millimeter resolution can result in studies that exceed 150 images. Review of image sets of this size in multiple window settings can be unwieldy on film. For this reason, digital review on a PACS workstation is a more time-efficient method to review these large datasets. Moreover, since the datasets are volumetric and isotropic, reformatted images can be produced that are of the same resolution as the original dataset.

MRI

Magnetic resonance imaging (MRI) has had a tremendous impact on the clinical evaluation of spinal and spinal cord injured patients. In the era of radiography, assessment of the bony axis was used to predict the integrity of the surrounding soft tissues (e.g. intervertebral disks, ligaments) as these structures are not visible on radiography. Besides evaluation of bony alignment, assessment of the stability of the injury (e.g. malalignment produced by normal motion) is an integral part of the initial analysis of the injury [2]. Spinal instability is dependant upon the integrity of the ligamentous complexes. Stability of the injured segment may be suggested by inference based upon the degree of bony injury seen on radiography. A number of the fracture classification systems based on radiography were used to give the probability of ligamentous rupture. While CT improved our ability to identify and characterize subtle fractures and large soft tissue abnormalities (e.g. large paravertebral hematomas), most of the soft tissue abnormalities remained hidden.

MRI has changed the way radiologists and clinicians view spinal injury because it depicts the entire spectrum of injury, notably the entire soft tissue component of injury. An understanding of the soft tissue characteristics of the injury is essential to diagnosis but it is imperative in surgical planning. Moreover, MRI is the only imaging modality that reveals the internal architecture of the spinal cord. Since the spinal cord is regularly evaluated when the spine is imaged, the clinical focus has changed from the spine to the spinal cord.

The diagnostic MR spectrum of spinal injury can be divided into six separate distinct categories: bony injury, disk disruption or herniation, ligamentous injury, vascular injury, epidural or paravertebral fluid collections, and spinal cord injury.

Osseous Injury

While there is no replacement for plain radiography or CT for the detection of fractures, MRI has certain unique advantages in the setting of spinal trauma. Multidetector CT with multiplanar reformations is the most complete and sensitive method for characterizing fractures. Cortical discontinuity can be difficult to identify on MRI without obvious loss of stature of the vertebral body or buckling of the cortical margin. However, a principal shortcoming of both radiography and CT is their inability to predict the age or chronicity of a fracture deformity. Acute fractures and significant compressive injuries to bone without obvious fracture produce injury to the trabecular network of bone, resulting in microhemorrhages. Because MRI is uniquely sensitive to subtle changes in water content, it can be used to locate subtle areas of fracture or compressive injury [3, 4]. The abnormal marrow in the injured vertebral body is of lower signal intensity on T1-weighted images, reverting to hyperintensity on T2-weighted images. MRI has proven useful in distinguishing chronic and acute insufficiency fractures in addition to identifying "damaged" vertebral levels that have endured the compressive effects of injury [5].

Ligamentous Injury

The ligamentous complexes that encase the vertebral column provide stability to the spine and are the critical components that allow the rigid bony components the characteristic of mobility while maintaining stability. As the ligaments are not visible on radiography and poorly delineated on CT, they are not routinely assessable with these modalities. Therefore, fracture classification schemas were devised to predict the integrity of the ligamentous complexes based on the pattern of bony injury to predict the probability of stability for a particular injury type [6, 7]. MRI is the only imaging modality which allows direct visual inspection of the ligaments and their relationship to the adjacent bony elements. The connective tissues that comprise the ligaments are of low signal intensity on all pulse sequences. The anterior and posterior longitudinal ligaments form a long, low-signal continuous band along the ventral and dorsal surfaces, respectively, of the vertebral bodies. The ligamentum flavum defines a continuous undulating low signal band along the ventral surface of the lamina. The posterior ligamentous complex (intraspinous and supraspinous ligaments) bridges the spinous processes. Ligament disruption is characterized by a discontinuity in the contour of ligament that is best identified on the sagittal T2-weighted images. Fat suppression is useful to augment the signal changes from damage to these connective tissues. The disrupted ligament may be identified in association with a prevertebral fluid collection in the setting of an anterior longitudinal ligament disruption or increased signal in the posterior paraspinal musculature in association with a posterior ligamentous complex disruption. Ligamentous disruption on MRI has a high correlation with surgical evaluation in thoracolumbar injuries [8].

Disk Injury and Herniation

Post-traumatic disk abnormalities are classified as injuries and herniations. Simple disk injuries occur as a result of tearing of the annulus or nuclear fibers. The disk exhibits abnormal, increased signal intensity on T2-weighted images relative to the adjacent disk spaces. Frequently, the disk space will be asymmetrically widened as a secondary sign of injury. Post-traumatic disk herniations have a similar appearance to disk herniations from a degenerative etiology; a polypoid extension of disk material in a subligamentous location. The incidence of post-traumatic disk herniation is quite varied in the published literature [9, 10]. However, the incidence of disk herniations overall is greater since MRI has come into general use.

Epidural Hemorrhage

Post-traumatic extra-axial hemorrhages in the spine occur in up to 40% of all cases of spine trauma. The most frequent cause is tearing of the epidural venous plexus resulting in a epidural hematoma. The epidural space offers no relative resistance to the spread of the hemorrhage, so that the hematoma usually extends over many vertebral levels. Therefore, even when large in volume, spinal epidural hematomas frequently are clinically insignificant as they do not compress the spinal cord. In certain circumstances, the hematoma may compress the thecal sac enough to warrant emergent surgical evacuation. Patients with intrinsic coagulopathy and ankylosing spondylitis have a higher incidence of dorsal epidural hematomas.

Vertebral Artery Injury

Vertebral artery dissection with thrombosis is a relatively common complication associated with cervical spinal injury. Rotational and translational forces applied to the fixed portions of the vertebral artery (contained within the foramen transversarium) damage the vascular intima during cervical injury. The reported incidence of vertebral artery injury is variable. Some arteriographic studies suggested that the vertebral artery is damaged in over 50% of all cervical spine fractures [11, 12]. Studies that use magnetic resonance angiography (MRA) suggested that post-traumatic thrombosis of the vertebral artery occurs in almost 25% of cases. In the majority of cases, the injury is clinically asymptomatic. Therefore, addressing this associated injury therapeutically remains controversial.

Spinal Cord Injury

MRI offers the only evaluation of spinal cord injury. MRI has been shown to be highly sensitive to a broad range of injury patterns in both humans and animal models of SCI. There are three fundamental MRI findings of SCI: spinal cord swelling, edema and hemorrhage. Collectively, the presence and extent of these injury patterns highly correlate to the neurologic deficit and prognosis for clinical recovery.

Spinal cord swelling is the non-specific enlargement of the caliber of the spinal cord at the level of injury. Since this finding refers to an alteration in shape of the spinal cord, it is visible on all pulse sequences. The length of spinal cord that exhibits swelling is directly proportional to the degree of neurologic deficit.

Spinal cord edema on MRI correlates to an increase in intramedullary fluid (intracellular or extracellular) in the injured tissues. This appears as a spindle-shaped area of increased signal intensity on T2-weighted images. The edema spans a variable length of the spinal cord in proportion to the severity of the neurologic deficit. Edema is invariably present in all cases where post-traumatic myelopathy is present. The entire cervical spinal cord may be edematous in the most severe neurologic deficits. The length of the initial injury is inversely proportional

to the degree of neurologic recovery at 12 months in the upper and lower extremities [13-16].

Post-traumatic spinal cord hemorrhage on MRI correlates histologically with coalescent areas of hemorrhagic necrosis after injury. Although hemorrhage is always identified on histologic preparations of spinal cord injury, it is only identified on clinical MRI when a focal clot is produced. The hemorrhage has a propensity to collect in the central gray matter of the spinal cord. On MRI, hemorrhagic features of SCI appear as foci of low signal intensity on T2-weighted and gradient-echo pulse sequences. The hemorrhage is generally found at the geographic epicenter of the spinal cord injury with the edema spanning a variable distance above and below the epicenter. The anatomic location of the hemorrhage correlates to the neurologic level of injury better than either edema or swelling. Hemorrhage correlates with the most severe neurologic injuries. Moreover, the presence of a focal hemorrhage at the injury epicenter portends for a poor neurologic recovery at one year [13-16].

Chronic Spinal Cord Injury Evaluation

Neurologic recovery following SCI is variable and is dependant on a multitude of factors including: the severity of the initial neurologic deficit, mechanism of injury, injuries associated with the central nervous system (CNS), level of multidisciplinary expertise in caring for SCI patients, early restoration and fixation of spinal alignment (controversial), administration of steroids (controversial) and aggressive rehabilitation. In the majority of cases, the full extent of potential neurologic recovery will be realized within a year after injury. The phenomenon of acute neurologic deterioration following a stable period of a persistent neurologic deficit is known as post-traumatic progressive myelopathy (PTPM). The imaging manifestations of this clinical syndrome are varied and include: progressive spinal cord atrophy, myclomalacia, syringomyelia and tethering. The latter two entities are the conditions amenable to surgical intervention. Surgery can halt the progression of the myelopathy and, in some instances, restore the patient to their former neurologic state [17, 18].

Future Applications

MRI will continue to play a major role in the acute and chronic evaluation of spinal and spinal cord injury. MRI plays an integral role in the clinical evaluation and surgical decision process at all SCI centers. The application of functional MRI techniques to diseases of the spinal cord is just being realized. This is technically challenging due to the small inherent size of the target (less than 1 cm in diameter) and the associated problems from cerebrospinal fluid (CSF) pulsation and proximity to bone, which tend to degrade image quality. As the physiologic techniques of diffusion, spectroscopy and BOLD (fMRI) for the spine become more clinically accessible, physicians will be able to gauge the degree of salvageable tissue with greater precision. MRI has already shown promise is assessing viability of spinal cord transplants. Diffusion tensor imaging (DTI) techniques and tractography may ultimately prove to be the most robust methods for gauging the proportion of survivable neurons and for assessing response to new therapies (e.g. transplants) [19-21].

References

1. – (2000) Spinal cord injury: facts and figures at a glance. J Spinal Cord Med 23:51-53
2. White AA III, Panjabi MM (1978) Clinical biomechanics of the spine. JB Lippincott, Philadelphia
3. Levitt MA, Flanders AE (1991) Diagnostic capabilities of magnetic resonance imaging and computed tomography in acute cervical spinal column injury. Am J Emerg Med 9(2):131-135
4. Tarr RW, Drolshagen LF, Kerner TC, Allen JH, Partain CL, James AE (1987) MRI imaging of recent spinal trauma. J Comput Assist Tomogr 11(3):412-417
5. Baker LL, Goodman SB, Perkash I, Lane B, Enzmann DR (1990) Benign versus pathologic compression fractures of vertebral bodies: assessment with conventional spin-echo, chemical shift, and STIR MRI imaging. Radiology 174:495-502
6. Holdsworth F (1970) Fractures, dislocations and fracture-dislocations of the spine. J Bone Joint Surg Am 52:1534-1551
7. Denis F (1983) The three column spine and its significance in the classification of acute thoracolumbar spinal injuries. Spine 8:817-831
8. Lee HM, Kim HS, Kim DJ, Suk KS, Park Jo, Kim NH (2000) Reliability of magnetic resonance imaging in detecting posterior ligament complex injury in thoracolumbar spinal fractures. Spine 25(16):2079-2084
9. Rizzolo SJ, Piazza MRI, Cotler JM, Balderston RA, Schaefer DM, Flanders AE (1991) Intervertebral disc injury complicating cervical spine trauma. Spine 16(6):187-189
10. Harrington JF, Likavec MJ, Smith AS (1991) Disc herniation in cervical fracture subluxation. Neurosurgery 29:374-379
11. Friedman DP, Flanders AE (1992) Unusual dissection of the proximal vertebral artery: description of three cases. AJNR Am J Neuroradiol 13:283-286
12. Friedman DP, Flanders AE, Thomas C, Millar W (1995) Vertebral artery injury after acute cervical spine trauma: rate of occurrence as detected by MR angiography and assessment of clinical consequences. AJR Am J Roentgenol 164:443-447
13. Marciello M, Flanders AE, Herbison GJ, Schaefer DM, Friedman DP, Lane JI (1993) Magnetic resonance imaging related to neurologic outcome in cervical spinal cord injury. Arch Phys Med Rehabil 74:940-946
14. Flanders AE, Spettell CM, Tartaglino LM, Friedman DP, Herbison GJ (1996) Forecasting motor recovery after cervical spinal cord injury: value of MR imaging. Radiology 201:649-55
15. Schaefer DM, Flanders AE, Osterholm JL, Northrup BE (1992) Prognostic significance of magnetic resonance imaging in the acute phase of cervical spine injury. J Neurosurg 76(2):218-223
16. Flanders AE, Spettell CM, Friedman DP, Marino RJ, Herbison GJ (1999) The relationship between the functional abilities of patients with cervical spinal cord injury and the severity of damage revealed by MR imaging. AJNR Am J Neuroradiol 20:926-934
17. Barnett HJM, Botterell EH, Jousse AT, Wynn-Jones M (1966) Progressive myelopathy as a sequel to traumatic paraplegia. Brain 89:159-173
18. Rossier AB, Foo D, Shillito J et al (1981) Progressive late post-traumatic syringomyelia. Paraplegia 19:96-97
19. Ford JC, Hackney DB, Alsop DC et al (1994) MRI characterization of diffusion coefficients in a rat spinal cord injury model. Magn Reson Med 31:488-494
20. Schwartz ED, Yezierski RP, Pattany PM, Quencer RM, Weaver RG (1999) Diffusion-weighted MR imaging in a rat model of syringomyelia after excitotoxic spinal cord injury. AJNR Am J Neuroradiol 20(8):1422-1428
21. Madi S, Vinitski S, Flanders AE, Nissanov J (2001) Functional imaging of the human spinal cord. AJNR Am J Neuroradiol 22(9):1768-1774

Spinal Inflammation and Demyelinating Diseases

C. Manelfe

Department of Diagnostic and Therapeutic Neuroradiology, Hôpital Purpan, Toulouse, France

Introduction

Clinical presentation and imaging findings of spinal inflammatory and demyelinating diseases are protean and often non-specific. They may mimic neoplastic lesions either clinically or radiologically. Magnetic resonance imaging (MRI) is the best imaging modality to screen patients who are clinically suspected of having myelitis.

The most challenging imaging presentation is that of an enlarged spinal cord. Enlargement or gadolinium enhancement of the spine are not synonymous with spinal cord tumor and can be observed in patients with myelitis, myelopathy or syringohydromyelia.

The words *myelitis* and *myelopathy* are often used interchangeably, are not specific and describe various pathologic conditions of the spinal cord. Myelopathy usually indicates a noninflammatory, degenerative disorder of the spinal cord resulting from compressive, vascular, toxic or metabolic insults. Myelitis results from inflammatory or infectious disorders (mainly viral), or presumed autoimmune or idiopathic conditions [1, 2].

The clinical presentation of the patient, anamnesis, mode of onset, and duration can orient the diagnosis:

– An *acute or rapidly progressive clinical onset* may have a vascular, infectious, viral or inflammatory origin;
– A *slowly progressive onset* is more likely due to compression, demyelination, vascular, metabolic or toxic etiologies.

Serologic and culture examinations of blood and cerebrospinal fluid (CSF), and biopsy specimens (skin, lymph nodes, etc.) may obviate surgical biopsy of the spinal cord.

Imaging Techniques

Among the various imaging modalities, MRI is the best technique due to its multiplanar capabilities and superior tissue sensitivity. MRI allows clinicians to answer the following questions: (1) Is the spinal cord normal or not? (2) Is the lesion localized to the cord (focal or diffuse) or to the whole neuraxis (brain, nerve roots, etc.)? (3) How is the signal? Is there an enhancement or not?

Some of the most common sequences are herein described:

– Sagittal and axial T1- and T2-weighted fast spin echo (FSE) sequences are the most frequently used. Spin echo (SE) sequences are superior to gradient echo (GE) sequences except when associated acute hemorrhage is suspected. The study of patients with suspected intramedullary lesions (mainly from multiple sclerosis) is improved by including separate sagittal proton density-weighted FSE scans which generally confirm the lesions suspected on the T2-weighted sequences and frequently may detect additional cord lesions [3].
– FSE sequences with longer repetition time (TR=3000 ms) and echo time (TE=150 ms) have poorer lesion-cord contrast than those with more moderate parameters (TR=2500 ms, TE=90 ms) [4]. Slice thickness must be 3 mm or less when a spinal cord lesion is suspected.
– SE sequences with short time inversion recovery (STIR) technique (TR=3000 ms; TE=40 ms; inversion time, TI=140-160 ms) are well suited for detecting intramedullary lesions and are particularly helpful in detecting multiple sclerosis plaque [3, 4].
– Sequences with long TI (e.g. FLAIR with TR=10 000 ms, TE=180 ms and TI=2000 ms) are less sensitive in detecting intramedullary lesions but can be useful to differentiate intramedullary cyst from myelomalacia or edema.
– In the axial plane, T2-weighted SE sequences are more sensitive to flow artifacts, while T2*-weighted GE sequences are more efficient, mainly at the cervical level.
– Gadolinium injection increases lesion conspicuity and imaging specificity, and improves localization and detection of subtle areas of infection or inflammation. Post-gadolinium fat-suppressed T1-weighted sequences are useful for imaging not only bone marrow and epidural space, but also spinal cord and nerve roots.
– Magnetic resonance angiography (MRA), also called black blood technique, of the spinal cord needs increased spatial resolution and presently, cannot replace spinal cord angiography when medullary vessels are not dilated. Gadolinium-enhanced MRA has increased spatial resolution and is giving promising results [4].

– Magnetic resonance myelography (MRM) using ultrafast techniques such as HASTE (half Fourier acquisition single shot turbo spin echo) sequence or CISS (constructive interference steady state) 3D sequence is a valuable method to explore spine and spinal cord pathology. It is, however, less useful in imaging intramedullary pathology than intra-extradural lesions (e.g. tumors, degenerative disk disease, spinal stenosis).

– Diffusion-weighted imaging (DWI) is still in evaluation. Anisotropic diffusion shows the microscopic architecture of the parenchyma and depicts losses of anisotropy probably due to axonal loss at an early stage. In the future, DWI may be used to detect or evaluate spinal cord ischemia, spondylotic myelopathy and cord trauma [5].

Intramedullary lesions represent the most difficult situation for the clinician and the radiologist. Myelitis may mimic spinal cord tumor and vice versa [2, 6]. As causes of myelitis, demyelinating and viral diseases are the most frequent. MRI is sensitive but lacks specificity: most lesions feature high signal intensity on T2-weighted images. Gadolinium injection improves specificity but a lack of enhancement does not definitely rule out tumor.

Demyelinating Diseases

Multiple Sclerosis

Multiple sclerosis (MS) is the most frequent demyelinating disease of the central nervous system of autoimmune origin. MS affects young adults and has 3 main clinical forms: (a) relapsing-remitting, (b) secondary progressive, and (c) primary progressive. Diagnosis is based on clinical history, physical examination and paraclinical tests, such as CSF analysis, cortical evoked responses and MRI findings. MRI is advantageous in that it demonstrates lesions in vivo; previously these lesions could only be show at autopsy [7-9].

Approximately 10%-15% of patients with spinal cord plaques have no intracranial disease. MS affects mainly the cervicothoracic cord: plaques are elongated, extend over 1-2 vertebral segments, and do not respect boundaries between tracts of gray and white matter. Cord enlargement may be noted in acute lesions and gadolinium enhancement may be observed. On axial sections, plaques are located at the periphery of the cord mainly in the posterior (41%) and lateral (25%) aspects. More than half of cord plaques longer than two vertebral segments are accompanied by cord atrophy or, alternatively, by cord swelling [4, 7].

Diffuse cord abnormalities seem to correlate with primary or secondary progressive clinical MS subtypes. Diffuse disease is more frequently associated with cord atrophy and has a weak but significant correlation with clinical disability [10].

The magnetization transfer ratio (MTR) in cervical cord of MS patients may be reduced compared to that in normal controls, even in the absence of detectable cord lesions on T2-weighted sequences [11].

Differential diagnosis with neoplasm, granulomatous infections and viral diseases may be difficult. The disappearance of enhancing lesions on follow-up examinations and associated brain lesions suggest the diagnosis of MS.

Acute Disseminated Encephalomyelitis

Acute disseminated encephalomyelitis (ADEM) is an acute or subacute demyelinating process of autoimmune origin mediated by antibody-antigen complexes. It has a monophasic course, typically following a specific viral illness, vaccination or non-specific respiratory infection. The mortality rate is approximately 10%-20% in the acute phase, but 60% of patients recover completely [12]. Pathological analysis shows perivenous demyelination with variable inflammatory cell infiltration of the white matter.

MRI of patients with ADEM gives non-specific results, showing extended and multifocal high signal intensity on T2-weighted images in the white matter. In the brain, lesions are usually bilateral, asymmetric, widely distributed without mass effect. Involvement of the basal ganglia and thalami has been reported [13]. A monophasic course of disease and gadolinium enhancement of all lesions help to differentiate ADEM from MS [12].

Granulomatous Diseases

Sarcoidosis is an idiopathic, multisystemic, noninfectious granulomatous disease. Spinal cord involvement is present in 6%-8% of cases of neurosarcoidosis. The clinical picture is non-specific and clinical and laboratory tests are mandatory (e.g. Kvein skin test, serum levels of angiotensin-converting enzyme (ACE), CSF studies, chest radiography). Histologic examination of biopsies of skin, nasal mucosa and lymph nodes is of great value and can obviate the need for cord biopsy. As in MS, cervical cord involvement is frequent in spinal sarcoidosis. T1- and T2-weighted images are not specific, and show an enlarged cord and hyperintensity on T2-weighted images, mimicking a tumor or an MS plaque [2, 6]. Four patterns of enhancement [14] correspond to different stages of the disease: (a) linear, leptomeningeal; (b) parenchymal, associated with cord swelling; (c) focal or multifocal with abnormal cord; and (d) atrophy. Associated leptomeningeal cranial involvement is helpful for the diagnosis of sarcoidosis but may also be present in tuberculosis or non-Hodgkin's lymphoma.

Involvement of the spinal cord in Lyme disease, due to *Borrelia burgdorferi* infection, is rare. Lymphocytic meningoradiculitis and acute transverse myelopathy (discussed later) are the most common clinical presentations. Leptomeningeal enhancement of the spinal cord, nerve roots and cranial nerves is usual [15].

Other infectious granulomatous diseases, such as tuberculosis and syphilis, give MRI findings similar to those of sarcoidosis.

Nongranulomatous Diseases

The class of nongranulomatous diseases comprises viral, bacterial and parasitic infections as well as toxic myelopathies.

Acute Transverse Myelitis

The clinical picture is frequently represented by an acute transverse myelitis (ATM) which can result from autoimmune or allergic response, vasculitis, direct viral invasion or demyelination [9]. Transverse myelitis is an inflammatory or infectious process involving the entire cross-sectional area of the cord at a particular level. The most prominent findings on histopathological examination are found in the blood vessels and the perivascular spaces of the gray and white matter: hyperemia, perivascular cellular exudate and edema, and hemorrhage [16]. Acute paraparesis, with motor, sensory and sphincter disorders, is the most common clinical presentation. In children, ATM is commonly preceded by infection (e.g. herpes, rabies, varicella, mumps, rubeola) or vaccination. In adults, the most frequent causes of ATM are acquired immune deficiency syndrome (AIDS), vasculitis (lupus) and paraneoplastic syndromes.

The MRI appearance of transverse myelitis is non-specific. Focal or extended cord enlargement is present in 40% of case and gadolinium enhancement is seen in 60%. On axial sections, the high signal intensity on T2-weighted images occupies more than two-thirds of the cross section of the cord [17].

AIDS Myelopathies

Patients infected with human immunodeficiency virus (HIV) frequently experience vacuolar myelopathy, HIV myelitis, opportunistic infections, lymphomas, and vascular and metabolic disorders [18].

Vacuolar myelopathy is the most common spinal cord disease in patients with AIDS (30%-50% in autopsy studies [19, 20]). It is characterized by a spongy degeneration of spinal white matter, affecting predominantly the lateral and posterior columns of the thoracic cord. Histopathological features are similar to those of subacute combined degeneration of the spinal cord secondary to vitamin B12 deficiency [19, 21]. Common clinical manifestations are progressive spastic paraparesis, incontinence and ataxia. Dementia is observed in 70% of cases [19, 20]. MRI usually shows diffuse and symmetric hyperintensities on T2-weighted images on the dorsal columns in a normal or atrophic spinal cord, more often without gadolinium enhancement.

HIV myelitis occurs in 5%-8% of AIDS patients and is caused by direct HIV infection. Lesions are focal, have high signal intensity on T2-weighted images, and predominate in the central gray matter.

Opportunistic infections in AIDS patients may be caused by cytomegalovirus (CMV), fungi, herpes simplex virus and varicella-zoster virus (VZV); other common opportunistic infections are tuberculosis, toxoplasmosis, syphilis and progressive multifocal leucoencephalopathy [20-22]. CMV infection, the most common opportunistic infection, frequently involves the conus and cauda equina [4, 20, 22]. Back and radicular pain, flaccid paraparesis, urinary retention, saddle anesthesia and inflammatory CSF profile (polymorphonuclear pleocytosis, low sugar and high protein contents), are usual [4, 16]. VZV myelitis may follow cutaneous vesicular eruption. Infection involves the posterior horns and dorsal root ganglia.

In AIDS patients, when focal spinal cord enlargement with gadolinium enhancement is present, toxoplasmic myelitis and lymphoma should be considered; brain involvement is present in both conditions, but a positive thallium-201 SPECT scan makes a diagnosis of lymphoma more likely [20]. When spinal cord enlargement and abnormal signal (hyperintensity on T2-weighted images) are associated with meningeal enhancement, CMV infection and tuberculosis should be considered [17].

Tropical Spastic Paraparesis

Infection with human T-cell lymphotrophic virus type I (HTLV-I), endemic in the Carribean and in some parts of Africa, is called tropical spastic paraparesis (TSP) [23]. In Japan, this myelopathy was found to be associated with leukemia and was thus called HTLV-I-associated myelopathy [23]. Neuropathology reveals demyelination in the lateral and dorsal tracts as well as axonal loss. Clinical presentation usually consists of progressive weakness of the lower limbs with paresthesias.

MRI may show either diffuse atrophy and abnormal signal intensity on T2-weighted images or, at the acute stage, spinal cord swelling with peripheral gadolinium enhancement [24]. Associated white matter lesions in the brain have been reported [16].

Bacterial and Parasitic Infections

Bacterial infections and abscesses of the spinal cord are extremely rare [25]. Clinical presentation can be acute, subacute or chronic; the infection may mimic tumor. Predisposing factors include cardiopulmonary infections, immunosuppression and drug abuse [26]. The most common causative agent is *Staphylococcus aureus*. Cord swelling and extensive edema are present at the initial stage (phlegmon). A rim-enhancing cavity is seen atat the abscess stage. *Listeria monocytogenes* can cause abscesses in the brain stem and upper cervical cord.

Parasitic infections such as schistosomal myelitis, toxocariasis, bilharziosis, and cysticercosis are suspected in patients who have been in countries where these diseases are endemic, and in patients who have hypereosinophilia (in blood or CSF). Spinal cord lesions are far less frequent than brain lesions.

MRI shows non-specific focal mass effect, low signal intensity on T1-weighted images and high signal intensity on T2-weighted images. Cysts in the subarachnoid spaces compressing the spinal cord or nerve roots are seen in neurocysticercosis; their mobility in the CSF can be helpful for the diagnosis of cysticercosis.

Metabolic and Nutritional Deficiency Myelitis

Subacute combined degeneration of the cord is due to vitamin B12 deficiency and is often associated with megaloblastic anemia [16]. Degenerative and demyelinating changes occur in the white matter of the dorsal and lateral columns of the spinal cord. MRI shows hyperintensity on T2-weighted images in the dorsal columns (mainly cervical and thoracic) with or without cord enlargement or gadolinium enhancement [27]. Following vitamin B12 supplementation, improvement is seen clinically and on MRI.

Radiation Myelitis

Atrophy is the most common appearance of radiation myelitis. It can mimic, however, tumoral infiltration when transient enlargement of the cord with high signal intensity on T2-weighted images is present. Focal enhancement after gadolinium administration may be seen. The thoracic cord is more sensitive to radiation. A spinal lesion attributed to radiation myelitis should lie in the radiation portal and appear at least 6 or 12 months after radiotherapy. Associated bony changes (e.g. fatty degeneration of the vertebral bodies) in the radiation portal help in differentiating myelitis from tumor. Overall, 82% of cases of radiation myelitis are related to tumors of the head and neck [6].

References

1. Plum F, Olson ME (1973) Myelitis and myelopathy. In: Baker AB, Baker LH (eds) Clinical neurology. Harper Row, Hagerstown, pp 1-52
2. Manelfe C (1992) Imaging of the spine and spinal cord. Raven, New York
3. Dietemann JL, Thibaut-Menard A, Warter JM et al (2000) MRI in multiple sclerosis of the spinal cord: evaluation of fast short inversion-recovery and spin-echo sequences. Neuroradiology 42:810-813
4. Finelli DA, Ross JS (2000) MR imaging of intrinsic inflammatory myelopathies. Magn Reson Imaging Clin N Am 8:541-560
5. Pattany PM, Puckett WR, Klose KJ et al (1997) High resolution diffusion-weighted MR of fresh and fixed cat spinal cords: evaluation of diffusion coefficients and anisotropy. AJNR Am J Neuroradiol 18:1049-1056
6. Balériaux D, Parizel P, Bank WO (1992) Intraspinal and intramedullary pathology. In: Manelfe C (ed) Imaging of the spine and spinal cord. Raven, New York, pp 513-564
7. Tartaglino LM, Friedman DP, Flanders AE et al (1995) Multiple sclerosis in the spinal cord: MR appearance and correlation with clinical parameters. Radiology 195:725-732
8. Thielen KR, Miller GM (1996) Multiple sclerosis of the spinal cord: magnetic resonance appearance. J Comput Assist Tomogr 20:434-438
9. Tartaglino LM, Croul SE, Flanders AE, Sweeney JD, Schwartzmann RJ, Liem M (1996) Idiopathic acute transverse myelitis: MR imaging findings. Radiology 201:661-669
10. Lyclama a Nijeholft GJ, Barkhof F, Scheltens P et al (1997) MR of the spinal cord in multiple sclerosis: relation to clinical subtype and disability. AJNR Am J Neuroradiol 18:1041-1048
11. Silver NC, Barker GJ, Losseff NA et al (1997) Magnetization transfer ratio measurements in the cervical spinal cord: a preliminary study in multiple sclerosis. Neuroradiology 39:441-445
12. Kesserling J, Miller DH, Robb SA, Kendall BE, Moseley IF, Kingsley D, Du Boulay EPGH, McDonald WI (1990) Acute disseminated encephalomyelitis: MRI findings and the distinction from multiple sclerosis. Brain 113:291-302
13. Caldemeyer KS, Smith RR, Harris TM, Edwards MK (1994) MRI in acute disseminated encephalomyelitis. Neuroradiology 36:216-220
14. Junger SS, Stern BJ, Levine SR, Sipos E, Marti-Masso F (1993) Intramedullary spinal sarcoidosis: clinical and magnetic resonance imaging characteristics. Neurology 43:333-337
15. Mantienne C, Albucher JF, Catalaâ I, Sévely A, Cognard C, Manelfe C (2001) MRI in Lyme disease of the spinal cord. Neuroradiology 43:485-488
16. Byrne TN, Benzel EC, Wasman SG (2000) Diseases of the spine and spinal cord. Oxford University, Oxford, pp 266-313
17. Choi KH, Lee KS, Chung So et al (1996) Idiopathic transverse myelitis: MR characteristics. AJNR Am J Neuroradiol 20:1412-1416
18. Barakos JA, Mark AS, Dillon WP, Norman D (1990) MR imaging of acute transverse myelitis and AIDS myelopathy. J Comput Assist Tomogr 14:45-50
19. Petito CK (1997) The neuropathology of human immunodeficiency virus infection in the spinal cord. In: Berger JR, Levy RM (eds) AIDS and the nervous system, 2nd edn. Lippincott-Raven, Philadelphia, pp 451-459
20. Quencer RM, Post MJD (1997) Spinal cord lesions in patients with AIDS. Neuroimaging Clin N Am 7:359-373
21. Santosh CG, Bell JE, Best JJK (1995) Spinal tract pathology in AIDS: postmortem MRI correlation with neuropathology. Neuroradiology 3:134-138
22. Turnher MM, Post MJD, Jinkins JR (2000) MRI of infections and neoplasms of the spine and spinal cord in 55 patients with AIDS. Neuroradiology 42:551-563
23. Vernant JC, Maurs L, Gessain A et al (1987) Endemic tropical spastic paraparesis associated with human T-lymphotropic virus type 1: a clinical and seroepidemiological study of 25 cases. Ann Neurol 21:123-130
24. Shakudo M, Inoue Y, Tsutada T (1999) HTLV-1 associated myelopathy: acute progression and atypical MR findings. AJNR Am J Neuroradiol 20:1417-1421
25. D'Angelo CM, Whisler W (1978) Bacterial infections of the spinal cord and its coverings. In: Vinken PJ, Bruyn GW (eds) Handbook of Clinical Neurology, vol. 33. Infections of the Nervous System, part I. North-Holland, Amsterdam, pp 187-194
26. Sverzut JM, Laval C, Smadja P, Gigaud M, Sevely A, Manelfe C (1998) Spinal cord abscess in a heroin addict: case report. Neuroradiology 40:455-458
27. Timms SR, Cure JK, Kurent JE (1993) Subacute combined degeneration of the spinal cord: MR findings. AJNR Am J Neuroradiol 14:1224-1227

Spinal Inflammation and Demyelinating Diseases

M. Leonardi, M. Maffei

Neuroradiology Service, Bellaria Hospital, Bologna, Italy

Introduction

Diagnosis of spinal inflammatory disease is a complex process requiring an appraisal of clinical, laboratory and neuroradiological findings. Spinal inflammation can be divided into two groups: diseases affecting the vertebral bodies and intervertebral disks, and diseases of the spinal cord.

Vertebral and Disk Space Infection

Tuberculosis

Tuberculosis (Figs. 1-5) is the most common cause of vertebral body infection; 75% of cases of tuberculous spondylitis occur prior to age 20 years. In most instances, vertebral body involvement is secondary to hematogenous spread of Mycobacterium tuberculosis from a pulmonary source, which more often than not remains quiescent. Disease onset is insidious and its course is more benign than that of pyogenic osteomyelitis. Clinical presentation is usually non-specific. Patients describe long-term back pain. Vague abdominal pain related to involvement of sympathetic nerves by a paravertebral mass may be the only symptom. Spinal cord and root compression with associated neurologic deficit due to epidural spread of the disease occurs in 10%-20% of patients. Paraplegia developing into Pott's disease is usually less severe and carries a better prognosis than that of pyogenic infections. The lower half of the spine is commonly involved.

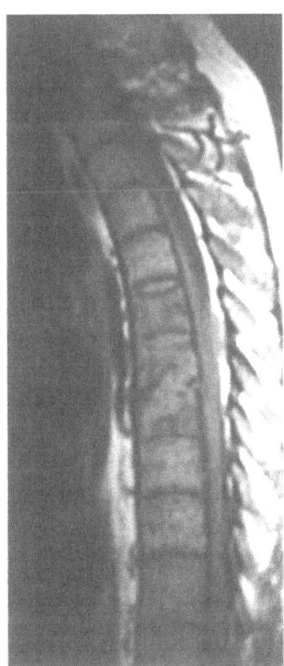

Fig. 1. Tuberculosis. Sagittal MR, T1-weighted image: signal intensity alteration of two vertebral bodies and of the disc space

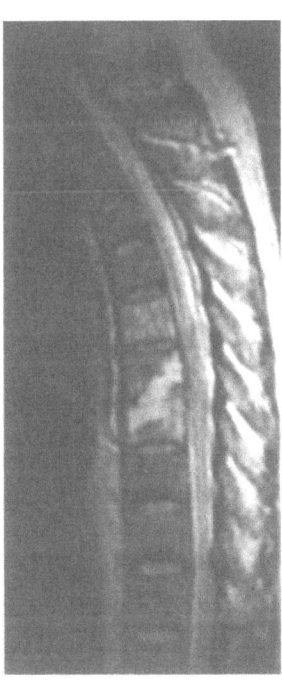

Fig. 2. Tuberculosis. Sagittal MR, T2-weighted image: hyperintensity of vertebral bodies and of the disc space

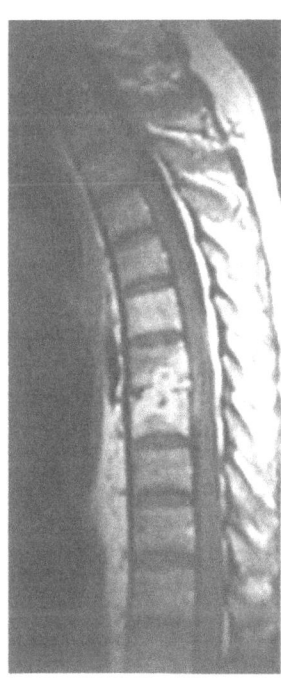

Fig. 3. Tuberculosis. Sagittal MR, T1-weighted postgadolinium image: marked enhancement of the granulomatous tissue

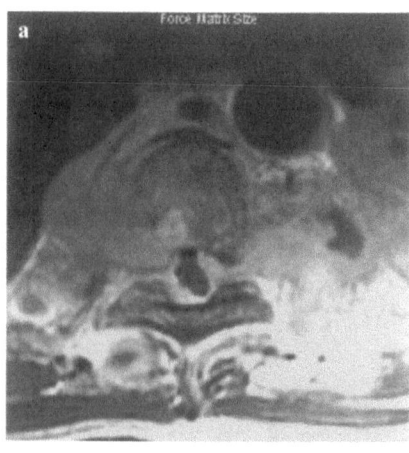
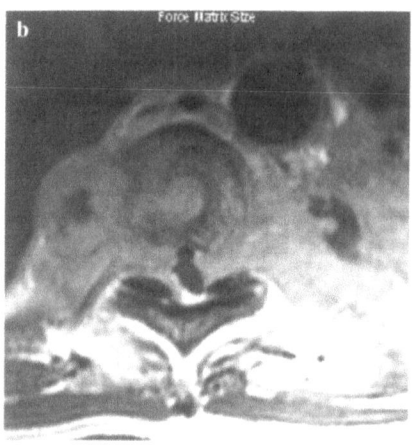
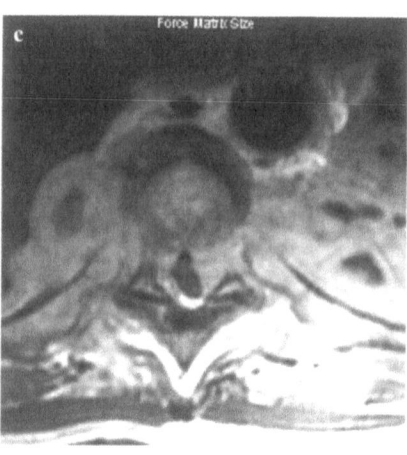
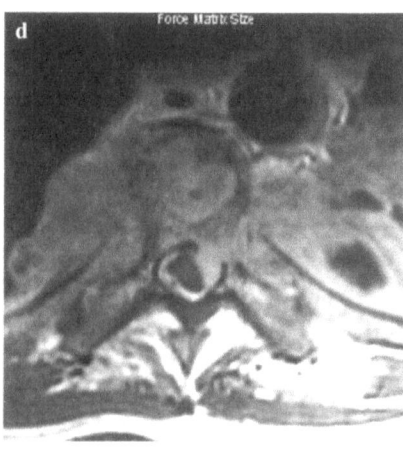

Fig. 4a-d. Tuberculosis. Axial MR, T1-weighted postgadolinium images: the granulomatous tissue involves the paravertebral structures and medially the epidural space

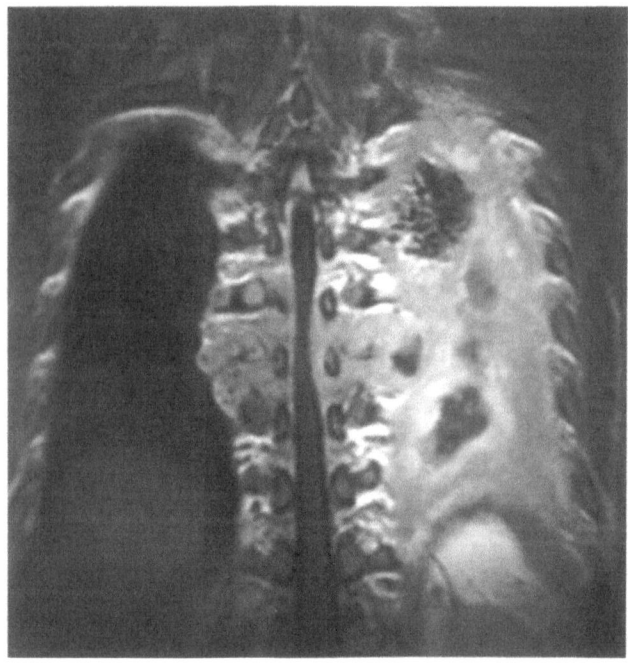

Fig. 5. Coronal MR, T1-weighted image of tuberculosis

The infection first appears in the anterior parts of the vertebral body adjacent to a disk space. In about 50% of cases, the infection spreads through the disk space to an adjacent vertebral body. Nonadjacent vertebral bodies can become involved secondarily to paraspinous or subligamentous spread of infection. In tuberculous spondylitis, involvement of posterior elements is much less common than in pyogenic or fungal infection. New bone formation is more characteristic of pyogenic infection than tuberculosis. The massive bone destruction in tuberculous spondylitis frequently results in gibbus deformity. Large often partially calcified paraspinal masses are a common feature of tuberculous spondylitis, reflecting the protracted course of the disease. Bilateral psoas abscesses typically accompany tuberculous spondylitis. Hallmarks identified on computed tomography (CT) or magnetic resonance imaging (MRI) include fragmentation and destruction of the anterior aspect of one or two adjacent vertebral bodies, disk space narrowing, and paraspinal abscesses containing small calcifications. T1 and T2 relaxation times of the disk space and vertebral bodies involved are prolonged.

In the early stages that present only signal intensity alteration and disk space narrowing, it may be difficult to distinguish between pyogenic and tuberculous osteomyelitis. Culture of aspirated or biopsied material is essential, particularly when the appearance is not typical. Once a gibbus has developed, MRI is far superior to CT in disclosing the presence and degree of spinal cord compression.

Intradural and intramedullary tuberculomas are rare. Clinical symptoms and imaging characteristics are indistinguishable from spinal neoplasms.

Pyogenic Infections

Pyogenic involvement of the vertebral body accounts for only 2%-4% of all cases of pyogenic osteomyelitis and usually arises in the lumbar region. Infection primarily involves the disk space in children and the vertebral body in adults. A disk space infection will rarely extend to the epidural and paravertebral spaces.

Staphylococcus aureus accounts for approximately 60% of adult infections, while Enterobacteriaceae, common agents of urinary tract infection, account for about 30%. The most frequent strain is Escherichia coli, followed by Pseudomonas aeruginosa and Klebsiella species.

The earliest findings detectable on CT examination are irregularity and erosion of contiguous end plates associated with narrowing of the disk space and diminished attenuation of the vertebral body. The posterior elements are seldom involved. Later in the process, usually beginning at 10-12 weeks, an osteoblastic response may develop with sclerotic new bone formation. Progression of the osteoblastic response may result in eburnation of the vertebral bodies and subsequent fusion. If treatment is improper or incomplete, collapse of the vertebral affected bodies may ensue with resulting gibbus deformity and instability of the vertebral column.

Paravertebral soft tissue extension is observed in about 20% of patients with pyogenic osteomyelitis and diskitis.

MRI is the most sensitive technique for detection of osteomyelitis and diskitis, and is the procedure of choice in evaluation of patients with suspected spine infection. Sagittal images are the most useful for demonstrating disk space and adjacent vertebral body involvement, whereas axial views demonstrate paravertebral soft tissue extension. The disk space and portions of the vertebral bodies adjacent to the disk exhibit low signal intensity on images with long repetition time (TR) and echo time (TE). With progressive involvement of the vertebral bodies, there is loss of the normal, well-delineated low signal of the vertebral end plates, and progressive loss of disk space height. Morphologic distinction between the disk and vertebral body becomes increasingly difficult. Gd-DTPA administration is important for evaluating diskitis or osteomyelitis. Infection evokes intense uptake of contrast material by both the disk and adjacent vertebral bodies and soft tissue. Any epidural or soft tissue spread is delineated in greater detail than in noncontrast studies.

Intramedullary Inflammatory Lesions

Multiple Sclerosis

Multiple sclerosis (MS) is a common demyelinating disease of the central nervous system affecting white matter of the brain and spinal cord. MRI is the best imaging modality for direct visualization of intramedullary demyelinating plaques in MS. Spinal MS lesions can present one of three appearances: segmental fusiform enlargement of the cord, most often in the cervical spine, an area of hyperintense signal on T2-weighted images without any changes in cord width, and cord atrophy. These three different appearances may represent the same lesion at three different stages. The segmental, usually subtle, enlargement of the spinal cord and high signal intensity seen on T2-weighted images in the acute phase can be linked to perivenous inflammation, interstitial edema, or microglial proliferation.

The appearance of cord atrophy may correspond to the endstage of the disease. The yield of positive spinal MR scans is higher in acute (82%) than in chronic (61%) spinal cord syndromes; it is also higher in the cervical region (86%) than in the thoracic (6%) and lumbar spine. Gd-DTPA administration has been used to differentiate active from inactive plaques. Delayed contrast enhancement of the lesions was seen in patients with clinically active disease, but no uptake could be detected in patients with stable disease.

Transverse Myelitis

Transverse myelitis, a condition generally encountered in younger age groups, characteristically develops as a rapidly progressing myelopathy. Generally, the myelitis regresses in 1-2 months, although in some patients a neurological deficit may persist. In many cases, transverse myelitis is related to a viral infection (herpes virus) and may also arise in patients with acquired immune deficiency syndrome (AIDS). MRI emphasizes diffuse cord enlargement but conflicting signal features are depicted on T2-weighted sequences. In all cases, areas of signal change show variable contrast uptake depending on acute stage and type of treatment. Lesion distribution results from the neurotropism of the causative virus and may help to identify the agent responsible. In any case, diagnosis of myelitis is confirmed by isolation of the viral strain from the CSF (Figs. 6-8).

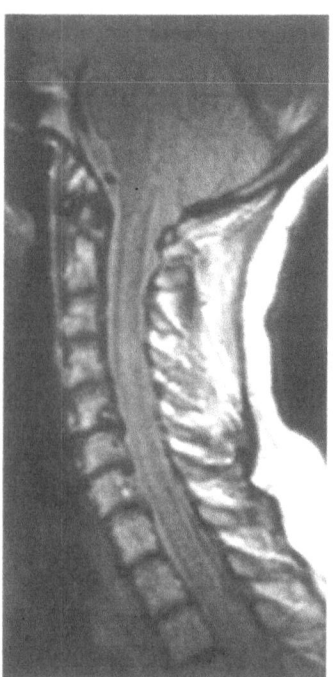

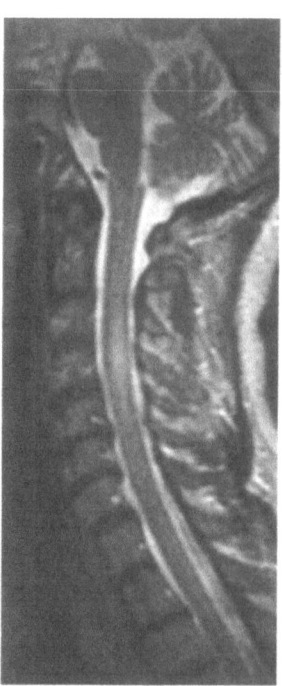

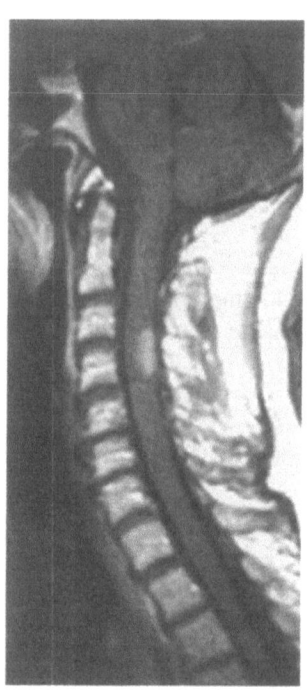

Fig. 6. Transverse myelitis. Sagittal MR, PD-weighted image: hyperintensity in mid-cervical cord; the cervical cord is moderately enlarged

Fig. 7. Transverse myelitis. Sagittal MR, T2-weighted image: confirmation of the hyperintensity in midcervical cord

Fig. 8. Transverse myelitis. Sagittal MR, T1-weighted postgadolinium image: marked enhancement of the lesion

Sarcoidosis

This multisystem, noncaseating granulomatous disease of unknown origin involves the central nervous system in approximately 5% of cases. Spinal cord involvement is much rarer. Intramedullary involvement is seen in 35%, extramedullary involvement in 35%, involvement of both in 23%, and extradural involvement in 2%.

Intramedullary swelling of the cervical and upper thoracic cord is the most common finding on imaging studies. This condition usually mimics intramedullary neoplasm and is often confused with gliomas at surgery. Spinal sarcoidosis usually involves the leptomeninges.

Neuro-Lupus and Neuro-Behçet's Disease

Although neurological complications arise in 20%-50% of patients with systemic lupus erythematosus (SLE), myelitis is rare and only arises many years after diagnosis of the disease. Neuropathologcal examination discloses areas of vacuolar degeneration in the spinal cord white matter, usually in the middle or lower thoracic spine, without clear signs of vasculitis. MRI features of spinal cord involvement in SLE are aspecific with single or multiple signal alterations on T2-weighted turbo spin echo (TSE) sequences.

Behçet's syndrome is a multisystem disease of unknown cause. Neuropathological changes of the central nervous system (CNS) include areas of demyelination and glial proliferation associated with perivascular lympho-cyte infiltrate and wallerian degeneration. As there are no specific laboratory or instrumental tests for Behçet's disease, diagnosis is based on major and minor clinical criteria, namely recurrent aphthous-type oral and genital ulceration and iritis with various skin lesions. CNS involvement is rare at onset, but may occur in 10%-50% of patients. Neuro-Behçet is characterized by a relapsing and remitting course similar to that of MS. Spinal cord involvement is clinically present in 10%-20% of cases. MRI findings are similar to those of MS and SLE myelitis and differential diagnosis cannot be based on imaging alone.

Guillain-Barré Syndrome

This acute inflammatory polyradiculoneuropathy affects people of all ages, but has a peak incidence between 50 and 70 years of age. In 60% of patients, there is a history of mild respiratory or gastrointestinal infection 1-3 weeks before onset of neurological symptoms. Sensory symptoms predominate with paresthesia, hypoesthesia, weakness and pain in the limb muscles commencing distally and ascending to involve the trunk, neck and head.

CSF analysis shows markedly elevated protein levels. Clinical features resolve spontaneously with full recovery in most cases although recurrences and a chronic progressive course have been described.

Contrast medium administration is essential to disclose the MRI features of Guillain-Barré syndrome, consisting of varying degrees of diffuse symmetrical intradural root enhancement.